D1519566

Obsessive-Compulsive Disorders

Compliments of

Solvay Pharmaceuticals, Inc.
and
The Pharmacia & Upjohn Company

Medical Psychiatry

Series Editor

William A. Frosch, M.D.

Cornell University Medical College
New York, New York

ADDITIONAL VOLUMES IN PREPARATION

Obsessive-Compulsive Disorders

Diagnosis · Etiology · Treatment

edited by

Eric Hollander
The Mount Sinai School of Medicine
New York, New York

Dan J. Stein
University of Stellenbosch
Tygerberg, South Africa

MARCEL DEKKER, INC.   NEW YORK · BASEL · HONG KONG

Library of Congress Cataloging-in-Publication Data

Obsessive-compulsive disorders : diagnosis, etiology, treatment /
    edited by Eric Hollander, Dan J. Stein.
            p.   cm. -- (Medical psychiatry ; 6)
        Includes index.
        ISBN 0-8247-9856-2 (alk. paper)
        1. Obsessive-compulsive disorder.   I. Hollander, Eric.
    II. Stein, Dan J.   III. Series.
        [DNLM: 1. Obsessive-Compulsive Disorder--diagnosis.   2. Obsessive
    -Compulsive Disorder--etiology.   3. Obsessive-Compulsive Disorder-
    -therapy.   W1 ME421SM v.6 1997 / WM 176 0143 1997]
    RC533.0276   1997
    616.85 ' 227--dc21
    DNLM/DLC
    for Library of Congress   97-11363
                                                                          CIP

The publisher offers discounts on this book when ordered in bulk quantities. For more information, write to Special Sales/Professional Marketing at the address below.

This book is printed on acid-free paper.

Marcel Dekker, Inc.
270 Madison Avenue, New York, New York 10016
http://www.dekker.com

Current printing (last digit):
10 9 8 7 6 5 4 3 2

PRINTED IN THE UNITED STATES OF AMERICA

Series Introduction

Thirty-five years ago, when I was just entering psychiatry, obsessive-compulsive neurosis (sic) was something we read about in Freud and heard about from our elders, but did not see in practice. It was rare and elusive; some thought it illusory, merely a symptom of impending schizophrenia. We did see bits and pieces of it—normal phase-related obsessiveness in young children, character traits of orderliness and hyperscrupulosity, and quasidelusional preoccupations that at that time were always interpreted as features of psychosis.

When we evaluated the frequency of obsessive-compulsive disease, we underrated the impact of the ego-alien qualities of the symptoms. Truly delusional patients believe in the reality of their experience, and are often willing to talk about it. On the other hand, obsessive-compulsive patients know that their thoughts and acts are "senseless" and "crazy," and they feel shame and humiliation and hesitate to tell family members, friends, physicians, or others what they are compelled to think or do.

As Drs. Hollander and Stein describe, it is now understood that there is a biology of the illness, and we are beginning to accumulate some knowledge of the details of that biology. Thus, it does not surprise us that we have discovered a number of effective biological treatments. However, it is also true that there are a number of focused psychotherapeutic treatments that appear to be more or less equivalently effective. It may be that the old biopsychosocial model of psychopathology will turn out to be correct! These findings have uncovered a significant population of previously undiagnosed, formerly untreatable, and certainly untreated patients. Seeing numbers of such patients impresses us with the always significant, and sometimes devastating, effects of this illness on quality of life. The contributors to this book help us through the morass of diagnosis, etiology, and treatment of this important illness. Now that we have an effective armamentarium, it is essential that we all learn when and how to use it.

William A. Frosch, M.D.

Preface

There has been a sea change in our understanding of obsessive-compulsive disorder (OCD) and related disorders over the past decade. Three myths about OCD continued to be promoted even as recently as a decade ago: that OCD was a rare, untreatable, and psychologically driven disorder. Nowadays, we consider OCD to be very common, affecting 2–3% of the U.S. population, or 5 million Americans; to be highly treatable, with a selective efficacy of serotonin-reuptake inhibitors (SRIs) and specific behavioral therapies; and to be mediated by specific biological mechanisms, involving serotonergic and select neurotransmitter/neuropeptide systems, and certain well-described neural circuits.

Contrary to earlier beliefs, OCD is certainly not a trivial illness. Recent survey studies of Obsessive-Compulsive Foundation members revealed a substantial impact of the illness on quality-of-life measures, including education, work, relationships, and suicide attempts. In addition, a 17-year treatment gap was discovered between onset of symptoms (age 14.5 years) and appropriate treatment (age 31.5 years). While specific treatment approaches, such as SRIs, behavior therapy, and reading about OCD were found to be highly effective, nonspecific treatment approaches such as psychoanalysis and hypnosis were reported to be ineffective.

OCD clearly differs from other affective and anxiety disorders, given the highly selective efficacy of the SRIs and the fact that other antidepressant/antianxiety treatments are generally ineffective. This makes the accurate diagnosis of OCD particularly critical, since misdiagnosis has important treatment implications, namely, the possible use of inappropriate and ineffective treatments.

The survey data reflect the fact that OCD continues to be a hidden epidemic. Clearly, the unusual obsessional symptoms may be considered "crazy" thoughts by the individual, associated with shame and humiliation, and thus symptoms may not be reported to family, friends, or medical or mental health professionals. This contributes to the 17-year time lag between onset of symptoms and appropriate treatment. Nevertheless, both the public and the medical/mental health profession need to be fully educated regarding presenting symptoms, screening questions, and the fact that OCD is a treatable illness. Further, OCD is more common and more treatable than other well-recognized medical conditions but remains less recognized by the medical profession.

During this time, we have also gained an understanding of the relationship between OCD and a group of related or spectrum disorders. These other diagnostic entities are certainly not OCD but may share certain key features: obsessional thoughts or compulsive repetitive behaviors; associated symptoms such as age at onset, clinical course, and co-morbidity; neurobiological markers or familial links; and selective efficacy to antiobsessional treatments. These disorders may include somatoform (body dysmorphic disorder, hypochondriasis), dissociative (depersonalization), eating (anorexia, binge eating disorder), schizo-obsessive, neurological (Tourette's syndorme, Sydenham's chorea, Huntington's disease, autism, and Asperger's syndrome), and impulse-control (pathological gambling, trichotillomania, self-injurious behavior, kleptomania, compulsive shopping, and sexually compulsive) disorders. These spectrum disorders may also be conceptualized as encompassing three overarching clusters, namely, those that involve preoccupations with bodily sensations or appearance, neurological disorders with compulsive symptoms, and the impulsive cluster of disorders.

This is of interest, since conceptually this group of disorders may affect up to 10% of the U.S. population. Further, these disorders tend to be overlooked and misdiagnosed, and frequently present to primary care and other medical specialists, rather than mental health specialists. Reflecting an increased interest in this area by medical professionals and consumers, the *Journal of CNS Spectrum Disorders: First in Obsessive-Compulsive & Neuropsychiatric Medicine* was recently launched.

This book focuses on new insights regarding etiology, diagnosis, and treatment of OCD. With the development of DSM-IV, ICD-10, and new assessment instruments, our ability to define and assess OCD has become further refined. In Chapter 1, Drs. Niehaus and Stein review current issues in diagnosis and assessment of OCD.

Etiological models have further refined the serotonin hypothesis, evaluated other systems including dopamine and oxytocin, probed auto-immune models, developed new neuropsychiatric perspectives and neural circuits, and proposed better animal models for OCD and specific spectrum disorders. Drs. Stein, Simeon, and Hollander update the reader on recent understanding of the neurochemistry of OCD; Drs. Cohen, Stein, and Hollander describe neuropsychiatric components of OCD; and Drs. Dodman, Moon-Fanelli, Mertens, Pflueger, and Stein explore veterinary and animal models of OCD.

New selective serotonin-reuptake inhibitors (SSRIs) have received indications for OCD from the FDA. However, treatment-resistant patients remain a problem. Thus, new pharmacological alternatives and augmentation strategies have been developed. To highlight pharmacological treatments, Drs. Dougherty and Rauch review SRIs; Dr. Hewlett describes novel pharmacological treatments; and Drs. McDougle and Goodman discuss combination pharmacological treatment strategies.

There has also been rapid growth in the development of nonpharmacological or behavioral treatments of OCD. While traditional cognitive-behavioral psychotherapy has a proven track record in OCD, other alternatives including group and family approaches or alternative or nontraditional therapies (e.g., yogic techniques) may also be helpful. New techniques such as PET may demonstrate specific metabolic changes associated with OC symptom improvement secondary to these behavioral approaches. Mr. Silvestre and Dr. Aronowitz describe psychotherapeutic approaches to OCD, including cognitive-behavior therapy. Dr. Schwartz describes a mind–brain interaction paradigm based on metabolic changes resulting from cognitive behavioral self-treatment; Mr. Shannahoff-Khalsa describes the effect of yogic techniques on OCD; and Ms. Van Noppen and Drs. Steketee and Pato update the role of group and family behavioral therapy for OCD.

Also, the exploration of subtypes and spectrums has blossomed in recent years. The role of developmental stages and causative factors in OCD has recently been addressed. Thus, Drs. Piacentini and Graae address childhood OCD, and Drs. Cohen, Stein, Simeon, and Hollander detail the OCD spectrum.

Finally, OCD sufferers have become empowered by gaining knowledge, realizing they are not alone, and organizing support groups and becoming involved in the OC Foundation. Mr. Broatch describes how support groups are an essential ingredient in recovery.

In reviewing the past decade, one is struck by the broad range of developments in OCD research and treatment. Clearly, much remains to be done. However, this book brings together diverse approaches and

developments in assessing where the field is today and where it needs
to go in the future.

Eric Hollander
Dan J. Stein

Contents

Contributors

Bonnie R. Aronowitz, Ph.D. Private Practice and Assistant Professor of Psychology in Psychiatry, The Mount Sinai Medical Center, New York, New York

James W. Broatch, M.S.W. Executive Director, Obsessive-Compulsive Foundation, Milford, Connecticut

Lisa J. Cohen, Ph.D. Supervising Psychologist and Assistant Professor of Psychiatry, Beth Israel Medical Center/Albert Einstein College of Medicine, New York, New York

N. H. Dodman, B.V.M.S., M.R.C.V.S., D.V.A., M.A.P.B.C. Professor and Head, Sections of Anesthesia and Animal Behavior, Tufts University School of Veterinary Medicine, North Grafton, Massachusetts

Darin Dougherty, M.D. Chief Resident, Psychopharmacology Clinic, Department of Psychiatry, Massachusetts General Hospital, and Clinical Fellow in Psychiatry, Harvard Medical School, Boston, Massachusetts

Wayne K. Goodman, M.D. Professor, Department of Psychiatry, University of Florida College of Medicine, Gainesville, Florida

Flemming Graae, M.D.* Department of Psychiatry, Cornell University Medical Center—The New York Hospital, New York, New York

Current affiliation: Assistant Professor and Director, OCD and Anxiety Disorder Service, and Associate Director, Department of Psychiatry, Division of Child Psychiatry, New York Hospital—Westchester Division, White Plains, New York.

William A. Hewlett, Ph.D., M.D. Director, OCD/Tourette Program, Department of Psychiatry, and Department of Pharmacology, Vanderbilt University School of Medicine, Nashville, Tennessee

Eric Hollander, M.D. Vice-Chairman, Department of Psychiatry, The Mount Sinai School of Medicine, New York, New York

Christopher J. McDougle, M.D. Associate Professor of Psychiatry and Child and Adolescent Psychiatry, Clinical Neuroscience Research Unit and Child Study Center, Yale University School of Medicine, New Haven, Connecticut

P. A. Mertens, D.V.M., Dr.med.vet.* Tufts University School of Veterinary Medicine, North Grafton, Massachusetts

A. Moon-Fanelli, Ph.D. Clinical Assistant Professor, Department of Surgery, Tufts University School of Veterinary Medicine, North Grafton, Massachusetts

Dana J. H. Niehaus, M.B. Fellow in Psychiatry Research, Department of Psychiatry, University of Stellenbosch, Tygerberg, South Africa

Michele Pato, M.D. Director of Outpatient Psychiatry and Residency Training Director, State University of New York at Buffalo, Buffalo, New York

S. Pflueger Director of Medical Genetics and Assistant Professor of Obstetrics and Gynecology, Tufts University School of Medicine, Boston, and Department of Pathology, Baystate Medical Center, Springfield, Massachusetts

John Piacentini, Ph.D. Director, Child and Adolescent OCD Program, and Assistant Professor, Division of Child and Adolescent Psychiatry, Department of Psychiatry and Biobehavioral Sciences, UCLA School of Medicine, Los Angeles, California

Scott L. Rauch, M.D. Director, Psychiatric Neuroimaging Research, Departments of Psychiatry and Radiology, Massachusetts General Hospital, and Assistant Professor of Psychiatry, Harvard Medical School, Boston, Massachusetts

**Current affiliation:* Institute for Ethology and Animal Welfare, Veterinary School, Ludwig-Maximilians-Universität, Munich, Germany.

Jeffrey M. Schwartz, M.D. Associate Research Professor, Department of Psychiatry, UCLA School of Medicine, Los Angeles, California

David S. Shannahoff-Khalsa Director, The Research Group for Mind–Body Dynamics, Institute for Nonlinear Science, University of California, San Diego, La Jolla, and President, The Khalsa Foundation for Medical Science, Del Mar, California

Joao Silvestre, C.S.W. Private Practice and Research Scientist, Anxiety Disorders Clinic, New York State Psychiatric Institute, New York, New York

Daphne Simeon, M.D. Assistant Professor, Department of Psychiatry, The Mount Sinai School of Medicine, New York, New York

Dan J. Stein, M.B. Director of Research, Department of Psychiatry, University of Stellenbosch, Tygerberg, South Africa

Gail Steketee, Ph.D. Professor and Associate Dean, Boston University School of Social Work, Boston, Massachusetts

Barbara Van Noppen, M.S.W. Clinical Research Associate, Butler Hospital and Brown University, Providence, Rhode Island

Obsessive-Compulsive Disorder

Diagnosis and Assessment

Dana J. H. Niehaus and Dan J. Stein

University of Stellenbosch
Tygerberg, South Africa

INTRODUCTION

Since the early case descriptions by Janet, Freud, and others, understanding of obsessive-compulsive disorder (OCD) has improved dramatically. In particular, there have been significant advances in the epidemiology, diagnosis, and treatment of OCD.

Current epidemiological data suggest that OCD is the fourth most common mental disorder. Only phobias, substance abuse, and depression are more common, and OCD is nearly as common as asthma and diabetes mellitus. Although this contradicts the original view that OCD is a rare psychiatric affliction, the latter notion—together with the often secretive nature of the disorder—continues to impede diagnosis.

Secretiveness may often result from feelings of shame or embarrassment about symptoms, and is sometimes a direct result of obsessions such as the fear of going "insane." It is not strange, then, that many OCD patients do not reveal their symptoms unless specifically asked (1). Depressive and anxiety-linked complaints often act as a disguise (2,3). The development of diagnostic criteria for OCD has, however, enabled physicians to distinguish these entities from OCD. Current diagnostic criteria for OCD in the DSM-IV reflect the results of an extensive field trial.

Accurate diagnosis of OCD has become increasingly important given advances in available treatments. The development of effective pharmacotherapeutic and cognitive–behavioral interventions for the management of OCD has encouraged the development of more reliable and sensitive symptom-assessment scales to monitor symptom change. The development of such scales in turn contributes to treatment research.

This chapter provides an overview of current issues in the epidemiology, diagnosis, and assessment of OCD.

EPIDEMIOLOGY

Prevalence

Two major studies have facilitated the recognition of OCD as a common psychiatric disorder. Data from the National Epidemiology Catchment Area (ECA) Survey suggest that the lifetime prevalence of OCD in the general population is on the order of 2.5%. This is almost 50 times greater than previously believed (4–6). Weismann et al. (7) undertook a second major study, the Cross National Epidemiological Study, at six additional sites: Canada; Puerto Rico; Germany; Taiwan; Korea; and New Zealand. Using the same diagnostic interview as in the ECA Survey, they found that the lifetime prevalence rate of OCD varied little between countries, with only Taiwan having a low incidence of both OCD and other psychiatric illnesses.

Criticism has been leveled at these studies, because the Diagnostic Interview Schedule (DIS) used to assess symptoms was designed for administration by lay interviewers rather than psychiatrists. Since studies using psychiatrists as interviewers have found lower rates of OCD, a more likely figure may be between 1 and 2% (1,9,10). Even so, it seems incontestable that OCD is a highly prevalent disorder in many countries. Further research is necessary, however, to ascertain the epidemiology of OCD in some countries, such as those on the African continent, for which little data exist.

Marital Status, Intelligence and Sex and Age distribution

Early clinical reports suggested an almost equal sex ratio in patients with OCD, as well as marital maladjustment and higher than average intelligence (11). The ECA study indicated, however, that females are somewhat more prone to development of OCD. OCD was also not exclusively associated with any level of educational attainment or marital status

(4,12). The Cross National Epidemiological Study confirmed that the female-to-male sex ratio varies between 1.6 and 1.2 (7). Among children, however, more males than females may present for treatment (14).

The mean age of onset has a wide range, between 21.9 and 35.5 years (7). Most patients (65%) develop OCD before the age of 25 years, with only a small percentage (15%) after the age of 35 years (11). Males seem to present with an earlier age of onset than females (17.5 versus 20.8 years) (11). Such differences between male and female OCD patients may provide clues to investigating underlying neurobiological processes in this disorder.

Course

Most patients describe a gradual onset with no clear precipitant. However, a subset of patients present with sudden onset of OCD after infection, and some cases of OCD in women develop after pregnancy (15–17).

OCD typically appears to be a chronic disorder with a waxing and waning course. Eighty-five percent of patients experience chronic impairment (1). A retrospective study of 62 patients fulfilling the ICD-8/9 criteria for OCD differentiated five courses: continuous and unchanging (27.4%), continuous with deterioration (9.7%), continuous with improvement (24.4%), episodic with partial remission (24.2%), and episodic with full remission (11.3%) (18).

An early study found that the mean time to first health-care contact for an affected person was 7.5 years (20). Despite advances in community education and awareness, the waiting period between onset and treatment remains significant.

DIAGNOSTIC CRITERIA

DSM-IV criteria for OCD note that either obsessions or compulsions must be present. These symptoms cause marked distress or impairment and are not due to the direct effect of a substance or general medical condition (21). The DSM-IV defines obsessions as persistent, intrusive, and inappropriate thoughts, impulses, ideas, or images. The individual realizes that they are not imposed from without (thought insertion) but are a product of his or her own mind. The person typically tries to suppress, ignore, or neutralize the obsessions with compulsive behavior. Compulsions are characterized as overt repetitive behaviors or mental acts performed to reduce distress caused by the obsessions (21).

The DSM-IV field trial of OCD contributed to a number of changes in diagnostic criteria (Table 1) (22). First, the majority of patients had mental compulsions, and these usually had a functional relationship to obsessions. The definition of compulsions was changed to emphasize the inclusion of mental acts as compulsions. Examples of such mental acts include counting, praying, and repeating of words silently. Thus, whereas obsessions cause marked anxiety or distress, compulsions (including mental acts) prevent or reduce anxiety or distress.

The DSM-IV field trial also addressed the DSM-III-R requirement that OCD symptoms be viewed by the patient as excessive or unreasonable (22). Several studies have indicated that some patients with OCD are uncertain about whether their symptoms are unreasonable or excessive; OCD is in fact characterized by a broad range of insight (23–25). Similarly, the field trial found that most OCD patients were uncertain to various degrees about whether their obsessions and compulsions were senseless, and that about 5% lacked insight into the senselessness of symptoms. To alert clinicians to this latter group of patients, the DSM-IV includes a subtype of OCD "with poor insight" (22). This lack of insight into unreasonable or excessive symptoms must be present most of the time during the current episode.

The DSM-IV notes that obsessions "are not simply excessive worries about real-life problems" (21), thus providing a differentiation between the symptoms of OCD and those of generalized anxiety disorder (38). Indeed, research has suggested that having unpleasant and unwanted thoughts is a frequent experience in both normal and clinical populations (31). In study populations, 80–99% of subjects experience cognitive intrusions, with no age or sex differences (32,33). Normal or subclinical obsessions may share some common themes with pathological obsessions, such as harm, death, disease, and sex (32,34). However, they differ with respect to the threshold of acceptability, which is higher for abnormal obsessions. Normal obsessions are easier to dismiss, less intense, shorter in duration, and less frequent. The abnormal/clinical obsessions are likely to have a specific onset and provoke urges to neutralize them. In short, they differ in frequency, intensity, and consequences.

SUBTYPING

The identification of homogeneous subgroups of patients with OCD has been an important goal. A better understanding of the heterogeneous nature of OCD may yield valuable clues to variance in neurobiological parameters and treatment response of OCD patients. Different

Table 1   Diagnostic Criteria for Obsessive-Compulsive Disorder (300.3)

A. Either obsessions or compulsions:
Obsessions as defined by (1), (2), (3), and (4)
  (1) Recurrent and persistent thoughts, impulses, or images that are experienced, at some time during the disturbance, as intrusive and inappropriate and that cause marked anxiety or distress.
  (2) The thoughts, impulses, or images are not simply excessive worries about real-life problems.
  (3) The person attempts to ignore or suppress such thoughts, impulses, or images, or to neutralize them with some other thought or action.
  (4) The person recognizes that the obsessional thoughts, impulses, or images are a product of his or her own mind (not imposed from without as in thought insertion).
Compulsions as defined by (1) and (2)
  (1) Repetitive behaviors (e.g., hand washing, ordering, checking) or mental acts (e.g., praying, counting repeating words silently) that the person feels driven to perform in response to an obsession, or according to rules that must be applied rigidly.
  (2) The behaviors or mental acts are aimed at preventing or reducing distress or preventing some dreaded event or situation; however, these behaviors or mental acts either are not connected in a realistic way with what they are designed to neutralize or prevent or are clearly excessive.
B. At some point during the course of the disorder, the person has recognized that the obsessions or compulsions are excessive or unreasonable. Note: This does not apply to children.
C. The obsession or compulsions cause marked distress, are time consuming (take more than 1 hour a day), or significantly interfere with the person's normal routine, occupational (or academic) functioning, or usual social activities or relationships.
D. If another Axis 1 disorder is present, the content of the obsessions or compulsions is not restricted to it (e.g., preoccupation with food in the presence of an Eating Disorder; hair pulling in the presence of Trichotillomania; concern with appearance in the presence of body Dysmorphic Disorder; preoccupation with drugs in the presence of Substance Use Disorder; preoccupation with having a serious illness in the presence of Hypochondriasis; preoccupation with sexual urges or fantasies in the presence of a Paraphilia; or guilty ruminations in the presence of Major Depressive Disorder).
E. The disturbance is not due to the direct physiological effects of a substance (e.g., a drug of abuse, a medication) or a general medical condition.
Specify if:
With Poor Insight: if, for most of the time during the current episode, the person does not recognize that the obsessions and compulsions are excessive or unreasonable.

Source: Ref. 22.

OCD subgroups may have different symptoms, course of illness, and prognosis.

Various types and forms of obsessions and compulsions exist (1,28,29). Rasmussen and Eisen (1) found that the most common obsessions in a large group of OCD patients were contamination fear (45%), pathological doubt (42%), and somatic obsessions (36%). Checking (63%), washing (50%), and counting (36%) were the most common compulsions. They also found that 60% of subjects had multiple obsessions and 48% multiple compulsions. This pattern seems to vary only slightly between different samples of OCD patients.

In a study of 412 subjects with OCD, the sociodemographic and clinical variables of washers and checkers were studied over a period of 9 years. Three groups were delineated: those with only checking behavior, those with only washing behavior, and a mixed group. Checkers were more likely to be single males with an earlier age of onset and first consultation. The mixed group, on the other hand, was female-dominated and appeared to be a variant of the checkers group (39).

Factor-analysis studies have also been used to subtype OCD. Baer (40) identified three factors of importance. The first referred to symmetry or hoarding symptoms. Patients with these symptoms experience a feeling of incompleteness (41). This factor was related to comorbid obsessive-compulsive personality disorder, Tourette's syndrome, and chronic tic disorder. Patients scoring higher on this factor had a relative risk 8.56 times greater for suffering from comorbid tic disorder. The second factor consisted of contamination fear and checking behavior, while the last was pure obsessions. These subtypes were not mutually exclusive, however, and a patient may express varying degrees of these three symptom subtypes (40).

Grouping on the grounds of OCD with or without Tourette's syndrome has revealed phenomenological differences between the groups. George et al. (42) found that patients suffering from concurrent OCD and Tourette's syndrome had significantly more violent, sexual, and symmetrical obsessions. This group of patients also had more touching, blinking, counting, and self-damaging compulsions. The group without comorbid Tourette's had more contamination obsessions and cleaning compulsions. The latter group's compulsions were frequently preceded by cognition, while those with OCD and Tourette's syndrome reported that their compulsions arose spontaneously (42,43).

Obsessional slowness is regarded as an uncommon but severely disabling subgroup of OCD (44). Slowness of performance may be specific to compulsive checkers since no significant correlation with other

MOCI subscales was found (45). It might, however, best be regarded as a secondary effect of OCD (44).

Identification of subgroups may have important implications for neurobiological and treatment studies. For example, Stein and colleagues (47) found that those OCD patients with high neurological soft signs had ventricular-brain ratios significantly greater than those of controls. McDougle and colleagues (46) have provided strong evidence that neuroleptic augmentation of serotonergic agents is particularly useful in OCD patients with comorbid tics.

FAMILY AND CHILDHOOD HISTORY

Rasmussen and Tsuang (48) identified eight traits characteristic of the childhood histories of OCD patients: separation anxiety, resistance to change or novelty, risk aversion, ambivalence, excessive devotion to work, magical thinking, high level of morality, and perfectionism. A total of 810 adults were also examined by psychiatrists in the second stage of the Eastern Baltimore Mental Health Survey (10). OCD patients were significantly more likely to report having had childhood fears, learning disabilities, and a family history of alcoholism and suicidal behavior.

Data from recent studies seem to indicate that some forms of OCD are familial (49). Relatives of OCD patients have significantly higher rates of OCD and subthreshold OCD. The rate of tics (Tourette's disorder and chronic tics) was also significantly greater among the relatives of the patients than among control subjects (49).

The precise role of familial transmission in OCD is still unclear. Molecular studies have not identified the genotype associated with OCD (49). The identification of a causative mutation or alteration may ultimately be a paramount contribution to the subtyping of OCD.

In obtaining a family history, the clinician should also note the effects of the patient's illness on the family, and the family's response. A recent study (50) evaluated burden of illness in 90 families—30 each with dysthymia, generalized anxiety disorder, and OCD. Burden was felt in four principal areas: financial issues and disruption of family routine, leisure, and interactions. All the groups showed this pattern. The burden was significantly greater in cases of married patients, married relatives, housewives, and employed patients. Families may differ significantly in the way that they respond to members who have OCD, and such reactions may in turn constitute an important factor in determing the course of the illness.

COMORBIDITY

It has become increasingly apparent that OCD is often comorbid with several other Axis I diagnoses, particularly mood and anxiety disorders. Indeed, more than 50% of OCD patients report a comorbid Axis I disorder (51). This high comorbidity may lead to difficulty in deciding whether OCD is the primary diagnosis, especially when the chronic waxing and waning course often found in OCD is considered.

In particular, OCD is often accompanied by depression; figures of up to 70% with lifetime major depressive episodes (MDE) have been reported (7,11,30,52,53). This makes MDE the most common comorbid disorder in OCD, and at any given time 30–38% of OCD patients meet diagnostic criteria for both disorders (51). Despite the high comorbidity, studies on treatment response and course of illness suggest that the depressive illness is probably not merely a secondary feature of OCD (51).

The other common comorbid conditions in OCD are anxiety disorders, eating disorders, substance abuse, and Tourette's syndrome (11,51). Studies indicate that 40 to 60% of OCD patients will at some time meet the criteria for an anxiety disorder (51). The most prevalent lifetime comorbid anxiety diagnoses are simple phobia (22%), social phobia (18%), and panic disorder (17%) (24,53,54).

Several studies suggest extensive comorbidity between OCD and eating disorders, with lifetime prevalence rates of 10–17% for anorexia nervosa and 5–20% for bulimia nervosa in OCD patients (51). Conversely, a high prevalence of OCD symptoms is found in patients with the primary diagnosis of anorexia and bulimia nervosa (51,56). This high prevalence may be correlated with the severity of the eating disorder (57).

OCD may also be found in patients with certain disorders possibly related to OCD, such as hypochondriasis (58), body dysmorphic disorder, trichotillomania, and Tourette's syndrome (55,59). The lifetime prevalence rates in patients with primary OCD may be as high as 18% for trichotillomania and 7% for Tourette's syndrome (51). Conversely, many OCD patients may exhibit tics (43,48). Indeed, Pitman et al. (43) found that tics were more useful than obsessions and compulsions in distinguishing relatives of OCD patients from relatives of controls.

Although comorbidity patterns indicate that most of the OCD spectrum disorders are associated with mood disorders, the impulse-control disorders such as kleptomania are more strongly associated with bipolar disorder than is OCD (61). The impulse-control disorders may also be characterized by higher rates of substance abuse and dependency than in OCD.

The relationship between OCD and schizophrenia has been disputed for years. Nevertheless, recent research strongly supports the conclusion that OCD and schizophrenia are quite separate entities (11,55). It has been found that OCD patients only rarely develop schizophrenia, and that patients with schizophrenia exhibit OCD symptoms in only about 10% of cases (11,62,63). However, a number of authors have emphasized the need for further research on schizophrenia patients with OCD symptoms and note that the prevalence may be higher than previously thought (55).

Personality disorders are highly prevalent among patients with OCD (11,41,51,64). A majority of OCD patients have at least one Axis II diagnosis according to studies based on DSM-III personality disorder criteria (51,65). Personality disorders identified as being frequent in OCD are obsessive-compulsive, dependent, avoidant, histrionic, borderline, and schizotypal (66,67). While studies have been conducted using different measures, there has been general agreement that cluster C disorders are most prevalent in OCD (51,65,66,68).

Psychoanalytical theory has long proposed that OCD and obsessive-compulsive personality disorder (OCPD) are on a spectrum. However, comorbidity research does not confirm this hypothesis (55). On the contrary, some evidence suggests that OCPD may be secondary to OCD (55). Swedo et al. (14) hypothesized that some children may develop compulsive personality traits as an adaptive mechanism to deal with OCD. This hypothesis is in accord with the finding of Baer and Jenike (65) that OCD often predates compulsive personality disorder and that mixed personality disorder may develop over time, possibly secondary to OCD. In their sample of 96 adult patients with OCD, mixed personality disorder was more likely with longer duration of OCD. The development of pathological personality traits may be related to behavioral and lifestyle changes that are secondary to OCD. Successful treatment of OCD may lead to a decrease in such traits.

The influence of an Axis II disorder on the outcome of OCD treatment is one of the reasons for the interest in this field. Studies suggest that comorbid personality disorders may inhibit the response to treatment (69). This poorer outcome of OCD appears more consistently so with comorbid schizotypal personality disorder (65).

Comorbid conditions are common in OCD, and their presence may present a viable way to divide OCD patients into homogeneous groups. In this regard, Rasmussen and colleagues (41) suggest that the comorbid conditions be grouped according to two core features of OCD: altered risk assessment and a prominent feeling of incompleteness. OCD patients with high lifetime prevalence rates of anxiety disorders, eating disorders, hypochondriasis, or body dysmorphic disorder probably have a deficit in risk assessment. A prominent feeling of incompleteness is expected if high lifetime prevalences of Tourette's syndrome, trichotillomania, or other "habit disorders" are found (51).

DIFFERENTIAL DIAGNOSIS

Distinguishing OCD from other disorders can be challenging. The differential diagnoses of OCD include mood disorders, anxiety disorders, OCD spectrum disorders, impulsive spectrum disorders, OCPD, and delusional disorders.

A careful history, however, usually allows accurate diagnosis. For example, individuals with OCPD do not have obsessions or compulsions. Rather, there is a chronic and pervasive preoccupation with orderliness, perfectionism, and control. This preoccupation is essentially ego-syntonic, although OCPD patients may be aware of the negative consequences of their traits (55).

Although there is phenomenological overlap between the anxiety disorders, treatment regimen and response differ (70,71). Optimal treatment therefore necessitates an accurate diagnosis. Some OCD patients experience panic attacks, but these are usually secondary to their obsessional fears (24). Since spontaneous panic attacks are necessary to meet the DSM-IV criteria for panic disorder, and few panic patients exhibit rituals, the distinction from OCD can be readily made (25).

Major depressive episodes often form part of the differential diagnosis of OCD. Depression can certainly be accompanied by ruminations that may have an obsessive nature. However, these occur on the background of depressed mood, and within that context they differ from the senseless intrusions of OCD obsessions (72–74).

OCD spectrum disorders are described in detail in Chapter 3 of this volume. Patients with trichotillomania, for example, appear to have only this one symptom rather than the multiple obsessions and compulsions often found in OCD (75). Although hair-pulling and other impulsive symptoms are associated with a sense of relief, they typically are not closely related to obsessional thoughts such as the prevention of a future event (55).

A recent case report (76) describes the misdiagnosis of vivid, intrusive, obsessional images as "flashbacks" of repressed childhood trauma. Conversely, patients with borderline personality disorder who experience strong thoughts and feelings about a particular theme may present complaining that these are symptoms of OCD.

While the delusions of schizophrenia can resemble particular obsessional concerns, there is typically markedly less insight in these patients. Similarly, the rituals of schizophrenia are often without purpose or in response to a force that is perceived as external. Other core positive and negative symptoms of schizophrenia are also not present in OCD.

ASSESSMENT TOOLS

Rasmussen and Eisen (1) suggest that the primary-care physician ask at least two screening questions to rule out OCD: "Are you bothered by thoughts that come into your mind, that make you anxious, and that you are unable to get rid of?" and "Are there certain behaviors you have to do repeatedly that may seem silly to you or others, but that you feel you just have to do?" These questions are the basis of a thorough investigation into the possibility of OCD as a diagnosis. In addition, the notion of an obsessive-compulsive spectrum of disorders is extremely valuable. It reminds the practitioner to inquire about a range of symptoms that are often ignored.

Several scales are available to assist in the diagnosis of OCD and the measurement of treatment efficacy. These include self-rating and rater-administered scales. Each group of scales has advantages and disadvantages.

Self-Rating Scales

The benefits of self-rating scales are that they save valuable professional time and expense and provide the clinician with an assessment of the patient's inner state (77). On the other hand, such scales rely on the patient's self-perception, which may not always be accurate in OCD (36,78). Self-rating may itself become ritualized, complicating management (79).

The three most widely used self-rating scales are the Leyton Obsessional Inventory (LOI), the Maudsley Obsessive Compulsive Inventory (MOCI), and the Hopkins Symptom checklist (HSCL and SCL-90).

The Maudsley Obsessive Compulsive Inventory

The MOCI consists of 30 questions designed to yield a total score and four subscale scores (36). A patient with OCD according to DSM-III criteria will usually have a score of at least 18 out of 30. Questions are balanced for true and false answers, and reliability can be partially assessed by looking at consistency of the patient's responses. Four pairs of questions have the same answers (2/8, 3/7, 10/12, 17/21), and two pairs of question have opposite answers (6/22, 16/26). If fewer than three of these pairs correspond, the responses can be considered suspect (78). This scale allows the therapist to explore the most common symptoms of OCD; data suggest that the MOCI is a valid instrument for identification of obsessions and compulsions. This also seemed to hold true in a nonclinical sample (80). Unfortunately, the MOCI has a disadvantage in that, because it relies on specific symptom sets, sometimes the chief obsessions of an individual are not listed. Furthermore, the MOCI cannot be graded. The subscales also seem to have no useful discriminative value (77).

The Leyton Obsessional Inventory

The LOI was originally developed to differentiate between normals, house-proud housewives, and obsessional patients. It consists of 69 yes–no questions (81). These questions are divided into two sets: 46 on symptoms and 23 on traits. The symptom questions comprise 10 categories, including unpleasant recurring thoughts, checking, household cleanliness and tidiness, order and routine, repetition, and indecision. The eight categories of trait questions include hoarding, cleanliness, irritability and nervousness, rigidity, and punctuality (82). Resistance and interference are evaluated for the yes answers and indicated on a 0–3 scale. The LOI scale would appear to have some construct validity and test–retest reliability, but the content validity may be compromised because the scale does not cover unpleasant obsessional thoughts and more florid bizarre symptoms (77). The questions are also oriented more toward the home and cleaning (77). The LOI seems acceptable as a screening tool since it is relatively easy to administer, but it may not be a good indicator of severity (83).

Symptom Checklist

The SCL-90 is an expanded version of the original HSCL, which covered only five symptom dimensions. The SCL-90 now consists of nine dimensions: obsessions-compulsions, anxiety, depression, somatization, interpersonal sensitivity, hostility, phobic anxiety, paranoid ideation, and psychoticism (84,85). Each item is rated according to a 0–4 scale of distress in frequency and/or intensity. Although this instrument has shown good test–retest reliability and internal consistency, it may not be sufficiently robust to act as a measure of change in symptoms (86).

Self-Rated Scale for Obsessive-Compulsive Disorder

The Self-Rated Scale for Obsessive-Compulsive Disorder is a 35-item questionnaire developed to measure the severity of OCD (87). This scale evaluates distressing thoughts, rituals, perfectionism, and fear of contamination as separate dimensions. A cross-validation study found high internal consistency and significant correlations between this scale and two clinician-rated measures of OCD. Although this scale is advocated as being psychometrically sound for the measurement of severity in OCD (87), it probably has the same limitations as the MOCI.

Computer-Assisted Evaluation

An apparently reliable and low-cost alternative to pencil-and-paper measures is a computer-assisted telephone system. Such a system might use digitized human speech to administer rating scales for OCD. Scores derived with such systems are comparable to those obtained with human administration of the scales (88).

Rater-Administered Scales

Yale-Brown Obsessive-Compulsive Rating Scale

The Y-BOCS—the best instrument available for assessment of change in severity of OCD—consists of 16 items. The sum of the first 10 questions is ordinarily used. These 10 questions are divided into two sets of five questions covering obsessions and compulsions. The questions assess time spent on obsession or compulsion, interference, distress, resistance, and control. Each is rated on a 0–4 scale correlating to severity (0 = no symptoms; 4 = extreme symptoms). Scores between 20 and 35 out of 40 are typical pretreatment values (89).

The Y-BOCS differs from other rater-administered scales in how it assesses resistance. Instead of evaluating distress, resistance, and control as a single item, it separates these entities and therefore affords a more sensitive measurement. Interrater reliability, internal consistency, and test–retest reliability are good (89). However, the performance of subscale items based on data from 204 patients with OCD suggested that the resistance items are not as sensitive to changes in OCD symptoms as the rest of the Y-BOCS items (91). This scale is currently used extensively in treatment evaluation. A form for children is now also available (77).

Comprehensive Psychopathological Rating Scale

The CPRS is a factor-analyzed scale, intended to cover a wide range of psychiatric symptoms and signs (93). It consists of several subscales, with the OCD subscale containing eight items: rituals, inner tension, compulsive thoughts, concentration difficulties, worry over trifles, sadness, lassitude, and indecision. Each item is scored on a 0–3 scale of severity. The fact that four of the items are also found on the depression subscale probably diminishes its discriminative validity (93). This is not as efficient a tool as the Y-BOCS for assessing OCD symptom severity.

NIMH Global Obsessive-Compulsive Scale and Clinical Global Improvement Subscale

The NIMH-GOCS is a rater-administered point scale (1–15 points). This scale comprises five severity categories (1–3-normal; 4–6-subclinical OCD; 7–9-clinical OCD; 10–12-severe, 13–15-very severe) (77).

The CGI scales come in many varieties, including 1–7 number ratings and analog scales. The CGI-OC has shown good correlation with the Y-BOCS and the NIMH-GOCS (83,89,90,93).

A limitation of all single-item global measures is that they cannot be resolved into smaller components. The analysis of different components with the multi-item Y-BOCS makes it more suitable as a primary measure of outcome, with a global scale as a secondary outcome measure (92).

Other Scales

Brown Assessment of Beliefs Scale

Eisen et al. (94) developed this scale to assess the degree of insight. This is a semistructured interview consisting of 18 items, each with probes and anchors. The items focus on features of delusional content, e.g., conviction, perception of others' views, and fixity of beliefs. It also assesses the degree of preoccupation and impairment secondary to the beliefs. Interrater reliability for the first 15 items is good, and a larger study is currently under way (77). Degree of insight might be important in predicting the outcome of treatment (95).

Challenge Scales

These scales are used mainly in research settings. The short time intervals in pharmacological challenge studies require the use of short, easy-to-administer scales for the sensitive rating of change (77).

CONCLUSION

It seems clear that OCD is a highly prevalent disorder in a number of countries. Further research is necessary, however, to determine the epidemiology of OCD in developing countries and to further assess interethnic variation in OCD. Epidemiological study of OCD-related disorders also warrants further attention.

Given the high morbidity of OCD and the existence of effective treatment, accurate diagnosis and thorough assessment of this disorder are essential. The DSM-IV field trial has supported such alterations in the diagnostic criteria as the inclusion of mental compulsions and the inclusion of a category for "poor insight." DSM-IV continues to place OCD and the OCD spectrum disorders in separate diagnostic categories; further research is necessary to elucidate the relationship between these entities.

The assessment of OCD is helped by the availability of valid and reliable clinician- and self-rated measures of OCD. Data from several studies suggest that the Y-BOCS is a reliable and valid clinician-rated scale. The Y-BOCS and the NIMH-GOCS seem suitable for monitoring changes in OCD symptoms and outcome in drug trials. Neither confuses trait with state, and final scores on both scales are not influenced directly by the type or number of obsessions and compulsions present.

Currently available patient-rated instruments such as the MOCI and LOI suffer from serious shortcomings, including insensitivity to change and poor representation of monosymptomatic clinical pictures (e.g., hoarding alone). In spite of these shortcomings, they can still be used as a quick and inexpensive diagnostic tool. Computer administration of rating scales such as the Y-BOCS shows particular promise.

At times, aspects of the disorder themselves interfere with diagnosis and evaluation of OCD. For example, fear of going insane or exaggerated responsibility may bias patient reports. Nevertheless, within a supportive relationship, patients are typically able to describe their symptoms fully and accurately. Obtaining an accurate and comprehensive evaluation is the first step toward effective management of OCD.

REFERENCES

1. Rasmussen SA, Eisen JL. Clinical features and phenomenology of obsessive compulsive disorder. Psychiatric Ann Feb 1989; 19(2):67–73.
2. Dysken MW, Davis JM. Obsessive compulsive disorder. Psychiatric Ann Feb 1989; 19(2):63–64.
3. Nymberg JH, Van Noppen B. Obsessive-compulsive disorder: a concealed

diagnosis. Am Fam Physician (U.S.) Apr 1994; 49(5):1129–1137, 1142–1149.

4. Karno M, Golding JM. Obsessive-compulsive disorders. In: Robins LN, Regier DA, eds. Psychiatric Disorders in America: The Epidemiology Catchment Area Study. New York: The Free Press, 1991:204–219.

5. Myers JK, Weisman MM, Tischler GL, et al. Six month prevalence of psychiatric disorders in three sites. Arch Gen Psychiatry 1984; 41:959–971.

6. Robins LN, Helzer JE, Weisman MM, et al. Lifetime prevalence of specific psychiatric disorders in three sites. Arch Gen Psychiatry 1984; 41:949–959.

7. Weismann MM, Bland RC, Canino GJ, Greenwald S, et al: The Cross National Collaborative Group. The Cross National Epidemiology of Obsessive-Compulsive Disorder. J Clin Psychiatry 1994; 55(3 suppl)5–10.

8. Khanna S, Gururay G, Sriram TG. Epidemiology of obsessive compulsive disorder in India. First International Obsessive-Compulsive Congress, Capri, Italy, March 1993.

9. Flament M, Whitaker A, Rappoport J, et al. Obsessive compulsive disorder in adolescence: an epidemiologic study. J Am Acad Child Adolesc Psychiatry 1988; 27:764–771.

10. Nestadt G, Samuels JF, Romanoski AJ, et al. Obsessions and compulsions in the community. Acta Psychiatr Scand (Denmark) Apr 1994; 89(4):219–224.

11. Rasmussen SA, Eisen JL. Epidemiology and clinical features of obsessive-compulsive disorder. In: Jenike MA, Baer L, Minilchiello WE, eds. Obsessive-Compulsive Disorders: Theory and Management. Chicago: Year Book 1990:10–27.

12. Karno M, Golding JM, Sorenson SB, et al. The epidemiology of obsessive-compulsive disorder in five US communities. Arch Gen Psychiatry 1988; 45:1094–1099.

13. Thomsen PH, Jensen J. Obsessive-compulsive disorder: admission patterns and diagnostic stability. A case-register study. Acta Psychiatr Scand (Denmark) Jul 1994; 90(1):19–24.

14. Swedo SE, Rapoport JL, Leonard H, et al. Obsessive-compulsive disorder in children and adolescents: clinical phenomenology of 70 consecutive cases. Arch Gen Psychiatry 1989; 46:335–341.

15. Sichel DA, Cohen LS, Rosenbaum JF, et al. Postpartum onset of obsessive-compulsive disorder. Psychosomatics (U.S.) May–Jun 1993; 34(3):277–279.

16. Neziroglu F, Anemone R, Yaryura-Tobias JA. Onset of obsessive-compulsive disorder in pregnancy. Am J Psychiatry Jul 1992; 149(7):947–950.

17. Swedo SE, Leonard HL. Childhood movement disorders and obsessive compulsive disorder. J Clin Psychiatry (U.S.) Mar 1994; 55(suppl):32–37.

18. Demal U, Lenz G, Mayrhofer A, et al. Obsessive-compulsive disorder and depression: a retrospective study on course and interaction. Psychopathology (Switzerland) 1993; 26(3–4):145–150.

19. Eisen JL, Rasmussen SA. Obsessive compulsive disorder with psychotic features. J Clin Psychiatry (U.S.) Oct 1993; 54(10):373–379.

20. Politts J. Natural history of obsessional states. Br Med J 1957; 1:194–198.

21. American Psychiatric Association. The Diagnostic and Statistical Manual of Mental Disorders. 4th ed. Washington, DC: American Psychiatric Press, 1994.

22. Foa EB, Kozak MJ. DSM-IV field trial: obsessive-compulsive disorder. Am J Psychiatry Jan 1995; 152(1):90–96.

23. Insel TR, Akiskal HS. Obsessive-compulsive disorder with psychotic features: a phenomenological analysis. Am J Psychiatry 1986; 143:1527–1533.

24. Rasmussen SA, Eisen JL. The epidemiology and differential diagnosis of obsessive compulsive disorder. J Clin Psychiatry Oct 1994; 55(10 suppl):5–10.

25. Kozak MJ, Foa EB. Obsessions, overvalued ideas, and delusions in obsessive-compulsive disorder. Behav Res Ther (England) March 1994; 32(3):343–353.

26. Marks IM. Fears, phobias and rituals: panic, anxiety and their disorders. New York: Oxford University Press, 1978.

27. Rasmussen SA, Eisen JL. Clinical and epidemiologic findings of significance to neuropharmacologic trials in OCD. Psychopharmacol Bull 1988; 24:466–470.

28. Mavissakalian MR, Barlow DH. Assesment of obsessive-compulsive disorders. In: Barlow DH, ed. Behavioral Assessment of Adult Disorders. New York: Guilford Press, 1981.

29. Akhtar S, Wig NN, Verma VJ, et al. A phenomenological analysis of symptoms in obsessive compulsive neurosis. Br J Psychiatry 1975; 127:342–348.

30. Okasha A, Saad A, Khalil AH, et al. Phenomenology of obsessive-compulsive disorder: a transcultural study. Compr Psychiatry (U.S.) May–Jun 1994; 35(3):191–197.

31. Wells A, Davies MI. The Thought Control Questionnaire: a measure of individual differences in the control of unwanted thoughts. Behav Res Ther (England) Nov 1994; 32(8):871–878.

32. Rachman S, de Silva P. Abnormal and normal obsessions. Behav Res Ther 1978; 16:233–248.

33. Niler ER, Beck SJ. The relationship among guilt, dysphoria, anxiety and obsessions in a normal population. Behav Res Ther (England) 1989; 27(3):213–220.

34. Edwards S, Dickerson M. Intrusive unwanted thoughts: a two-stage model of control. Br J Med Psychol Dec 1987; 60(4):317–328.

35. Frost RO, Sher KJ, Geen T. Psychopathology and personality characteristics of nonclinical compulsive checkers. Behav Res Ther (England) 1986; 24(2):133–143.

36. Rachman SJ, Hodgson RJ. Obsessions and compulsions. Englewood Cliffs, NJ: Prentice-Hall, 1980.

37. Insel TR. Obsessive compulsive disorder—five clinical questions and a suggested approach. Compr Psychiatry (U.S.) May–Jun 1982; 23(3):241–251.

18 Niehaus and Stein

38. MacKenzie TB, Christenson G, Kroll J. Obsession or worry? [letter]. Am J Psychiatry Nov 1990; 147(11):1573.
39. Khanna S, Mukherjee D. Checkers and washers: valid subtypes of obsessive compulsive disorder. Psychopathology (Switzerland) 1992; 25(5):283–288.
40. Baer L. Factor analysis of symptom subtypes of obsessive-compulsive disorder and their relation to personality and tic disorders. J Clin Psychiatry March 1994; 55(3 suppl):18–23.
41. Rasmussen S, Eisen J. Assessment of core features, conviction and psychosocial function in OCD. In: 1st International OCD Conference Abstracts, Isle of Capri, Italy, March 9–12, 1993:32–33.
42. George MS, Trimble MR, Ring HA, et al. Obsessions in obsessive-compulsive disorder with and without Gilles de la Tourette's syndrome. Am J Psychiatry Jan 1993; 150(1):93–97.
43. Pitman RK, Green RC, Jenike MA, et al. Clinical comparison of Tourette's disorder and obsessive-compulsive disorder. Am J Psychiatry 1987; 144:1166–1171.
44. Veale D. Classification and treatment of obsessional slowness. Br J Psychiatry Feb 1993; 162:198–203.
45. Frost RO, Lahart CM, Dugas KM. Information processing among non-clinical compulsives. Behav Res Ther (England) 1988; 26:275–277.
46. Holzer JC, Goodman WK, McDougle CJ, et al. Obsessive-compulsive disorder with and without a chronic tic disorder: a comparison of symptoms in 70 patients. Br J Psychiatry Apr 1994; 164:469–473.
47. Stein DJ, Hollander E, Chan S, et al. Computed tomography and neurological soft signs in obsessive-compulsive disorder. Psychiatry Res (Ireland) Oct 1993; 50(3):143–150.
48. Rasmussen SA, Tsuang MT. Clinical characteristics and family history in DSM-III obsessive-compulsive disorder. Am J Psychiatry 1986; 143:317–322.
49. Pauls DL, Alsobrook II JP, Phil M, et al. A family study of obsessive-compulsive disorder. Am J Psychiatry 1995; 152:76–84.
50. Chakrabarti S, Kulhara P, Verma SK. The pattern of burden in families of neurotic patients. Soc Psychiatr Epidemiol (Germany) Aug 1993; 28(4):172–177.
51. Pigott TA, L'Hereux F, Dubbert B, et al. Obsessive compulsive disorder: comorbid conditions. J Clin Psychiatry Oct 1994; 55(10 suppl):15–27.
52. Breier A, Charney DS. The diagnostic validity of anxiety disorders and their relationship to depressive illness. Am J Psychiatry 1985; 142:787–797.
53. Breier A, Charney DS, Heninger GR. Agoraphobia with panic attacks. Arch Gen Psychiatry 1986; 43:1029–1036.
54. Barlow DH. The dimensions of anxiety disorders. In: Tuma AH, Maser JD, eds. Anxiety and the Anxiety Disorders. Hillsdale, NJ: Lawrence Erlbaum Publishers, 1985.
55. Stein DJ, Hollander E. The spectrum of obsessive-compulsive related disorders. In: Hollander E, ed. Obsessive-Compulsive Related Disorders. Washington, DC: American Psychiatric Press, 1993.

56. Kaye WH, Weltzin TE, Hsu LK, et al. Patients with anorexia nervosa have elevated scores on the Y-BOCS. Int J Eating Disord 1992; 12:57–62.

57. Thiel A, Broocks A, Ohlmeier M, et al. Obsessive-compulsive disorder among patients with anorexia nervosa and bulimia nervosa. Am J Psychiatry Jan 1995; 152(1):72–75.

58. Barsky AJ. Hypochondriasis and obsessive compulsive disorder. Psychiatr Clin North Am Dec 1992; 15(4):791–801.

59. Stein DJ, Hollander E, Mullen L, et al. Compulsive and impulsive symptoms and traits in the obsessive-compulsive realted disorders. Biol Psychiatry 1992; 31:267A.

60. Hoehn-Saric R, Barksdale VC. Impulsiveness in obsessive-compulsive patients. Br J Psychiatry 1983; 143:177–182.

61. McElroy SL, Phillips KA, Keck PE. Obsessive compulsive spectrum disorder. J Clin Psychiatry Oct 1994; 55(10 suppl):33–51.

62. Boyd JH, Burke JD, Gruenberg E, et al. Exclusion criteria of DSM-III. Arch Gen Psychiatry 1984; 41:983–989.

63. Goodwin DW, Guze SB, Robins E, et al. Follow-up studies in obsessional neurosis. Arch Gen Psychiatry 1969; 20:182–187.

64. Stein DJ, Hollander E. Personality disorders and obsessive-compulsive disorder. In: Hollander E, Zohar J, Marazzati D, Olivier B, eds. Current Insights in Obsessive-Compulsive Disorder. New York: John Wiley, 1994.

65. Baer L, Jenike MA. Personality disorders in obsessive compulsive disorder. Psychiatr Clin North Am Dec 1992; 15(4):803–812.

66. Baer L, Jenike MA, Ricciardi JN, et al. Standardized assessment of personality disorders in obsessive-compulsive disorder. Arch Gen Psychiatry 1990; 47:826–830.

67. Black L, Jenike M. Personality disorders in OCD. Psychiatr Clin North Am 1992; 15(4):803–812.

68. Black DW, Noyes R Jr, Pfohl B, et al. Personality disorder in obsessive-compulsive volunteers, well comparison subjects, and their first-degree relatives. Am J Psychiatry Aug 1993; 150(8):1226–1232.

69. AuBuchon PG, Malatesta VJ. Obsessive compulsive patients with comorbid personality disorder: associated problems and response to a comprehensive behavior therapy. J Clin Psychiatry Oct 1994; 55(10):448–453.

70. Zohar J, Insel T. Obsessive-compulsive disorder: psychobiological approaches to diagnosis, treatment, and pathophysiology. Biol Psychiatry 1987; 22:667–687.

71. Leonard H, Swedo S, Rapoport JL, et al. Treatment of childhood obsessive-compulsive disorder with clomipramine and desmethylimipramine: a double-blind crossover comparison. Psychopharmacol Bull (U.S.) 1988; 24(1):93–95.

72. Peselow ED, Robins C, Block P, et al. Dysfunctional attitudes in depressed patients before and after clinical treatment and in normal control subjects. Am J Psychiatry 1990; 147(4):439–444.

73. Vaughan M. The relationship between obsessional personality, obsessions

in depression and symptoms of depression. Br J Psychiatry July 1976; 129:36–39.

74. Martin LL, Tesser A. Toward a motivational and structural theory of ruminative thought. In: Uleman JS, Bargh JA, eds. Unintended Thought. New York: Guilford Press.

75. Jenike MA, Hyman S, Baer L, et al. Clomipramine versus fluoxetine in obsessive-compulsive disorder: a retrospective comparison of side effects and efficacy. J Clin Psychopharmacol 1990; 10:122–124.

76. Lipinski JF Jr, Pope HG Jr. Do "flashbacks" represent obsessional imagery? Compr Psychiatry (U.S.) Jul–Aug 1994; 35(4):245–247.

77. Pato MT, Eisen JL, Pato CN. Rating scales for obsessive compulsive disorder. In: Hollander E, Zohar J, Marazzati D, Olivier B. Current Insights in Obsessive-Compulsive Disorder. New York: John Wiley, 1994:77–91.

78. Hodgson RJ, Rachman S. Obsessional-compulsive complaints. Behav Res Ther 1977; 15:389–395.

79. Insel T, Murphy D, Cohen R, et al. Obsessive compulsive disorder: A double-blind trail of clomipramine and clorgyline. Arch Gen Psychiatry 1983; 40:605.

80. Sternberger LG, Burns GL. Obsessions and compulsions: psychometric properties of the Padua Inventory with an American college population. Behav Res Ther (England) 1990; 28(4):341–345.

81. Cooper J. The Leyton obsessional inventory. Psychiatr Med 1970; 1:48.

82. Cooper J, Kelleher M. The Leyton obsessional inventory: A principal component analysis on normal subjects. Psychiatr Med 1973; 3:204.

83. Kim S, Dysken M, Kuskowski M. The Yale-Brown obsessive compulsive scale: a reliability and validity study. Psychiatric Res 1990; 34(1):94–106.

84. Derogatis L, Lipman R, Covi L. The SCL-90: An outpatient psychiatric rating scale. Psychopharmacol Bull 1973; 9:13.

85. Guy W. ECDEU assessment manual for psychopharmacology. Publication 76–338. US Department of Health, Education and Welfare. Washington, DC: US Goverment Printing Office, 1976.

86. Steketee G, Doppelt H. Measurement of obsessive compulsive symptomatology: Utility of the Hopkins symptom checklist. Psychiatry Res 1986; 19:135–145.

87. Kaplan SL. A self-rated scale for obsessive-compulsive disorder. J Clin Psychol (U.S.) July 1994; 50(4):564–567.

88. Baer L, Brown-Beasley MW, Sorce J, et al. Computer-assisted telephone administration of a structured interview for obsessive-compulsive disorder. Am J Psychiatry Nov 1993; 150(11):1737–1738.

89. Goodman WK, Price LH, Rasmussen SA, et al. The Yale-Brown Obsessive Compulsive Scale. I. Development, use, and reliability. Arch Gen Psychiatry (U.S.) Nov 1989; 46(11):1006–1011.

90. Goodman W, Price L, Rasmussen S, et al. The Yale-Brown Obsessive Compulsive Scale. II. Validity. Arch Gen Psychiatry (U.S.) Nov 1989; 46(11):1012–1016.

91. Kim SW, Dysken MW, Pheley AM, et al. The Yale-Brown Obsessive-Compulsive Scale: measures of internal consistency. Psychiatry Res (Ireland) Feb 1994; 51(2):203–211.
92. Goodman W, Price L. Assessment of severity and change in obsessive compulsive disorder. Psychiatr Clin North Am 1992; 15(4):861–869.
93. Asberg M, Montgomery S, Perris C, et al. A comprehensive psychopathological rating scale. Acta Psychiatr Scand 1978; 271(suppl):5.
94. Eisen JL, Phillips KA, Beer D, et al. Assessment of Insight in Obsessions and Delusions. San Francisco: New Research APA, 1993.
95. Foa EB. Failures in treating obsessive compulsives. Behav Res Ther 1979; 17:169–176.

2

Childhood OCD

John Piacentini
UCLA School of Medicine
Los Angeles, California

Flemming Graae
Cornell University Medical Center—The New York Hospital
New York, New York

EPIDEMIOLOGY OF CHILD AND ADOLESCENT OCD

Prevalence

Until the last decade, obsessive-compulsive disorder (OCD) was thought to be rare in children and adolescents. The Isle of Wight Study (1) identified only seven of 2000 youngsters as having an "obsessional/anxiety disorder" and five children as having "disease or dirt phobias," for a total point prevalence of 0.7%. Hollingsworth et al. (2), in a chart review of over 8000 child psychiatry inpatient and outpatient charts, found a clinic prevalence rate of only 0.2%. Moreover, even though Flament et al. (3) found a weighted current prevalence for OCD of 1.0% in a community sample of 5600 high school students, only four of 20 (20%) identified adolescents were in treatment and none had received a clinical diagnosis of OCD. Over the past few years, there has been a substantial upward revision in the prevalence rate for OCD in young people. This increase can be attributed to several factors, including the finding that many adults with OCD report an onset of the disorder in childhood (4,5), the development of more sophisticated assessment and survey methodology, and an increasing public and professional awareness of the disorder. Although national prevalence data do not exist, recent epidemiological studies suggest a lifetime prevalence for OCD in children and adolescents of between 2% and 3% (3,6–8), indicating that the disorder is approximately as common in children as it is in adults (9,10).

Age of Onset

Most studies report a mean age of onset for childhood OCD ranging from 9 to 11 years, although onset age appears to be bimodally distributed, with peaks in early childhood and early adolescence (11–14). Youngsters with an early onset of OCD are more likely to be male (12,14) and to have a family history of OCD (14) than those with later onset, suggesting that genetic factors may be more likely to play a role in the development of the early-versus late-onset subtype (14).

Gender Effects

The evidence for a gender difference in OCD rates among children and adolescents is mixed. Data from most clinic-based studies suggest a male preponderance in childhood, ranging from 1.5:1 to 3:1 (11,2,15,14). In the most well-studied pediatric cohort to date, a consecutive series of 70 youngsters (mean age 13.7 years) seen prospectively at the National Institute of Mental Health (NIMH) between 1977 and 1987, males outnumbered females by a margin of 2:1 (47 males to 23 females) (14). This male overrepresentation, however, has not been replicated in community-based studies of mostly older adolescent samples (16,3,6,8). Thus, it is not clear whether the male preponderance seen in children but not adolescents is the result of a developmental phenomenon or due to an ascertainment bias. The NIMH group's observation that an early age of onset was associated with a higher male-to-female ratio, however, offers some support for the former hypothesis (14). Referral bias may also account for the underrepresentation of minorities and families from lower socioeconomic strata in clinical samples of OCD youth (13,14).

PHENOMENOLOGY OF CHILD AND ADOLESCENT OCD

Diagnosis

According to the *Diagnostic and Statistical Manual of Mental Disorders,* fourth edition–revised (DSM-IV) (17), OCD is characterized by recurrent obsessions or compulsions that are severe enough to be time-consuming (at least one hour per day), cause marked distress, or are associated with significant impairment. Obsessions are persistent thoughts, ideas, impulses, or images that are experienced, at least initially, as intrusive or inappropriate (i.e., ego-dystonic). Although the obsessions are often anxiety-provoking or distressing, they are not simply excess worries about real-life problems (such as school, social, or financial problems). The individual with OCD tries to ignore or suppress his or her obsessions, or neutralize them with another thought or action (i.e., a compulsion). Compulsions are repetitive behaviors or mental acts that are performed in response to an obsession or according to other rigidly applied rules. Compulsions are meant to reduce anxiety or distress or prevent some dreaded event but are clearly excessive or are not realistically connected with the triggering stimulus. To meet the diagnostic criteria for OCD, adults must recognize at some point that their OCD symptoms are excessive or unreasonable. However, given their typically lower levels of cognitive awareness and the fact that many youngsters are unable to recall periods of symptom-free functioning, the requirement that symptoms be experienced as ego-dystonic does not apply to children and adolescents.

Clinical Picture

The most common obsessions among children and adolescents tend to focus on germs or contamination, followed by fears of harm to self or others, concerns with symmetry, and excessive moralization or religiosity. The most common compulsions include excessive washing and bathing, repeating, checking, touching, counting, and ordering or arranging. Swedo et al. (14) reported the following symptom breakdown for their NIMH sample of OCD youngsters: excessive bathing or grooming (85%), repeating rituals (51%), excessive checking (46%), and rituals to remove contact with contaminants (23%). Less common symptoms include an inability to wear certain articles of clothing, getting "stuck" or being unable to move without assistance, needing to remember conversations or parts of conversations verbatim, seeking verbal reassurances from others, hoarding, and blinking or staring rituals. Community surveys of adolescents with OCD have yielded symptom patterns similar to those found for clinic patients (3). Like adults, the majority of youngsters with OCD have both obsessions and compulsions (3,13,14). Compulsions in the absence of anxiety-related or otherwise distress-inducing obsessions are most commonly found in younger children, who typically describe their rituals as being performed in response to either an irresistible urge or an otherwise vague sensation (18,14). Pure obsessives are less common than pure ritualizers (3,14), although recent community studies found that approximately 50% of affected adolescents experienced either obssessions or compulsions only (8,19). Most youths with OCD report that although the absolute number of symptoms remains relatively constant, the pattern and type of symptoms tend to shift over time (11,20). There is also evidence to suggest that gender plays a role in some OCD symptom patterns, with obsessions more common in males and compulsions more common in females (20,21,8). OCD symptoms also tend to show a variable course throughout the day and in different settings and are often exacerbated by stress or change (14).

Given the typically strange and senseless nature of many OCD behaviors, most children and adolescents with OCD attempt to camouflage or hide their rituals and obsessions. Like individuals with Tourette's syndrome, children and adolescents with OCD are often able to inhibit or control their symptoms for short periods of time and with substantial effort, especially in social situations or at school (18). These episodes of symptom suppression may lead to a rebound effect or an increased rate of symptom occurrence once the individual finds himself in a safe and/ or private environment (e.g., at home or with family members). Except in severe cases, teachers, friends, and even family members may remain unaware of the child's problem for months or years, learning of it only in response to media or other outreach efforts or when the child becomes too overwhelmed to cope (22).

Not surprisingly, OCD in children and adolescents can lead to severe disruptions in social, familial, academic, and vocational functioning (23,24). Dressing and washing rituals may result in chronic lateness to school, while contamination fears often prevent the child's going to school, movies, restaurants, or other social events. Counting and checking rituals and intrusive thoughts can impair focus and concentration and interfere with reading and writing, adversely impacting school and job performance. In more severe cases, symptoms may also interfere with the child's ability to initiate and maintain friendships, and adversely impact the adolescent's attempts to develop heterosexual relationships.

Comorbidity

Comorbidity is the rule rather than the exception in children and adolescents with OCD. Lifetime rates for associated diagnoses range from 62% to 84%, with upward of 50% of OCD youths experiencing multiple comorbid conditions (16,3,11–14,8). The most frequent associated diagnoses include other anxiety disorders (26% to 75%), depressive disorders (25% to 62%), and disruptive behavior disorders (18% to 33%).

In most cases, the onset age for OCD precedes that for depression, suggesting that co-occurring mood disturbance may often be reactive. Substance-use disorders, learning disorders, and eating disorders also appear to be overrepresented (18). Rates for obsessive-compulsive personality disorder (OCPD) range from 11% to 14% (13,14) and are generally similar to findings from recent adult studies using structured diagnostic assessments (25,18). Of interest is the fact that the rates for comorbid depressive and substance-use disorders tend to be higher in community samples than in clinical samples (16,3,8). Although possibly due to the older mean age of the community samples, this difference may also reflect increased morbidity associated with the low identification and treatment rates characteristic of nonreferred youth.

Tic disorders (Tourette's syndrome, motor tics, vocal tics) have been reported in between 20% to 30% of youngsters with OCD (14,13,11). Certain features appear to distinguish individuals with OCD and Tourette's syndrome from those with OCD only. Comorbid youths are less likely to describe their compulsions as anxiety-driven; instead, they describe feeling a need to achieve a sense of something's looking or feeling "just right." As compared to uncomplicated OCD, adults with tic-related OCD are more likely to report compulsions involving touching, symmetry, blinking/staring, violent or religious obsessions, or other intrusive images, and less likely to report compulsions related to contamination, cleaning, or checking (26). Clinical experience suggests that this pattern applies to children and adolescents as well.

Course

Longitudinal studies attest to the chronicity of the disorder in childhood, as approximately 43% to 68% of OCD youth from community (27) and clinical (28–32) samples have been found to meet criteria for the disorder at 2- to 14-year follow-up. Flament et al. (30) found 68% (17/25) of a subsample of the NIMH sample met criteria for OCD 2 to 7 years after their initial presentation. although none of the subjects was deemed to have received satisfactory treatment for his obsessive-compulsive symptoms. Follow-up studies of more adequately treated cohorts have yielded slightly more positive outcomes (29,31,32). In the largest study to date, Leonard et al. (31) re-evaluated 54 youngsters who had participated in controlled trials of clomipramine at NIMH 2 to 7 years earlier and who had access to continued interim treatment. At follow-up, 43% of subjects still met diagnostic criteria for OCD, 70% were taking psychoactive medication, and only 6% were classified as complete remitters. Overall, however, the group as a whole was significantly improved, with only 19% of subjects rated as unchanged or worse. Given the advances in both behavioral and psychopharmacological interventions for childhood OCD, it is reasonable to conclude that the majority of youngsters with OCD will be able to experience significant improvement with adequate treatment over the course of their illness (33).

Substantial rates of comorbid psychiatric diagnoses have also been found at follow-up, with depression and other anxiety disorders being the most common (29–32). In a longitudinal study investigating the relationship between OCD and tic disorders, Leonard et al. (31) found that 59% of the NIMH Child OCD sample reported a lifetime incidence of tics at follow-up, even though the presence of Tourette's syndrome was an exclusionary criterion at baseline. Most follow-up studies have not had a sample large enough to examine predictors of outcome. Leonard et al. (31), however, found that a worse outcome at follow-up was predicted by a poor 5-week response to clomipramine, lifetime history of a tic disorder, and the presence of parental axis I psychiatric disorder.

Developmental Considerations

Obsessive thoughts and compulsive behaviors are normative during early childhood. These behaviors, which typically include bedtime or mealtime rituals, rigid or stereotypic rules for many activities, ritualistic play, and superstitious beliefs, often serve to enhance the young child's sense of mastery and control (34,33). Although some have speculated that OCD represents the extreme endpoint along a continuum of normal developmental rituals, OCD symptoms can be reliably distinguished from normal developmental phenomena on the basis of timing, content, and severity (34). From a clinical perspective, the level of associated distress and impairment, a family history of OCD or tic disorders, the extent to which the behaviors are controllable by the child, and any significant environmental stressors or other factors that may explain the behaviors in question may also be useful indicators for determining the significance of obsessive-compulsive behavior in young children.

Family History

Several studies suggest that a substantial proportion of childhood OCD cases may be familial in nature (35–37,13). Lenane et al. (36), studying a subset of the NIMH child and adolescent sample, reported that 25% of first-degree relatives and 17% of parents met criteria for OCD according to a structured assessment. Riddle et al. (13) reported that 71% of their pediatric OCD sample had a parent with either OCD (19%) or obsessive-compulsive symptoms (52%). Pauls et al. (37) found significantly higher rates of both OCD and tics among the relatives of 100 OCD probands as compared to nonpsychiatric controls. Further, increased risk for both OCD and tics was found in the relatives of probands with an earlier age of onset for OCD. No significant correlation has been found between the type of OCD symptoms experienced by probands and their affected family members, suggesting that modeling may not play a primary role in the intergenerational transmission of the disorder.

NEUROBIOLOGY OF OCD

The onset of OCD following encephalitis (38), head trauma (39), and epilepsy (40), and the association between OCD and increased abnormal birth events (41) Sydenham's chorea (42), Tourette's disorder (43), choreoathetoid movements (44), and toxic brain lesions (45) all serve to strengthen the understanding of OCD as a neurobiological disorder.

Neurophysiological Findings

Several pharmacological and biochemical challenge studies suggest that abnormalities in CNS serotonergic activity and/or sensitivity are related to OCD in at least a substantial proportion of cases. The most important evidence for this finding is the fact that highly potent serotonin (5-HT) reuptake blockers are currently the most effective treatments for OCD. Studies of both adult (46) and adolescent (47,48,49) samples have shown a relationship between OCD severity and treatment outcome and peripheral markers of serotonergic functioning. Flament et al. (47) reported a positive relationship between decreased platelet serotonin concentration and decreases in OCD symptomatology in clomipramine-treated adolescents. These authors also reported a negative correlation between baseline platelet serotonin content and clinical severity, although there was no overall difference between patients and controls at baseline. Hanna et al. (48) found a negative correlation between basal prolactin levels—an indirect measure of serotonergic activity—and both duration and severity of OCD symptoms in a group of children and adolescents with severe OCD. Treatment with clomipramine resulted in significant overall increases in basal prolactin levels over an 8-week period. Responders, however, demonstrated more distinct decreases than nonresponders during the second 4 weeks of treatment, although they remained above baseline levels, suggesting that treatment may have led to an adaptive hyporesponsivity of the serotonergic system. In a follow-up study, Hanna et al. (49) found a significant positive correlation between percentage change of whole blood serotonin and clinical change after 8 weeks of clomipramine treatment.

Although methodological complications, including seasonal changes in serotonergic functioning in normal controls (50,51) but not OCD patients (52), call for caution in interpreting the above data, these results are consistent with clinical observations regarding the time course of treatment response. Serotonergic reuptake blockers such as clomipramine and fluoxetine are not immediately effective (in fact, acute administration with too large a dose may lead to transient symptom exacerbation) but require up to 8 to 10 weeks or more for significant improvement. While acute administration of serotonin reuptake blockers results in increased synaptic serotonin, chronic administration may result in decreased presynaptic firing and/or postsynaptic desensitization. Thus, it is possible that OCD may be related to the hyperactivity and/or hypersensitivity of certain serotonergic pathways in the CNS, and serotonin reuptake blockers exert their therapeutic effects by "inoculating" patients against their own overactive serotonergic systems or helping them offset another biological derangement in these regulatory systems. The induction of transient obsessive-compulsive symptoms in psychotic patients by antipsychotic agents with antiserotonergic activity, such as clozapine (53,54) and clothiapine (55), provides further support for a serotonergic dysregulation hypothesis.

Additional support for a serotonergic dysregulation hypothesis of OCD comes from biochemical challenge studies in adults with the 5-HT agonist oral m-chlorophenylpiperazine (m-CPP). Administration of m-CPP in adults has been shown to result in a transient exacerbation of OCD symptoms in subsets of OCD patients that may last for several hours, with the worsening of symptoms paralleling m-CPP blood levels (56,57). Although m-CPP is anxiogenic, other anxiety-causing compounds, such as yohimbine and lactate, do not lead to exacerbation of OCD symptoms, suggesting some response specificity. Behavioral hypersensitivity to m-CPP and similar 5-HT agonists has been shown to disappear following successful treatment of OCD with such 5-HT reuptake blockers as clomipramine (58) and fluoxetine (59,60), suggesting that chronic treatment with serotonin reuptake blockers reduces baseline supersensitivity to endogenous serotonin.

In addition, various neuropeptides that produce hyperarousal and delayed extinction of conditioned behaviors in animals have also been implicated in the pathophysiology of at least some types of OCD. These include oxytocin and vasopressin (61), as well as corticotropin-releasing hormone, somatostatin, and monoamine metabolites (62). Continued work in this area will, hopefully, elucidate more fully the role these peptides play in the pathogenesis of OCD and may also lead to the development of newer, more specific pharmacological treatments for the disorder.

A possible subgroup of children with autoimmune OCD has been described by the NIMH group (63). These researchers hypothesize that, in a process analagous to the development of Sydenham's chorea, antineuronal antibodies formed against group A β-hemolytic streptococci interact with caudate nuclear tissue, resulting in caudate swelling. This swelling then leads to the initiation or exacerbation of pre-existing OCD. Four cases with abrupt, severe onset or worsening of OCD or tics were evaluated and found to have evidence of recent streptococcal or other viral infections. All four were treated with plasmapheresis, intravenous immunoglobulin, or immunosuppression, which led to clinically signficant improvement in each case (63).

Neuroanatomical and Neurological Findings

Imaging studies of adults with OCD implicate abnormalities in cortico-striatal-thalamocortical pathways (64–66). Positron emission tomography (PET) studies have found increased glucose metabolism in orbital frontal and prefrontal cortex, right caudate nucleus, and anterior cingulate gyrus (65,67–71). Moreover, successful treatment with either behavior therapy (65) or selective serotonin-reuptake inhibitor (SSRI) medication (68) has resulted in decreased activity in these areas as well as an attenuation of the correlations of activity between these regions. Magnetic resonance imaging (MRI) and volumetric computed tomography (CT) scan studies have also suggested frontal lobe and caudate nuclei abnormalities (72–74), and both increases and decreases in frontal and basal ganglia glucose metabolism have been observed with improvement of OCD after treatment, with most studies showing posttreatment metabolism changes in the direction of normalization (75–79).

From a functional perspective, the orbitofrontal cortex serves as a warning system that alerts the brain when something is awry (65). In patients with OCD, signals from an overactive orbitofrontal cortex may underscore the feeling that something is not right and lead to ritualistic behavior. Conversely, Insel (66) has postulated that orbitofrontal cortex may serve as the neural substrate for symptom resistance and that increased activity in this area is the result of intensive, yet unsuccessful, efforts to deal with intrusive urges and thoughts. In contrast, the caudate nucleus and cingulate gyrus are associated with the visceral and affective aspects, i.e., the dread and worry of the disorder. According to Baxter and colleagues (64), a high degree of intercorrelation of activity along the corticostriatal-thalamocortical pathway may lead to the circuits becoming "stuck," resulting in an escalating pattern of doubt and checking characteristic of many OCD patients. When successful, treatment may lead to symptom relief by reducing the correlation in activity rates among these different brain areas.

OCD has also been associated with higher rates of neurological soft signs in both adults (44) and children (80). One prospective follow-up study found the presence of neurological soft signs at age 7 to be related to the occurrence of obsessive-compulsive symptoms in adulthood (81). The findings from both neurological and neuropsychological studies have generally implicated greater right than left hemispheric dysfunction (44,80). These results are consistent with those of PET studies, which also appear to implicate greater dysfunction in the right hemisphere (67,65).

TREATMENT

Like many psychiatric disorders, the majority of treatment research for OCD has been conducted in adults. While psychodynamic and other insight-oriented therapies have shown limited efficacy for the treatment of OCD (82,83), the efficacy of SRIs and exposure plus response prevention (ERP) in treating adult OCD is well documented (84,85). Similarities in the clinical phenomenology of OCD across the agespan, however, suggest that treatment findings from the adult literature should also be applicable to children and adolescents with the disorder. The available evidence supports this hypothesis. Despite the fact that only clomipramine has FDA approval for use in childhood OCD, clomipramine, fluoxetine, and fluvoxamine have all been found effective in controlled studies with pediatric populations (86–89). As with adults, however, controlled trials show that from one-third to one-half of children with OCD do not respond to medication; of those that do, average symptom reduction ranges from 20% to 50%. Although data from controlled trials with adults imply that behavior therapy may lead to higher response rates and greater symptom reduction than medication (85), there are no controlled trials of behavior therapy for childhood OCD. Nevertheless, preliminary results from two small open behavioral trials with children suggest that ERP may be an effective and well-tolerated treatment option in this age group (90,91).

BEHAVIORAL INTERVENTIONS

Although there have been no controlled trials of behavior therapy for childhood OCD, results from several single-case reports and small case series have generally been promising (92,33). Similar to most childhood treatments, behavior therapy for childhood OCD is based closely on that for the adult disorder and centered on ERP (93).

The first step in ERP consists of developing a rank-ordered list of all the child's symptoms (both thoughts and rituals) along with the situations in which these symptoms are most likely to occur. Following this, patients are systematically exposed to these situations, the least difficult situations first, while being instructed to not engage in their ritualistic behaviors. Over repeated exposures, the associated anxiety dissipates through the process of autonomic habituation. In addition, when the feared consequences of not ritualizing fail to occur, patients' heightened expectations of harm disappear, reducing anxiety even further (94).

However, a number of development considerations serve to complicate the behavioral treatment of childhood OCD. The most important complications stem from the cognitive and motivational limitations of young children, for whom the motivating aspect of future improvement is likely to be heavily outweighed by the high degree of anxiety associated with the initial treatment exercises. Effective behavioral treatment programs for childhood OCD have addressed these issues through the use of metaphorical techniques to facilitate an understanding of the illness, an emphasis on therapist modeling, the use of cognitive coping strategies for helping patients deal with anxiety, an emphasis on visual or graphic feedback of progress, the incorporation of behavioral rewards for compliance with in-session and homework tasks, and family involvement in treatment (90,91). The increased rates of family conflict, family dysfunction, and parental OCD associated with childhood OCD (95,96) provide further support for the inclusion of a family therapy component in the child's treatment program (90,33,97).

March et al. (91) describes a manualized treatment program entitled "How I Ran OCD Off My Land," which uses several narrative, cartographic, and metaphorical techniques to facilitate compliance. In this protocol, a child's experience with OCD is diagrammed on a map, which is then used to generate a narrative-based visual-stimulus hierarchy and provide graphic feedback regarding progress over time. In addition, an anxiety-management training (AMT) "toolkit" consisting of guidelines for relaxation training, constructive self-talk, breathing techniques, and positive coping strategies is systematically presented and used to increase compliance with exposure tasks. An open trial of 15 OCD youngsters, all but one of whom also received other treatments, yielded a 60% response rate, with responders showing a 50% reduction in the Yale-Brown Obsessive-Compulsive Scale (Y-BOCS) from pre- to posttreatment (91).

Piacentini and colleagues (90) have developed a child and adolescent treatment protocol based on ERP that also includes concurrent family management sessions. The family sessions, which generally parallel and are closely integrated with the individual child treatment, aim to provide psychoeducation about OCD, establish guidelines to facilitate family members' disengagement from the child's OCD behaviors, and restructure family interactions free of impairment from the disorder. As treatment progresses, family members are taught to differentiate OCD-related behaviors from other inappropriate behaviors and to use contingency management systems to positively reshape problematic family interaction patterns. In a 12-week open trial, four of five patients were rated as treatment responders (clinician-rated CGI ≤ 2), with the entire sample showing a 58% mean reduction in children's Y-BOCS (CY-BOCS) scores over the treatment interval.

PSYCHOPHARMACOLOGICAL TREATMENTS

Clomipramine

The earliest U.S. psychopharmacology trials for childhood OCD were conducted using clomipramine, a tricyclic antidepressant. In a 10-week crossover design (5 weeks on each treatment) of 19 children, Flament et al. (98) found clomipramine significantly superior to placebo. After 5 weeks, clomipramine produced a 46% decrement in OCD symptoms, measured as a composite of preoccupation with obsessions or rituals, number of rituals, degree of interference in personal activities, and amount of time spent resisting compulsive urges and behaviors. Forty-two percent of the sample showed 50% or more symptom reduction and 74% of the sample showed at least 25% or more symptom reduction. Significant improvement was noted on most of the clinical outcome measures by the third week of active treatment. In the largest clomipramine trial for childhood OCD, 54 10–17-year-olds from five sites were studied in an 8-week, industry-sponsored, double-blind comparison of clomipramine and placebo (87). At the completion of treatment, approximately 60% of the clomipramine group was rated as significantly improved (CGI ≤ 2) versus only 17% on placebo. Although the effect size for clomipramine was nearly five times that for placebo

(37% vs. 8% decrease in CY-BOCS score), patients on average remained in the mildly to moderately ill range at the end of the trial. As with the results of Flament et al. (98), signficant between-group differences in the CY-BOCS and the NIMH Global scores emerged between the second and third weeks of treatment. Clomipramine side effects were typical of tricyclic antidepressants; they included dry mouth (63%), somnolence (46%), dizziness ((41%), fatigue (35%), tremor (33%), headache (28%), constipation (22%), and anorexia (22%). In a 1-year open-label continuation, clomipramine continued to be effective and well tolerated (87). Child and adolescent OCD appears to show the same pharmacological selectivity that has been found in adult OCD. Leonard et al. (99) compared clomipramine with desipramine (DMI), a primarily noradrenergic reuptake blocker, in a 10-week, placebo-controlled, double-blind crossover study with clomipramine increased to 3 mg/kg as tolerated. In the 48 subjects who entered, clomipramine appeared significantly more effective than DMI; the DMI effects were very similar to those of placebo in the authors' earlier study (98). Intravenous clomipramine has also been found effective in adolescent OCD cases (100).

Fluoxetine

The generally positive results from open trials and retrospective record reviews documenting the use of fluoxetine for childhood OCD have been supported by the findings from two controlled trials. Three open trials with a total of 31 patients aged 6 to 17 years found response rates ranging from 50% to 85% and mean effect sizes of 30% to 57% (101,102,13). However, in these studies, the majority of patients were comorbid for Tourette's syndrome and the average daily doses were less than 30 mg/day (101,13). A recent retrospective chart review reported a 74% response rate and a 47% effect size for 38 OCD children treated with an average daily fluoxetine dose of 50 mg (103).

In a placebo-controlled crossover study of 14 OCD youngsters aged 8 to 15 years, Riddle et al. (88) found fluoxetine superior to placebo, with the active treatment resulting in a mean average decrease of 44% in CY-BOCS score. The authors noted that symptom improvement in the fluoxetine condition was evident by week 4. An interim report from an ongoing double-blind, placebo-controlled trial of fluoxetine conducted by Clarvit and colleagues (86) found that 67% of youngsters randomized to fluoxetine were rated as much or very much improved on blind CGI ratings at week 8 (versus 30% rated as improved on placebo), with no significant adverse effects noted.

Fluvoxamine

Only two studies of fluvoxamine for childhood OCD have been published. Apter et al. (104) treated 13 adolescent inpatients with OCD in an 8-week, open-label trial, with daily doses ranging from 100 to 300 mg. Treatment resulted in a 29% mean decrease in CY-BOCS scores and was well tolerated. Preliminary results from a recent multicenter, double-blind, placebo-controlled trial of 120 8–17-year-olds with OCD (89) found fluvoxamine to be significantly more efficacious than placebo across multiple outcome measures, including the CY-BOCS and NIMH Global Scale. Insomnia and asthenia were the only side effects, occurring significantly more often in the fluoxetine than in the placebo condition. Moreover, only three fluvoxamine subjects terminated early as a result of side effects, none of which was considered serious. The FDA is currently considering an indication for fluvoxamine for OCD in children and adolescents down to 8 years of age.

Sertraline

There are no published reports of sertraline in children and adolescents with OCD, although the results from a large multicenter controlled study are pending. Preliminary results from one open-label trial for pediatric OCD in a sample of 6–17-year-olds indicated a 48% decrease in CY-BOCS ratings following 5 weeks of treatment (105). However, a retrospective chart review of 175 child and adolescent patients with various diagnoses (including 149 with a mood disorder but only 12 with OCD) found a 45% rate of adverse effects, with 13% of subjects experiencing activation and 7% (all with mood disorder) switching to bipolar disorder type I (106). Almost 25% of the sample (and half of patients experiencing adverse effects) discontinued the medication because of side effects. Although the authors suggest caution in using sertraline, the lack of data regarding dosing, induction rate, concurrent medication, and the breakdown of side effects by diagnosis make these data difficult to interpret, especially regarding the use of sertraline in OCD youth.

Other Medications

Open-label and case reports conducted primarily with adult samples have suggested that tryptophan (107), fenfluramine (108,109), lithium (110), buspirone (111), clonazepam (112,113), and risperidone (114) may have utility for OCD, alone or in combination with SSRIs or other drugs. Inositol was reported to show efficacy comparable to that of fluoxetine in one small controlled study of adult OCD (115). Although the putative efficacy of these agents is based on their reported serotonergic activity, all these substances have also been noted to be ineffective or associated with untoward events in other instances. There are no systematic studies of these substances, alone or in combination, for children and adolescents with OCD.

Combination drug therapy does appear to have a place in the treatment of children and adolescents with OCD, however, and clinical reports indicate that adult treatment-resistant patients may respond to a combination of either an SSRI plus one of the compounds listed above, an SSRI plus clomipramine, an SSRI plus another drug (e.g., clonidine, neuroleptic, tricyclic), or two SSRIs simultaneously. The successful use of a fluoxetine-clomipramine combination for adolescent OCD has also been described (116). Given the paucity of data, and therefore the potential for untoward drug interactions with combination therapy, such an approach should be used very conservatively, for treatment-resistant cases or when comorbid conditions justify additional medication.

OTHER MEDICAL INTERVENTIONS

Several other medical procedures have been used to treat OCD in adults and, less commonly, in adolescents. Case reports suggest that plasmapheresis and intravenous immunoglobulin is helpful for those adolescents with presumed infection-triggered autoimmune OCD and Tourette's syndrome (63). Both stereotactic radiosurgery (gamma-knife capsulotomy) (117) and bilateral stereotactic electrode lesioning of the anterior cingulate cortex have been successfully reported for severe, intractible OCD in adults, although these procedures carry a high risk of postsurgical morbidity. The only published study of psychosurgery in adolescents with OCD reported significant symptom reduction in five adolescents following stereotactic capsulotomy, although the course of postoperative rehabilitation was difficult (118). Although scattered reports exist describing the use of ECT, sleep deprivation, phototherapy, acupuncture, and biofeedback for adult OCD, the available data are sparse or inconsistent, and no information is available regarding the utility of these techniques with child and adolescent patients.

Combined Treatment Approaches

Even though the concurrent behavioral and psychopharmacological treatment of pediatric OCD has not been studied, the limited evidence available from the adult literature and clinical experience with children and adolescents may provide some support for the use of a combined treatment approach. As noted, most medication and behavior therapy responders experience continued significant OCD symptoms, and in adults combined treatment has been shown to afford greater symptom relief than ERP or medication alone (85). Moreover, in adults, medication has been shown to increase compliance with behavior therapy, whereas the addition of behavior therapy has been shown to minimize relapse upon medication holiday and breakthrough symptoms associated with prolonged medication use (119). This latter point is especially significant for youngsters, in whom the long-term effects of medication are not well known (22). As with adults, relapse is the norm when medication is decreased or stopped altogether. Leonard et al. (120) reported a near-universal relapse rate in children with severe OCD in response to a blind substitution of desipramine for clomipramine. It is possible, then, that in addition to offering the best chance for overall symptom reduction, combined treatment may also provide the only avenue for successful medication discontinuation. However, fully standardized and validated behavioral treatment protocols for childhood OCD are needed before these hypotheses can be systematically tested in this age group.

REFERENCES

1. Rutter M, Tizard J, Whitmore K. Education, Health, and Behavior. London: Longmans, 1970.
2. Hollingsworth CE, Tanguay PE, Grossman L, et al. Long-term outcome of obsessive-compulsive disorder in childhood. J Am Acad Child Adolesc Psychiatry 1980; 19:134–144.
3. Flament M, Whitaker A, Rapoport J, et al. Obsessive compulsive disorder in adolescence: an epidemiological study. J Am Acad Child Adolesc Psychiatry 1988; 27:764–771.
4. Rapoport JL, ed. Obsessive Compulsive Disorder in Children and Adolescents. Washington, DC: American Psychiatric Association, 1989.
5. Rasmussen SA, Tsuang MT. DSM-III obsessive compulsive disorder: clinical characteristics and family history. Am J Psychiatry 1986; 143:317–332.
6. Reinherz HZ, et al. Prevalence of psychiatric disorders in a community population of older adolescents. J Am Acad Child Adolesc Psychiatry 1993; 32:369–377.
7. Shaffer D, Fisher P, Dulcan M, Davies M, Piacentini J, Schwab-Stone M, Lahey B, Bourden K, Jensen P, Bird H, Canino G, Regier D. The NIMH Diagnostic Interview Schedule for Children (DISC-2): description, acceptability, prevalences, and performance in the MECA Study. J Am Acad Child Adolesc Psychiatry 1996; 35:865–877.
8. Valleni-Basile LA, et al. Frequency of obsessive-compulsive disorder in a community sample of young adolescents. J Am Acad Child Adolesc Psychiatry 1994; 33:782–791.

9. Karno M, et al. The epidemiology of obsessive compulsive disorder in five US communities. Arch Gen Psychiatry 1988; 45:1094–1099.

10. Robins LN, et al. Lifetime prevalence of specific psychiatric disorders in three sites. Arch Gen Psychiatry 1984; 41:949–958.

11. Hanna G. Demographic and clinical features of obsessive-compulsive disorder in children and adolescents. J Am Acad Child Adolesc Psychiatry 1995; 34:19–27.

12. Last CG, Perrin S, Hersen M, et al. DSM-III-R anxiety disorders in children: sociodemographic and clinical characteristics. J Am Acad Child Adolesc Psychiatry 1992; 31:1070–1076.

13. Riddle MA, Hardin MT, King R, et al. Fluoxetine treatment of children and adolescents with Tourette's and obsessive compulsive disorders: preliminary clinical experience. J Am Acad Child Adolesc Psychiatry 1990; 29:45–48.

14. Swedo SE, Rapoport JL, Leonard H, et al. Obsessive compulsive disorder in children and adolescents. Arch Gen Psychiatry 1989; 46:335–341.

15. Last CG, Strauss CC. Obsessive-compulsive disorder in childhood. J Anxiety Disord 1989; 3:295–302.

16. Douglass HM, Moffitt TE, Reuven D, et al. Obsessive-compulsive disorder in a birth cohort of 18-year-olds: prevalence and predictors. J Am Acad Child Adolesc Psychiatry 1995; 34:1424–1431.

17. American Psychiatric Association. Diagnostic and Statistical Manual of Mental Disorders. 4th ed. Washington, DC: American Psychiatric Association, 1994.

18. Rapoport J, Swedo S, Leonard H. Obsessive compulsive disorder. Child Adolesc Psychiatry 1993; 3:441–454.

19. Zohar AH, Ratzoni G, Pauls DL, et al. An epidemiological study of obsessive-compulsive disorder and related disorders in Israeli adolescents. J Am Acad Child Adolesc Psychiatry 1992; 31:1057–1061.

20. Rettew DC, Swedo SE, Leonard HL, et al. Obsessions and compulsions across time in 79 children and adolescents with obsessive-compulsive disorder. J Am Acad Child Adolesc Psychiatry 1992; 31:1050–1056.

21. Minichiello WE, Baer L, Jenike MA, et al. Age of onset of major subtypes of obsessive-compulsive disorder. J Anxiety Disord 1990; 4:147–150.

22. Piacentini J, Jaffer M, Gitow A, et al. Psychopharmacologic treatment of child and adolescent obsessive compulsive disorder. Psychiatr Clin North Am 1992; 15:87–107.

23. Piacentini J, Jaffer M, Liebowitz M, et al. Systematic assessment of impairment in youngsters with obsessive compulsive disorder: the OCD Impact Scale. Meeting of the Association for Advancement of Behavior Therapy, Boston, MA, Nov 1992.

24. Swedo SE, Rapoport JL. Phenomenology and differential diagnosis of obsessive compulsive disorder in children and adolescents. In: Rapoport JL, ed. Obsessive Compulsive Disorder in Children and Adolescents. Washington, DC: American Psychiatric Press, 1989:13–32.

25. Rasmussen SA, Eisen JL. The epidemiology and clinical features of obsessive compulsive disorder. Psychiatr Clin North Am 1992; 15:743–758.
26. Holzer JC, Goodman WK, et al. Obsessive-compulsive disorder with and without a chronic tic disorder: a comparison of symptoms in 70 patients. Br J Psychiatry 1994; 164:469–473.
27. Berg CZ, Rapoport JL, Whitaker A, et al. Childhood obsessive compulsive disorder: a two-year prospective follow-up of a community sample. J Am Acad Child Adolesc Psychiatry 1989; 28:528–533.
28. Allsop M, Verduyn C. A follow-up of adolescents with obsessive-compulsive disorder. Br J Psychiatry 1988; 154:829–834.
29. Bolton D, Luckie M, Steinberg D. Long-term course of obsessive-compulsive disorder treated in adolescence. J Am Acad Child Adolesc Psychiatry 1995; 34:1441–1450.
30. Flament M, Koby E, Rapoport J, et al. Childhood obsessive-compulsive disorder: a prospective follow-up study. J Child Psychol Psychiatry 1990; 31:363–380.
31. Leonard HL, Swedo SE, Lenane MC, et al. A two to seven year follow-up study of 54 obsessive compulsive children and adolescents. Arch Gen Psychiatry 1993; 50:429–439.
32. Thomsen PH, Mikkelsen HU. Course of obsessive-compulsive disorder in children and adolescents: a prospective follow-up study of 23 Danish cases. J Am Acad Child Adolesc Psychiatry 1995; 34:1432–1440.
33. March J, Leonard H, Swedo S. Obsessive compulsive disorder. In: March J, ed. Anxiety Disorders in Children and Adolescents. New York: Guilford Press, 1995:251–275.
34. Leonard H, Goldberger E, Rapoport J, et al. Childhood rituals: normal development or obsessive-compulsive symptoms. J Am Acad Child Adolesc Psychiatry 1990; 29:17–23.
35. Black DW, Noyes R Jr, Goldstien RB, Blum N. A family study of obsessive-compulsive disorder. Arch Gen Psychiatry 1992; 49:362–368.
36. Lenane M, Swedo S, Leonard HL, et al. Psychiatric disorders in first degree relatives of children and adolescents with obsessive compulsive disorder. J Am Acad Child Adolesc Psychiatry 1990; 29:407–412.
37. Pauls DL, Alsobrook JP II, Goodman W, Rasmussen S, Leckman JF. A family study of obsessive-compulsive disorder. American Journal of Psychiatry 1995; 152:76–84.
38. Schilder P. The organic background of obsessions and compulsions. Am J Psychiatry 1938; 94:1397.
39. McKeon J, McGuffin P, Robinson P. Obsessive-compulsive neurosis following a head injury: A report of four cases. Brit J Psychiatry 1984; 144:190–192.
40. Kettle PA, Marks M. Neurological factors in obsessive compulsive disorder: Two case reports and a review of the literature. Brit J Psychiatry 1986; 149:315–319.
41. Capstick N, Seldrup U. Obsessional states: A study in the relationship be-

tween abnormalities occurring at birth and subsequent development of obsessional symptoms. Acta Psychiatr Scand 1977; 56:427–439.

42. Swedo SE, Rapoport JL. Phenomenology and differential diagnosis of obsessive compulsive disorder in children and adolescents. In: Rapoport JL, ed. Obsessive Compulsive Disorder in Children & Adolescents. Washinton DC: American Psychiatric Press, 1989:13–32.

43. Swedo SE, Shapiro MB, Grady CL, et al. Cerebral glucose metabolism in childhood-onset obsessive-compulsive disorder. Arch Gen Psychiatry 1989; 46:518–523.

44. Hollander E, Schiffman E, Cohen B, et al. Signs of central nervous system dysfunction in obsessive-compulsive disorder. Arch Gen Psychiatry 1990; 47:27–32.

45. Laplane E, Baulac M, Widlocher D, et al. Pure psychic akinesia with bilateral lesions of the basal ganglia. J Neurol Neurosurg Psychiatry 1984; 47:337–385.

46. Thoren P, Ashberg M, Chronholm B, Jornestedt L, Tracskman L. Chlorimipramine treatment of obsessive compulsive disorder. Arch Gen Psychiatry 1980; 37:1281–1285.

47. Flament MF, Rapoport JL, Murphy DL, et al. Biochemical changes during clomipramine treatment of childhood obsessive-compulsive disorder. Arch Gen Psychiatry 1987; 44:219–225.

48. Hanna GL, McCracken JT, Cantwell DP. Prolactin in childhood obsessive-compulsive disorder: clinical correlates and response to clomipramine. J Acad Child Adolesc Psychiatry 1991; 30:173–178.

49. Hanna G, Yuwiler A, Cantwell D. Whole-blood serotonin during clomipramine treatment of juvenile obsessive-compulsive disorder. J Child Adolesc Psychopharmacol 1993; 3:223–229.

50. Wirz-Justice A, Freer H, Richter R. Circannual rhythm in human plasma free and total tryptophan, platelet serotonin, monoamine oxidase activity. Chronobiologia 1977; 4:165–166.

51. Corona G, Cucchi M, Santogostino G, Frattini P, Zerbi F, Fengolio L, Savoldi F. Blood nonadrenaline and 5-HT levels in depressed women during amitryptaline and lithium treatment. Psychopharmacology 1982; 77:236–241.

52. Brewerton T, Flament M, Rapoport J, et al. Seasonal effects on platelet 5-HT content in patients with OCD and controls. Arch Gen Psychiatry 1993; 50:409.

53. Baker RW, Chengappa KNR, Baird JW, Steingard S, Christ MAG, Schooler NR. Emergence of obsessive compulsive symptoms during treatment with clozapine. J Clin Psychiatry 1992; 53:439–442.

54. Patel B, Tandon R. Development of obsessive compulsive symptoms during clozapine treatment. Am J Psychiatry 1993; 150:836.

55. Toren P, Samuel E, Weizman R, Golomb A, Eldar S, Lao N. Case study: emergence of transient compulsive symptoms during treatment with clothiapine. J Am Acad Child Adolesc Psychiatry 1995; 34:1469–1472.

56. Hollander E, Fay M, Cohen B, et al. Serotogenic and nonadrenegic sensitiv-

ity in obsessive-compulsive disorder: behavioral findings. Am J Psychiatry 1988; 145:1015–1017.

57. Zohar J, Insel T. Obsessive compulsive disorder: psychobiological approaches to diagnosis, treatment and pathophysiology. Biolog Psychiatry 1987; 22:667–687.

58. Zohar J, Insel TR, Zohar-Kadouch RC, et al. Serotogenic responsivity in obsessive-compulsive disorder: effects of chronic clomipramine treatment. Arch Gen Psychiatry 1988; 45:197–172.

59. Hollander E, DeCaria C, Gulley R, et al. Effects of chronic fluoxetine treatment on behavioral and neuroendocrine response of m-CPP in obsessive-ciompulsive disorder. Psychiatric Res 1991; 36:1–17.

60. Bastani B, Nash FJ, Meltzer HY. Prolactin and cortisol responses to Mk-212, a serotonin agonist, in obsessive-compulsive disorder. Arch Gen Psychiatry 1990; 47:833–839.

61. Swedo SE, et al. Cerebral glucose metabolism in childhood-onset obsessive-compulsive disorder: revisualization during pharmacotherapy. Arch Gen Psychiatry 1992; 49:690–694.

62. Altemus M, Swedo S, Leonard H, Richter D, Rubinow D, Potter W, Rapoport J. Changes in cerebrospinal fluid neurochemistry during treatment of obsessive-compulsive disorder with clomipramine. Arch Gen Psychiatry 1994; 51:794–803.

63. Allen AJ, Leonard HL, Swedo SE. Case study: a new infection-triggered autoimmune subtype of pediatric OCD and Tourette's syndrome. J Am Acad Child Adolesc Psychiatry 1995; 34:307–311.

64. Baxter LR Jr, Schwartz JM, Bergman KS, et al. Caudate glucose metabolic rate changes with both drug and behavior therapy for obsessive-compulsive disorder. Arch Gen Psychiatry 1992; 49:681–689.

65. Schwartz J, Stoessel P, Baxter L, Martin K, Phelps M. Systematic cererbral glucose metabolic rate changes after successful behavior modification treatment of obsessive compulsive disorder. Arch Gen Psychiatry 1996; 53:109–113.

66. Insel TR. Toward a neuroanatomy of obsessive-compulsive disorder. Arch Gen Psychiatry 1992; 49:739–744.

67. Baxter LR Jr, et al. Caudate glucose metabolic rate changes with both drug and behavior therapy for obsessive-compulsive disorder. Arch Gen Psychiatry 1992; 49:681–689.

68. Swedo SE, Pietrini P, Leonard HL, Schapiro MB, Rettew DC, Goldberger EL, Rapoport SI, Rapoport JL, Grady CL. Cerebral glucose metabolism in childhood-onset obsessive-compulsive disorder: revisualization during pharmacotherapy. Arch Gen Psychiatry 1992; 49:690–694.

69. Baxter LR, Phelps ME, Mazziotta JC, et al. Local cerebral glucose metabolic rates in obsessive-compulsive disorder: a comparison with rates in unipolar depression and in normal controls. Arch Gen Psychiatry 1988; 44:211–218.

70. Swedo SE, Shapiro MB, Grady CL, et al. Cerebral glucose metabolism in childhood-onset obsessive-compulsive disorder. Arch Gen Psychiatry 1989; 46:518–523.

71. Nordahl TE, Benkelfat C, Semple WE, et al. Cerebral glucose metabolic rates in obsessive-compulsive disorder. Neuropsychopharmacology 1989; 2:23–28.
72. Garber HJ, Anath JV, Chiu LC, et al. Nuclear magnetic resonance study of obsessive-compulsive disorder. Am J Psychiatry 1989; 146:1001–1005.
73. Luxemberg JS, Swedo SE, Flament MF, et al. Neuroanatomic abnormalities in obsessive-compulsive disorder detected with quantitative x-ray computed tomography. Am J Psychiatry 1988; 145:1089–1094.
74. Weilburg JB, Mesulam MM, Weintraub S, et al. Focal striatal abnormalities in a patient with obsessive-compulsive disorder. Arch Neurol 1989; 46:233–235.
75. Baxter TL, Schwartz J, Guze B, et al. Trazadone treatment response in obseeeive-compulsive disorder correlated with shifts in glucose metabolism in the caudate nuclei. Psychopathology 1987; 20:114–122.
76. Benkelfat C, Nordahl TE, Semple WE, et al. Local cerebral glucose metabolic rates in obsessive-compulsive disorder: patients treated with clomipramine. Arch Gen Psychiatry 1990; 47:840–848.
77. Hamlin CL, Swayne LC, Liebowitz MR. Striatal IMP-SPECT decrease in obsessive-compulsive disorder, normalized by pharmacotherapy. Neuropsychiatry Neurophysiol Behav Neurol 1989; 2:290–300.
78. Martinot JL, Allilaire JF, Mazoyer BM, et al. Obsessive-compulsive disorder: a clinical, neuropsychological and positron emission tomography study. Acta Psychiatrica Scandanavia 1990; 82:233–242.
79. Mindus R, Ericson K, Greitz T, et al. Regional cerebral glucose metabolism in anxiety disorders studied with positron emission tomography before and after psychosurgical intervention. Radiolog Suppl 1986; 369:444–448.
80. Hooper SR, March JS. Neuropsychology. In: March JS, ed. Anxiety Disorders in Children and Adolescents. New York, Guilford Press: 1995:35–60.
81. Hollander E, DeCaria C, Aronowitz B, et al. A pilot follow-up study of childhood soft signs and the development of adult psychopathology. J Neuropsychiatry 1991; 3:186–189.
82. Rapoport J, Mikkelson E. Clinical controlled trial of chlorimipramine in adolescents with obsessive compulsive disorder. Psychopharmol Bull 1980; 16:61–63.
83. Salzman L, Thaler F. Obsessive compulsive disorders: a review of the literature. Am J Psychiatry 1981; 138:286–296.
84. Greist JH. An integrated approach to treatment of obsessive compulsive disorder. J Clin Psychiatry 1992; 53:38–41.
85. Steketee G. Treatment of Obsessive Compulsive Disorder. New York: Guilford Press, 1993.
86. Clarvit S, Davies S, DelBene D, Gitow A, Graae F, Jaffer M, Liebowitz M, Piacentini J, Schneier F, Tancer N. Double-blind, placebo-controlled study of fluoxetine for childhood/adolescent obsessive-compulsive disorder. Scientific Proceedings of The Annual Meeting of the American Academy of Child and Adolescent Psychiatry, 1994:10.
87. De Veaugh-Geiss J, Moroz G, Biederman J, et al. Clomipramine; hydro-

chloride in childhood and adolescent obsessive-compulsive disorder—a multicenter trial. J Am Acad Child Adolesc Psychiatry, 1992; 31:45–49.

88. Riddle MA, Scahill L, King R, et al. Double-blind crossover trial of fluoxetine and placebo in children and adolescents with obsessive-compulsive disorder. J Am Acad Child Adolesd Psychiatry 1992; 31:1062–1069.

89. Riddle MA, Claghorn J, Gaffney G, et al. A Controlled Trial of Fluvoxamine for OCD in Children and Adolescents. Biol Psychiatry 1996; 568.

90. Piacentini J, Gitow A, Jaffer M, Graae F, Whitaker A. Outpatient behavioral treatment of child and adolescent obsessive compulsive disorder. J Anxiety Dis 1994; 8:277–289.

91. March J, Mulle K, Herbel B. Behavioral psychotherapy for children and adolescents with OCD: an open trial of a new protocol driven treatment package. J Am Acad Child Adolesc Psychiatry 1994; 33:333–341.

92. Berg CZ, Rapoport JL, Wolff RP. Behavioral treatment for obsessive-compulsive disorder in children. In: Rapoport JL, ed. Obsessive Compulsive Disorder in Children and Adolescents. Washington, DC: American Psychiatric Press, 1989:169–185.

93. Meyer V. Modification of expectations in cases with obsessive rituals. Behav Res Ther 1966; 4:270–280.

94. Foa E, Kozac M. Emotional processing of fear: exposure to incorrect information. Psycholog Bull 1986; 99:450–472.

95. Hibbs ED, Hamburger SD, Lenane M, Rapoport JL, Kruesi MJ, Keysor CS, Goldstein MJ. Determinants of expressed emotion in families of disturbed and normal children. J Child Psychol Psychiatry Allied Disc 1991; 32:757–770.

96. Toro J, Cerevera M, Osejo E, Salamero M. Obsessive-compulsive disorder in childhood and adolesence: a clinical study. J Child Psychol Psychiatry Allied Disc 1992; 33:1025–1037.

97. Lenane MC. Family therapy for children with obsessive-compulsive disorder. In: Pato MT, Zohar J, eds. Current Treatments of Obsessive-Compulsive Disorder. Washington, DC: American Psychiatric Press, 1991:103–113.

98. Flament MF, Rapoport JL, Berg CJ, et al. Clomiprimine treatment of children with obsessive compulsive disorder. Arch Gen Psychiatry 1985; 42:977–979.

99. Leonard HS, Swedo S, Rapoport JL, et al. Treatment of childhood obsessive compulsive disorder with clomipramine and desmethylimipramine: a double blind crossover comparison. Psychopharmacol Bull 1988; 24:93–95.

100. Warneke LB. Intravenous chlorimipramine in the treatment of obsessional disorder in adolescence: Case report. J Clin Psychiatry 1985; 46:100–103.

101. Como PG, Kurlan R. An open-label trial of fluoxetine for obsessive-compulsive disorder in Gilles de la Tourette's syndrome. Neurology 1991; 41:872–874.

102. Liebowitz MR, Hollander E, Fairbanks J, Campeas R. Fluoxetine for ado-

lescents with obsessive compulsive disorder. Am J Psychiatry 1990; 147:370–371.

103. Geller DA, Biederman J, Reed ED, Spencer T, Wilens TE. Similarities in response to fluoxetine in the treatment of children and adolescents with obsessive-compulsive disorder. J Am Acad Child Adolesc Psychiatry 1995; 34:36.

104. Apter A, Ratzoni G, King RA, Weizman A, Iancu I, Binder M, Riddle MA. Fluvoxamine open-label treatment of adolescent inpatients with obsessive-compulsive disorder or depression. J Am Acad Child Adolesc Psychiatry 1994; 33:342–8.

105. Alderman JA, Wolkow R, Johnston HF. Sertraline Treatment in Children and Adolescents: Tolerability, Efficacy and Pharmacokinetics. Meeting of the American Psychiatric Association, Toronto, May 1996.

106. Tierney E, Joshi P, Llinas J, Freedman A. Adverse affects, behavioral activation, bipolar disorder with sertraline in 175 child and adolescent patients. Scientific Proceedings of the Annual Meeting of the American Academy of Child and Adolescent Psychiatry 1995; 11:129.

107. Mattes J. A pilot study of combined trazodone and tryptophan in obsessive-compulsive disorder. Int J Clin Psychopharmacol 1986; 1:170–173.

108. Hollander E, DeCaria C, Schneier F. Fenfluramine augmentation of serotonin reuptake blockade in anti-obsessional treatment. J Clin Psychiatry 1990; 51:119–123.

109. Judd F, Chua P, Lynch C, et al. Fenfluramine augmentation of clomipramine treatment of obsessive-compulsive disorder. Aust NZ J Psychiatry 1991; 25:412–414.

110. Ruegg R, Evans D, Comer W, et al. Lithium plus fluoxetine treatment of obsessive-compulsive disorder. Abstr NR 92:81. In: New Research Program and Abstracts of 143rd Annual Meeting of the American Psychiatric Association, New York, May 1990.

111. Alessi N, Bos T. Busiprone augmentation of fluoxetine in a depressed child with obsessive-compulsive disorder [letter]. Am J Psychiatry 1991; 148:1605–1606.

112. Leonard H, Topol D, Bukstein O, et al. Clonazepam as an augmenting agent in the treatment of childhood-onset obsessive-compulsive disorder. J Am Acad Child Adolesc Psychiatry 1994; 33:792–794.

113. Ross D, Piggot L. Clonazepam for OCD: a case report. J Am Acad Child Adolesc Psychiatry 1993; 32:470–471.

114. Jacobsen F. Risperidone in the treatment of effective illness and obsessive-compulsive disorder. J Clin Psychiatry 1995; 56.

115. Fux M, Levine J, Aviv A, Belmaker R. Inositol treatment of obsessive-compulsive disorder. Am J Psychiatry. In press.

116. Simeon J, Thatte S, Wiggins D. Treatment of adolescent obsessive-compulsive disorder with a clomipramine-fluoxetine combination. Psychopharm Bull 1990; 26:285–290.

117. Baer L, Rauch S, Ballantine H, et al. Cingulotomy for intractable obses-

sive-compulsive disorder: prospective long-term follow-up of 18 patients. Arch Gen Psychiatry 1995; 52:384–392.

118. Lopez Ibor J, Lopez Ibor-Alino J. Selection criteria for patients who should undergo psychiatric surgery. In: Sweet W, Obrador S, Martin-Rodriguez J, eds. Neurosurgical Treatment in Psychiatry. Baltimore: University Park Press, 1975.

119. Abel J. Exposure with response prevention and serotonergic antidepressives in the treatment of OCD. Behav Res Ther 1993; 31:463–478.

120. Leonard HL, Swedo SE, Lenane MC, et al. A double-blind desipramine substitution during long term clomipramine treatment in children and adolescents with obsessive-compulsive disorder. Arch Gen Psychiatry 1991; 48:922–927.

3

Obsessive-Compulsive Spectrum Disorders

Lisa J. Cohen

Beth Israel Medical Center/
Albert Einstein College of Medicine
New York, New York

Daphne Simeon and Eric Hollander

The Mount Sinai School of Medicine
New York, New York

Dan J. Stein

University of Stellenbosch
Tygerberg, South Africa

In recent years, a growing body of data has supported the notion of an obsessive-compulsive spectrum of disorders (OCSD). This conceptualization is based on similarities among disorders across several domains, including symptomatology, associated clinical features (age of onset, clinical course, comorbidity), possible etiology, familial transmission, and response to selective pharmacological or behavioral treatments (1–3). More recently, this conceptualization has been criticized as vague and overinclusive. A more stringent definition might characterize OCSDs by impairment in inhibition of repetetive behaviors or cognitions (4). Significant similarities with OCD are necessary, primarily in phenomenology but also in comorbidity, family history, and/or neurobiology (5).

  Phenomenologically, OCSDs are characterized by obsessive thoughts or preoccupations with the body (body dysmorphic disorder

[BDD], depersonalization, anorexia nervosa, hypochondriasis), stereo-typed motor or grooming behavior (Tourette's syndrome, Sydenham's chorea, trichotillomania, onychophagia, face picking), or driven forms of impulse dyscontrol (pathological gambling, sexual compulsions/addictions, borderline personality disorder). Biological models of OCSDs are supported by evidence from studies of neurotransmitter function (serotonin, in particular), brain imaging, neurological soft signs, and neuropsychological function. The serotonergic model has received particular attention in studies of OCD. Serotonin-reuptake inhibitors (SRIs) such as clomipramine (6), fluoxetine (7), and fluvoxamine (8) are effective in approximately 60% of OCD patients. Moreover, there is substantial indirect evidence of serotonergic dysregulation in OCSDs. Although there are few controlled trials to date, preliminary studies and case reports suggest that serotonin-reuptake blockers may also be effective in a number of OCSDs (1).

COMPULSIVE-IMPULSIVE SPECTRUM

Within the OCSDs several subclassifications have been proposed, including a habit spectrum, harm-avoidant spectrum, and a psychotic spectrum (9). The OC spectrum might also be viewed along a compulsive–impulsive dimension reflecting varying degrees of harm avoidance, with a compulsive risk-aversive endpoint (OCD, BDD, hypochondriasis) opposing an impulsive risk-seeking endpoint (pathological gambling, sexual impulsions, impulse-control disorders) (2,3,10). Compulsive disorders are characterized phenomenologically by an increased sense of harm avoidance, risk aversiveness, and anticipatory anxiety. These disorders may include OCD, BDD, anorexia nervosa, depersonalization disorder, hypochondriasis, and Tourette's syndrome. In these illnesses, ritualistic behaviors are often undertaken in an attempt to reduce anxiety and magically decrease the sense of harm or risk.

In contrast, impulsive disorders are characterized by risk-seeking behavior, a defect in harm avoidance, and little anticipatory anxiety. They may include disorders of impulse control, such as intermittent explosive disorder, pyromania, kleptomania, pathological gambling, and trichotillomania; paraphilias; and sexual acting-out behaviors. These disorders are characterized by pleasure-producing behaviors, although the consequences of such behavior may be painful. Whereas personality disorders characterized by impulsive aggression, such as Cluster B personality disorders (borderline, antisocial), may not meet stringent criteria for OCSDs, they are often included in studies of impulsivity.

This distinction, however, is not always so clear-cut. Some disorders may have both impulsive and compulsive features, or lie between these two poles. Thus, patients with trichotillomania and pathological gambling may have both compulsive and impulsive features, in that behavior may have a driven, tension-reducing quality as well as pleasurable characteristics.

In addition, a hallmark of OCSDs is the inability to delay or inhibit repetitive behaviors. In compulsive disorders such behaviors have a driven quality and function mainly to reduce anxiety or tension. Impulsive behaviors are usually experienced as pleasurable. However, the common feature involves the repetitive nature of the behavior and the impairment in inhibition.

PSYCHOBIOLOGY OF OBSESSIVE-COMPULSIVE-RELATED DISORDERS

The biological model of OCD was first suggested by the association of OCD with neurological insult and disease. Precipitation of OCD has been reported following numerous neurological disorders, such as seizure disorders (11), head trauma (12), diabetes insipidus (13), encephalitis (14), and multiple sclerosis (15). A number of neurological disorders specifically associated with basal ganglia disease have also been associated with OCD. These include Sydenham's chorea (16), disease of the globus pallidate (17), and head of the caudate (18).

Neurotransmitter Function

The serotonergic model of OCD followed the discovery of the selective efficacy of SRIs. Likewise, considerable evidence implicates serotonergic dysfunction in the neurobiology of OCSDs. Serotonergic (5-HT) function may be measured by cerebrospinal fluid (CSF) metabolites of 5-HT (5-hydroxyindoleacetic acid: 5-HIAA), by behavioral and neuroendocrine responses to serotonergic probes (m-CPP and others), and by treatment outcome to serotonin-reuptake blockers (fluoxetine, clomipramine, fluvoxamine, and others). Moreover, there is preliminary evidence that compulsive disorders may have increased serotonergic tone while impulsive disorders have decreased serotonergic tone. However, the complexity of neurotransmitter systems demands caution regarding any such hypotheses.

Elevated levels of CSF 5-HIAA have been demonstrated in a subgroup of OCD patients (19), as well as corresponding decreases following successful treatment with clomipramine (20). Other compulsive disorders such as anorexia nervosa (21) demonstrate increased 5-HIAA overall or in subgroups of patients responsive to 5-HT-reuptake blockers. On the other hand, patients with impulsive aggressive (22) and violent suicidal (23) behavior have decreased CSF 5-HIAA. Patients successfully completing violent suicide also have decreased 5-HT receptors in frontal cortex (24).

Acute challenges with serotonergic agents have provided further evidence of 5-HT involvement in OCD and have even pointed to specific 5-HT receptor sites. The partial agonist m-CPP has been reported to produce symptom exacerbation (25–27) and prolactin and cortisol abnormalities (25,28,29) in OCD patients, although these results are not always replicated (4,27). m-CPP acts as an agonist at 5-HT1 receptor sites, an antagonist at 5-HT3 receptor sites, and a mixed agonist/antagonist at 5-HT2 receptor sites. The fact that challenges with nonspecific 5-HT agents such as fenfluramine (4,25) and the 5-HT precursor tryptophan (29) do not produce behavioral or hormonal abnormalities in OCD patients supports the specific nature of 5-HT dysfunction in OCD.

Acute serotonergic challenges in OCSDs also show irregularities in 5-HT function. Moreover, compulsive and impulsive disorders may demonstrate opposing behavioral responses. In response to 5-HT agonists such as m-CPP, patients with compulsive disorder such as OCD (25,27), eating disorders (30), and Tourette's syndrome (Hollander et al., unpublished observations) show increased dysphoria and increased obsessional thoughts and compulsive urges. On the other hand, patients with impulsive disorders, such as impulsive personality disorders (31), pathological gambling (26), and trichotillomania (33), for the most part do not show a dysphoric response, but rather often have a "high" response to m-CPP. Neuroendocrine response is less clearly differentiated in impulsive and compulsive disorders. Neuroendocrine blunting in response to 5-HT agonists has been reported in OCD patients (25) as well as impulsive personality disorder patients (34), although pathological gamblers demonstrated increased prolactin response to challenge with m-CPP (32).

Neuropsychiatry

In OCD, localized abnormalities in brain function have been demonstrated in numerous brain imaging studies, utilizing positron emission tomography (PET), single photon emission computed tomography (SPECT), rCBF, and MRI. Fairly consistent findings point to abnormal activation of an orbital frontal–thalamic–basal ganglia loop (35).

Structural abnormalities have been assessed with CT scan and MRI. Increased ventricle-brain ratios (VBR) in OCD patients relative to controls have been demonstrated in some CT studies (36) but not others

(18,37), as have findings of decreased caudate volume (37,38). Both CT (18,36) and MRI (39) studies fail to reveal gross pathology of the frontal lobes, but abnormalities in frontal tissue (increased T1 signal) have been demonstrated on MRI (39). Robinson et al. (40) assessed the volume of the prefrontal cortex, caudate nucleus, and lateral and third ventricles on MRI in 26 OCD patients and 26 healthy controls. OCD patients demonstrated lower bilateral caudate volume than controls but nonsignificant differences in ventrical and prefrontal volume.

Functional abnormalities in the frontal cortex and basal ganglia have been well documented in OCD patients relative to normal controls. On PET, increased glucose metabolism was demonstrated in orbitofrontal cortex in many studies (41–44) but not all (45). Moreover, SPECT has documented increased blood flow (HMPAO uptake) in frontal cortex (46,47). Increased (41,42), decreased (45), and unchanged activity in the caudate (43,44) has been shown on PET studies. Decreased blood flow in the head of the caudate has been shown on SPECT (46).

Moreover, several studies have demonstrated correspondence between frontal-basal ganglia abnormalities and 5-HT function. In one study with [133]-Xe rCBF, the partial 5-HT agonist m-CPP increased OCD symptoms and frontal blood flow. Increase in frontal blood flow correlated with increase in OC symptoms (48). Following successful SRI or behavioral treatment, decreased metabolic activity on PET compared to baseline in the right caudate nucleus was demonstrated (49), decreased orbital frontal activity on PET was correlated with treatment (50), and reduction in both medial frontal HMPAO uptake on SPECT and OCD symptoms was documented (51).

Functional abnormalities have been demonstrated in other OCSDs. Increased frontal activity on SPECT has also been demonstrated in case reports of depersonalization disorder (52) and BDD (Cohen et al., unpublished observations). In the case of depersonalization disorder, left-temporal activation and decreased caudate perfusion were also demonstrated on SPECT (52). Notably, impulsive patients, such as those with borderline personality disorder, have decreased frontal glucose metabolic rates, and those with greater aggression have lower frontal activity (53).

Several recent imaging studies have documented structural and functional abnormalities in Tourette's patients that suggest overlap with OCD. Reduced basal ganglia volume in Tourette's patients has been shown in several MRI studies (54,55). Another MRI study demonstrated abnormal T2 relaxation time asymmetries in 14 adult Tourette's patients compared to 14 controls in the insular cortex and frontal white matter (56). On PET, 16 Tourette's patients demonstrated decreased glucose metabolism relative to 16 control subjects in orbitofrontal, inferior insular, and parahippocampal regions as well as striatal areas and the midbrain (57).

One study of 10 adult female trichotillomania patients and 20 matched controls demonstrated elevated glucose metabolism in right and left cerebellar and right parietal areas on PET. Improvement following treatment with CMI was negatively correlated with anterior cingulate and orbital frontal metabolism (58).

Neurological soft signs provide another measure of neuropsychiatric function. These are nonlocalizing signs of deviant performance on a motor or sensory test where no other sign of a neurological lesion is present (59). Abnormalities include disorders of coordination, involuntary movements, and sensory signs. Early studies demonstrated increased soft signs in emotionally unstable character disorder (60).

We found that a subgroup of OCD patients has increased neurological soft signs (61). OCD patients with increased neurological soft signs may have more severe illness (61), increased ventricular size on CT (38), greater familial transmission of soft signs (62), and a worse treatment outcome with serotonin-reuptake blockers (63). Follow-up studies of children with increased neurological soft signs have demonstrated the development of adult OCD and affective and anxiety disorders (64).

Studies of neurological soft signs in OCSDs have provided conflicting results. Social phobic patients demonstrate elevated soft signs relative to normal controls (65). While social phobia is not generally considered an OCSD per se, it is an anxiety disorder characterized by excessive harm avoidance. We also studied the relationship between soft signs and neurological functions in impulsive personality disorders (66). While patients had more left-sided soft signs than controls, those with a history of aggression had more right-sided soft signs than those without a history of aggression. Furthermore, right-sided soft signs predicted to measures of executive dysfunction. On the other hand, a study comparing female trichotillomania patients, OCD patients, and normal controls found no difference in number of soft signs (67), suggesting that soft signs may be more prevalent in males.

Neuropsychological research examines the cognitive manifestations of neurological impairment. Consistent findings of hyperfrontality on imaging studies might suggest neuropsychological dysfunction in frontal lobe–related executive tasks. While there is some suggestion of impaired executive function (ability to form, maintain, and switch cognitive sets) in OCD (36,45,68,69), findings are inconclusive (70–72) and measures often include strong visual-spatial components (36,45). Unfortunately, most measures of executive function are associated with presumed *hypofunction* of the frontal lobes, secondary to various etiologies, and thus may not be sensitive to *hyper*frontality, which may be more characteristic of OCD (41,43). There has, however, been, consistent evidence of impairment in visual-spatial functions, including visual memory and visual constructional function (68,70–72). This has been interpreted to reflect right-hemisphere dysfunction. Findings regarding impairment in memory and attention have been inconclusive (36,45, 69,70,72,73).

There is less data on neuropsychological function in other OCSDs. Social phobic patients, who show increased risk aversion regarding interpersonal evaluation although not otherwise considered to have an OCSD, have also demonstrated executive and visual-spatial dysfunction (74). In contrast to OCD patients, patients with impulsive personality disorders show greater impairment in verbal functions than in visual-spatial functions (75). Pathological gamblers also demonstrated visual-spatial (32) and higher-order attentional impairment (76) and may have elevated rates of childhood ADHD (76). Patients with Tourette's syndrome performed more than one standard deviation below standardized means only on tests of motor function (77), consistent with basal ganglia impairment. Although little has been published on neuropsychology in trichotillomania, one study compared 11 trichotillomania patients, 17 OCD patients, and 16 age- and education-matched controls on measures sensitive to neuropsychological impairment associated with Huntington's disease. Groups did not differ on measures of verbal fluency, visuoconstructional functioning (WAIS-R Block Design), egocentric spatial ability (Money's Road Map Test, the Room Test), and processing speed in visual search tasks. OCD patients differed from controls only on measures of verbal memory. The authors interpreted these findings to reflect neuropathological differences between Huntington's disease and OCD and trichotillomania, despite suggestion of common basal ganglial involvement (78).

Treatment

In OCD there is ample evidence of the specific efficacy of SRIs such as clomipramine (6), fluoxetine (7), fluvoxamine (79), and sertraline (80). Serotonin-reuptake blockers have also been shown to be effective in the treatment of several OCSDs, including BDD (81,82), sexual compulsions (83), anorexia nervosa (84), trichotillomania (85), hypochondriasis (86), depersonalization disorder (87), and impulsive personality disorders (88).

Although the data are far from conclusive, there is some preliminary evidence suggesting pharmacological dissection between impulsivity and compulsivity. Compulsive-style disorders such as OCD (2), BDD (81,82,89), hypochondriasis (86), depersonalization disorder (87), and anorexia nervosa (90) may respond preferentially to SRIs. Because SRIs function to stimulate 5-HT activity, symptoms may initially worsen following acute administration with high doses (91). Chronic treatment with these agents, however, may work to desensitize or down-regulate 5-HT receptors over time (92,93). Disorders with mixed impulsive and compulsive features, such as trichotillomania, show early improvement (85), although this effect has also been reported to wear off with time (94,95). It remains to be seen whether other impulsive-style disorders, such as pathological gambling (96), sexual compulsions and paraphilias (83), and impulsive-style personality disorders (88), have a similar response. For example, true sexual obsessions, a typical subtype of OCD, are highly responsive to serotonin-reuptake blocker treatment, whereas paraphilias and sexual impulsions have a less robust and shorter-lasting response to this treatment (83). Open pilot work in impulsive personality disorders shows some improvement early on (88) but this effect may also wear off with time and long-term follow-up studies are needed.

Despite advances in the treatment of compulsive disorders, however, most patients attain only partial relief from their symptoms. For example, about 40% of OCD patients remain refractory to a single trial of a standard selective SRI (SSRI).

Dopaminergic mechanisms may also be involved in OCSDs, particularly those with simple motor symptoms, such as Tourette's syndrome (97) or trichotillomania (95), or those with psychotic features, such as delusional OCD or BDD (81). Haloperidol and pimozide (97) are effective treatments for Tourette's syndrome, and augmentation of SSRIs with low-dose pimozide has been effective in trichotillomania (95).

Behavior therapy has also shown considerable success with certain OCSDs (98,99). The technique of exposure and response prevention (ERP) was first shown to be effective with OCD patients (100). This technique involves graduated exposure to the feared stimulus with simultaneous prevention of anxiety-reducing ritualistic behaviors. The patient thus becomes desensitized to the anxiety-provoking stimulus and no longer relies on the compulsions to regulate anxiety. ERP combined with cognitive therapy to decrease distortions in self-perceptions has also been found to be effective in a series of BDD patients (101). In trichotillomania, behavior-therapy techniques aim to increase patients' awareness of the symptomatic behavior in order to make it accessible to conscious control. Habit reversal—which involves identification of the behavioral antecedents and then substitution with a less problematic behavior, e.g., fist-clenching—has been reported to be effective with trichotillomanic patients (102). The different focus of the two techniques (increased awareness vs. decreased anticipatory anxiety) may reflect the impulsive features of trichotillomania.

SPECIFIC OCSDs

Body Dysmorphic Disorder

BDD, characterized by an excessive concern with imagined or overvalued defects in bodily appearance, is classified in DSM-IV as a somatoform disorder. Areas of concern focus primarily on the face and head but can also include the hands, feet, torso, and sexual body parts. Behaviors related to BDD involve mirror-checking, ritualized application of makeup, repeated requests for reassurance, avoidance of social and occupational situations for fear of exacerbating or exposing the perceived defect, and even multiple cosmetic surgical procedures. BDD ideation may vary along a continuum of insight. While beliefs of delusional intensity were an exclusion criterion for BDD in DSM-III-R, a number of investigators argued that many BDD patients have delusional certainty regarding the body defect (81,89,103). In DSM-IV, delusional BDD ideation earns a comorbid diagnosis of delusional disorder, somatic-type, in addition to a diagnosis of BDD. Although to date there are no controlled treatment studies, preliminary investigations point to a preferential response to SSRIs (81,82,79). In delusional patients, neuroleptic augmentation may be useful (81,103).

Findings from the DSM-IV Field Trial for OCD suggest that 12% of OCD patients also met DSM-III-R criteria for BDD (104). Family history of OCD was also found to be high in two series (Hollander et al., unpublished observations; 89). Thus, similarities in clinical symptoms, family history, and response to serotonin-reuptake blockers as well as evidence of high comorbidity with OCD support the classification of BDD as an OCSD.

The differences in symptomatology between the two disorders involve ideational content, complexity, and frequency of delusional beliefs. The content of BDD symptoms reflects a sense of self as ugly and unlovable while OCD symptoms involve fear of harm and danger. Because BDD symptoms concern body image, feelings of shame and lowered self-esteem are very frequent in these patients. Consequently, comorbid social phobia and depression are also common (89). Comorbid depression occurs in OCD as well, but OCD symptoms are less directly related to patients' self-esteem. While both BDD and OCD symptoms can involve highly complex ideational content, consistent with higher cortical involvement, OCD symptoms can also include simpler behaviors like touching or tapping that may implicate striatal involvement. BDD patients, however, are more likely to demonstrate overvalued ideas or delusional ideation (89,104,105). A study comparing 26 BDD patients with delusional ideation with 26 nondelusional BDD patients revealed little differences beyond lifetime history of psychotic diagnoses (105).

Although there are no controlled treatment studies of BDD to date, there are promising indications from case reports and exploratory studies that serotonin-reuptake blockers, such as clomipramine, fluoxetine, and fluvoxamine, are superior to standard tricyclics, neuroleptics, and benzodiazepines (81,89,106–108). Three of five BDD patients in one series (81) and five of seven in another (89) responded to clomipramine after failing to respond to neuroleptics, tricyclics, anticonvulsants, and/ or benzodiazepines. Ten of 19 patients (53%) in the latter series had a partial or full response to fluoxetine. In our retrospective study of 50 BDD patients, we found that BDD symptoms were much improved following clomipramine (average maximum dosage 188 mg/day; $n = 15$; CGI change score = 1.9), fluoxetine (57.8 mg/day; $n = 14$; CGI change = 2.0), and fluvoxamine (260 mg/day, $n = 6$; CGI change = 1.8), but did not change following tricyclics (178 mg/day; $n = 15$; CGI change = 3.9) (82). Again, treatment response is not seen in a proportion of patients. Vitello and DeLeon (109) reported one patient who did not respond to clomipramine. A double-blind, crossover study comparing CMI and DMI in BDD patients is under way in our laboratory.

Anorexia Nervosa

Anorexia nervosa, classified in DSM-IV as an eating disorder, is a serious and potentially fatal psychiatric disorder, characterized by disturbance in body image, obsessive fears of being fat, and compulsive, driven attempts to reduce weight via restricted eating, abuse of laxatives and/or diet pills, or excessive exercise.

A number of factors point to the inclusion of anorexia as an OCSD. First, there is evidence of elevated comorbidity between OCD and anorexia nervosa. There are increased rates of comorbid or prior anorexia in populations of OCD patients. Estimates have varied from 42% of a sample of 31 female OCD patients (110) to 11% of 105 female OCD patients (111) to 12.9% of 62 OCD patients of both sexes, 31 of each (112). Anorexia patients have also scored higher than normals on the Yale-Brown Obsessive Compulsive Scale (YBOCS), demonstrating obsessions and compulsions independent from the eating disorder (113). On the other hand, there was no difference in Maudsley Obsessive Compulsive Inventory scores among 29 anorexics, 77 bulimics, and normal controls (114).

Second, as with other compulsive disorders, anorexics show indications of increased 5-HT tone. Elevated levels of CSF 5-HIAA (21) as well as a blunted prolactin response to m-CPP challenge have been reported in anorexic patients (90). In an open trial, fluoxetine treatment resulted in good response in 10 anorexic patients, partial response in 17, and poor response in four (115). Restricted-eating anorexics showed greater benefit than bulimic-type anorexics, which is consistent with a putative distinction between impulsive and compulsive forms of eating disorders (115).

Trichotillomania

Trichotillomania, classified in DSM-IV as an impulse-control disorder, is characterized by an irresistible urge to pull out one's hair, accompanied by a buildup of tension and a subsequent sense of relief. The hair-pulling is usually ego-dystonic and may result in extensive, disfiguring hair loss.

There is debate over this classification, as trichotillomania presents compulsive as well as impulsive features (1,116,117). Compulsive features are suggested by similarities between trichotillomania and OCD in phenomenology and neurobiology. These include the inability to inhibit repetitive, ego-dystonic behavior (1,117), higher comorbidity between the two disorders than might be expected by chance (118,119), and possible serotonergic mediation (20,85).

Impulsive features in trichotillomanic patients include evidence of pleasurable feelings following symptomatic behavior (120), a high rate of comorbid personality disorders in some studies (121,122), and patterns of serotonergic function consistent with impulsive disorders, such as indication of early treatment response to SSRIs with long-term relapse (94) and a "high" response to 5-HT probes (33). Most trichotillomania studies document a chronic disorder, early age of onset, and higher prevalence in females (118).

In trichotillomania, hair is pulled from a variety of sites, most frequently from the scalp, but eyelashes, eyebrows, and body and pubic hair are also pulled, the consequent bald spots resulting in intense shame and embarassment (118,119,123). Hats, scarves, wigs, and makeup are often employed in attempts to hide hair loss (118). Associated behaviors may include nail-biting (124) (onycophagia) or eating of the hair (trichotillophagia) (125). Although symptoms often increase under stress, many patients report that hair-pulling is most frequent in conditions of relaxation, e.g., while watching television or reading (118). Some patients report pleasure associated with hair-pulling (126). Many patients report decreased tension following the act, but this may not be the case for all patients (118,127).

Available data also suggest considerable psychiatric comorbidity in trichotillomania, although there are few controlled studies on this. Comorbid axis I disorders include anxiety, affective, and obsessive-compulsive disorders, substance abuse, and eating disorders (118,120,121,123). Comorbid axis II disorders (118,121) and habit disorders (onycophagia, trichotillophagia) are also frequent. In a sample of 169 trichotillomanic patients, five (3%) also met criteria for BDD (128). The likelihood of a family history of mental disorders may also be elevated, particularly for OCD, affective disorder, and trichotillomania (123,129). Lenane et al. (129) found an age-corrected rate of 6.4% of first-degree relatives with OCD, which was marginally higher than that of controls.

Until recently, little was known about effective treatments for trichotillomania. Reports of successful trials with SRIs include a controlled trial of clomipramine (85) and two open trials with fluoxetine (130,131). However, a 6-week placebo-controlled crossover study with fluoxetine demonstrated no significant treatment effect (132). Furthermore, three of four patients showed relapse on 3-month follow-up of clomipramine (94). On the other hand, augmentation of standard SRIs with the neuroleptic pimozide restored treatment response in six of seven patients (95). An open trial of lithium also proved effective in eight of 10 patients (133). There is support for the efficacy of behavior therapy (134)—specifically, the technique of habit reversal (102), which involves identifying the behavioral antecedents and then substituting a less problematic behavior, e.g., fist-clenching (102).

Sexual Obsessions

Sexual disorders related to the OCD spectrum may be divided into three categories: sexual obsessions (intrusive sexual images that are subjectively experienced as being morally repugnant), paraphilias (exhibitionism, pedophilia, sexual masochism and sadism, transvestite fetishism, and voyeurism), and nonparaphilic sexual addictions (e.g., compulsive masturbation and promiscuous sexual behavior). It has been suggested that the term *addictions* be used when sexual interests and behaviors are culturally acceptable but have a frequency or intensity that interferes with the capacity for sexual intimacy (135).

While there are notable differences between some of these sexual disorders and OCD, their commonalities suggest inclusion among the

OCSDs. Typically, patients with OCD experience their symptoms as being intrusive or senseless whereas patients with sexual addictions experience their sexual urges and acts as being pleasurable. Whereas OCD patients may experience relief after completion of rituals, patients with paraphilias and sexual addictions may experience guilt or shame on completion of their behaviors. Nevertheless, OCD patients may have sexual obsessions involving animals, children, or homosexuality. These sexual images, however, are not experienced as being pleasurable but as intrusive, offensive, and morally repugnant. In addition, patients with sexual compulsions may have comorbid OCD (136). Furthermore, OCD patients do not always experience their symptoms as being senseless and may obtain a sense of relief from completion of rituals. Conversely, patients with sexual addictions can experience their urges as being alien to their self-concept and highly discomforting despite the pleasurable aspects.

In an open trial in 13 patients with sexual disorders, we found that response to clomipramine, fluoxetine, or fluvoxamine depended on the class of sexual disorder. Of the five patients diagnosed with nonparaphilic sexual addictions (sexual behaviors that have a frequency or intensity that interferes with normal sexual functioning), two patients showed improvement in compulsive masturbation. Two of three patients classified as having sexual obsessions showed improvement following SRI treatment. The results of this study suggest that sexual symptoms with compulsive and obsessional features are more likely to respond to SRIs than those with primarily impulsive symptoms (83). Nonetheless, there have been reports of successful treatment of paraphilias with serotonin-reuptake blockers. Kafka (135) reported successful treatment of paraphilic coercive disorder (a rapist) with fluoxetine. Other reports have been of fluoxetine treatment of voyeurism (137) and exhibitionism (138).

Depersonalization Disorder

Depersonalization disorder, classified in DSM-IV as a dissociative disorder, is characterized by a subjective sense of unreality or disconnection from one's own body, mentation, feelings, or action. Symptoms can include feeling detached from one's own body and feeling like an outside observer of one's own mental processes. All these symptoms are egodystonic and the person retains intact reality testing. While depersonalized states can occur in a variety of clinical syndromes, including depression (139), schizophrenia (140), seizure disorders (141), and anxiety disorders (142), depersonalization disorder is diagnosed only if the symptom is persistent and recurrent and causes distress. Depersonalized experiences are often associated with depression, anxiety, severe stress, or trauma (143). Depersonalization disorder has been conceptualized as an obsessive-compulsive-related disorder falling on the compulsive end of the impulsive–compulsive spectrum. Although depersonalization is not characterized by repetitive behaviors per se, obsessive-compulsive features include preoccupation with and repetitive experiences of altered sensory perceptions and feelings of detachment. Serotonergic involvement is suggested by reports of symptom precipitation following migraines or marijuana intoxication (143) as well as by positive response to SRIs (87,144). There is also evidence in depersonalization for neuropsychiatric impairment (manifested by soft signs, neuropsychological findings, electrophysiology, and SPECT) that may be similar to that found in OCD (52).

Previous case reports have documented improvement of depersonalization symptoms with antidepressants (145), stimulants (140), benzodiazepines and antiepileptics (141), and ECT (142). Although there has been a report of precipitation of depersonalization symptoms following acute administration of fluoxetine (146), chronic treatment with SSRIs may improve depersonalization (91). In a series of eight patients, Hollander et al. (87) found a preferential response of depersonalization symptoms to agents that manifest potent serotonin-reuptake blockade. Chronic depersonalization symptoms resolved in six of the eight patients treated with fluoxetine or fluvoxamine. Currently we are conducting a controlled trial on fluoxetine in depersonalization.

Hypochondriasis

Hypochondriasis is characterized by the preoccupying fear of having a serious disease, frequently based on the interpretation of physical sensations or signs as symptoms of illness. It is similar to OCD in its obsessional preoccupation with avoidance of harm (in the form of illness) and frequent checking in the form of requests for reassurance. Both OCD and hypochondriasis have an early age of onset, and both have a high rate of comorbid affective and anxiety disorders (147–149). In OCD the symptoms involve fears of becoming ill, whereas in hypochondriasis the patient fears that he or she is already ill, based on interpretation of physical signs and symptoms (86,103). In addition, hypochondriasis is generally ego-syntonic and OCD is ego-dystonic, although there is argument that some OCD patients have sufficient conviction in their obsessional beliefs to render them ego-syntonic. Like OCD, hypochondriasis may be responsive to behavior therapy (150).

Open clinical trials suggest efficacy of SRIs, such as fluoxetine and clomipramine (Josephson, unpublished observations; 151). Fallon et al. (151) reported six cases of hypochondriasis; two patients were treated with fluoxetine but the other patients declined treatment, mainly out of hypochondriacal concerns with medication side effects. One patient was much improved after 4 months of fluoxetine 60 mg/day. The other patient's hypochondriacal symptoms improved after 3 months of fluoxetine 60 mg/day, but comorbid symptoms of BDD developed, specifically a concern about sunken eyes. All symptoms resolved with the addition of clonazepam to fluoxetine treatment.

Pathological Gambling

Pathological gambling is classified in DSM-IV as an impulse-control disorder, not otherwise specified. There is debate over its appropriate classification. It has been diagnosed as a disorder of impulse control, a compulsive disorder, and an addiction. Pathological gambling is characterized by the pressing need to gamble and the inability to resist gambling urges in spite of damaging personal, social, and financial consequences. The gambling preoccupation, urge, and activity increase during periods of stress. Problems that arise as a result of the gambling lead to an intensification of the gambling behavior.

Pathological gambling presents features of both compulsivity and impulsivity. As with compulsive behavior, gambling behavior is preceded by mounting tension and arousal and is followed by a sense of release. While this tension is not pleasurable, the ensuing sense of relief may be experienced as being highly gratifying.

The impulsive nature of pathological gambling points to serotonergic dysfunction. While normal levels of CSF 5-HIAA were found in a sample of pathological gamblers (152), elevated prolactin response to acute challenge with m-CPP, the partial serotonin agonist, has also been reported (32). Noradrenergic hyperactivation, consistent with elevated novelty-seeking, is suggested by increased rates of CSF 3-methoxy-4-hydroxyphenylglycol (MHPG), a metabolite of norepinephrine (152), and increased GH response to clonidine challenge (32).

Although there are few controlled studies to date, there are some indications of the efficacy of serotonin-reuptake blockers in the treatment of pathological gambling. Hollander et al. (96) reported on a double-blind, placebo-controlled clomipramine trial (10 weeks in each phase) in a woman with pathological gambling. While gambling improved minimally during the placebo phase, there was marked improvement within 3 weeks of clomipramine treatment. The question remains, however, of long-term efficacy of SSRIs in impulsive disorders. Currently we are conducting a placebo-controlled, single-blind study of the efficacy of fluvoxamine in pathological gamblers. In addition, lithium carbonate has been reported to provide mild improvement in gamblers who also suffered from an affective disorder (153).

Tourette's Syndrome

Tourette's syndrome is characterized by motor and vocal tics, which are defined as sudden repetitive movements, gestures, or utterances that typically mimic normal behavioral sequences. There is a large literature addressing the overlap between Tourette's syndrome and OCD. In a 2- to 7-year follow-up of 554 childhood OCD patients, 59% developed tics (154). In addition, 30–40% of Tourette's syndrome patients have some OC features (155). Moreover, many Tourette's patients feel a need to perform tics until they are completed or "just right" (155).

Likewise, the neurobiology of Tourette's has several features in common with OCD. Basal ganglia dysfunction is implicated in Tourette's, with abnormal activation of the caudate demonstrated on neuroimaging studies (156). Visual-spatial dysfunction similar to that found in OCD has also been reported in Tourette's patients (77). Although dopaminergic dysregulation is strongly implicated in Tourette's, such that the effectiveness of neuroleptics such as haloperidol or pimozide are widely accepted (97), serotonergic dysfunction is also suggested. In OCD patients with tics, the ratio of serotonergic vs. dopaminergic measures (CSF 5-HIAA: homovanillic acid) was higher than that in OCD patients without tics (154). Nonetheless, SSRIs have been reported to reduce obsessive-compulsive symptoms associated with Tourette's, but not the tics themselves (157). However, neuroleptic addition of SSRIs is helpful in treatment-refractory OCD patients with a history of tics (158).

CONCLUSION

We have discussed the notion of OCSDs, a group of disorders that are frequently comorbid with OCD and that share numerous features with one another, including phenomenology, clinical features (age of onset, course), family history, neurobiology, and possible 5-HT mediation. Specifically, the concept of a compulsive–impulsive spectrum, with a compulsive, harm-avoidant pole opposing an impulsive, sensation-seeking pole, was considered. In addition, the literature on the psychobiology of OCD, including studies of neurobiology, neuropsychiatry, and treatment efficacy, was reviewed in view of related findings in OCSDs. Finally, literature on specific OCSDs was presented. Many of the findings on OCSDs are intriguing and offer significant new insights, but they nonetheless remain preliminary. It is important to note that the construct of an obsessive-compulsive spectrum has been criticized as being too vague and lacking in clear inclusion/exclusion criteria. As such, the notion of an OCSD is, at this point, useful primarily for heuristic purposes (116,159). Further controlled studies on the phenomenology, comorbidity, family history, treatment response, and neurobiology of specific OCSDs are necessary to strengthen our understanding of this important area of inquiry.

REFERENCES

1. Hollander E, ed. Obsessive-Compulsive Related Disorders. Washington, DC: American Psychiatric Press, 1993.
2. Hollander E, Cohen LJ. Psychobiology and Psychopharmacology of Compulsive Spectrum Disorders. In: Oldham J, Hollander E, Skodol AE, eds. Impulsivity and Compulsivity. Washington DC: American Psychiatric Press, 1996:167–195.
3. McElroy SL, Phillips KA, Keck PE. Obsessive-compulsive spectrum disorder. J Clin Psychiatry 1994; 55(suppl):33–51.
4. Rapoport JL. The "obsessive-compulsive spectrum": a useful concept? Encephale 1994; 20:677–680.
5. Hollander E, Phillips K, Eisen J, Aronowitz B, Black D, Decaria C, Cohen LJ, Grossman R, Neziroglu F, Yaryura-Tobias J. Is there a distinct OCD spectrum? Workshop presented at 2nd International Obsessive-Compulsive Disorder Conference, St. Francoise, Guadeloupe, Feb 16–17, 1996.
6. The Clomipramine Collaborative Study Group. Clomipramine in the treatment of patients with obsessive-compulsive disorder. Arch Gen Psychiatry 1991; 48:730–738.
7. Tollefson GD, Rampey AH, Potrin JH, et al. A multicenter investigation of fixed dose fluoxetine in the treatment of obsessive-compulsive disorder. Arch Gen Psychiatry 1994; 51:559–567.
8. Goodman WK, McDougle CJ, Delgado PL, Price LH. Pharmacologic challenges in obsessive-compulsive disorder. Am J Psychiatry 1989; 146:1350–1351.
9. Piggott TA, l'Heureux F, Dubbert B, Bernstein S, Murphy DL. Obsessive compulsive disorder: comorbid conditions. J Clin Psychiatry 1994; 55(suppl):15–27.
10. Stein DJ, Simeon D, Cohen LJ, Hollander E. Trichotillomania and obsessive-compulsive disorder. J Clin Psychiatry 1995; 56:28–35.
11. Levin BE, Duchowny MS. Association of childhood obsessive compulsive disorder and cingulate epilepsy. Biological Psychiatry 1991; 30:1049–1055.

12. McKeon J, McGuffin P, Robinson P. Obsessive-compulsive neurosis following head injury. A report of four cases. Br J Psychiatry 1984; 144:190–192.
13. Barton R. Diabetes insipidus and obsessional neurosis. Am J Psychiatry 1976; 133:235–236.
14. Johnson J, Lucey PA. Encephalitis lethargica, a contemporary cause of catatonic stupor, a report of two cases. Br J Psychiatry 1987; 151:550–552.
15. George MS, Kellner CH, Fossey MD. Obsessive-compulsive symptoms in a patient with multiple sclerosis. J Nerv Ment Dis 1989; 177:304–305.
16. Swedo SE, Rapoport JL, Cheslow DL, et al. High prevalence of obsessive compulsive symptoms in patients with Sydenham's chorea. Am J Psychiatry 1989; 146:246–249.
17. Laplane D, Levasseur M, Pillon B, Dubois B, Baulac M, Mazoyer B, Tran Dinh S, Sette G, Danze F, Baron JC. Obsessive-compulsive and other behavioural changes with bilateral basal ganglia lesions. Brain 1989; 112(3):699–725.
18. Insel TR, Donnelly ER, Lalakea ML, Alterman IS, Murphy DL. Neurological and neuropsychological studies of patients with obsessive-compulsive disorder. Biological Psychiatry 1983; 18:741–745.
19. Insel TR, Mueller EA, Alterman I, Linnoila M, Murphy DL. Obsessive-compulsive disorder and serotonin: is there a connection? Biological Psychiatry 1985; 20:1174–1188.
20. Thoren R, Asberg M, Bertilsson L, Mellstrom B, Syoquist F, Trachman L. Clomipramine treatment of obsessive-compulsive disorder. II. Biochemical aspects. Arch Gen Psychiatry 1980; 37:1289–1294.
21. Kaye WH, Gwirstman HE, George DT, Ebert MH. Altered serotonin activity in anorexia nervosa after long-term weight restoration: does elevated cerebrospinal fluid 5-hydroxyindoleacitic acid level correlate with rigid and obsessive behavior? Arch Gen Psychiatry 1991; 48:556–562.
22. Linnoila M, Virkkunen M, Scheinen M, Nuutila A, Rimon R, Goodwin FK. Low cerebrospinal fluid 5-hydroxyindoleacetic acid concentration differentiates impulsive from nonimpulsive violent behavior. Life Sci 1983; 33:2609–2514.
23. Asberg M, Traskin L, Thoren P. 5 HIAAA in the cerebrospinal fluid: a biochemical suicide predictor? Arch Gen Psychiatry 1976; 33:1193–1197.
24. Arora RC, Meltzer HY. Serotonergic measures in the brains of suicide victims: 5-HT2 binding sites in the frontal cortex of suicide victims and control subjects. Am J Psychiatry 1989; 146:730–736.
25. Hollander E, DeCaria C, Nitescu A, Gully R, Sucker RF, Cooper TB, Gorman JM, Klein DF, Liebowitz MR. Serotonergic function in obsessive-compulsive disorder: behavioral and neuroendocrine responses to oral m-CPP and fenfluramine in patients and healthy volunteers. Arch General Psychiatry 1992; 49:21–28.
26. Murphy DL, Zohar J, Benkelfat C, Pato MT, Pigott TA, Insel TR. Obsessive-compulsive disorder as a 5-HT subsystem-related behavioural disorder. Br J Psychiatry 1989; 155:15–24.

27. Zohar J, Mueller EA, Insel TR, Zohar-Kadouch RC, Murphy DL. Serotonergic responsivity in obsessive-compulsive disorder: comparison of patients and healthy controls. Arch Gen Psychiatry 1987; 44:946–951.

28. Hollander E, Cohen LJ, DeCaria C, Saoud JB, et al. Timing of neuroendocrine responses and effect of m-CPP and fenfluramine plasma levels in OCD and healthy subjects. Biological Psychiatry 1993; 34:407–413.

29. Charney DS, Heninger GR, Breier A. Serotonin function in obsessive-compulsive disorder: a comparison of the effects of tryptophan and m-CPP in pateints and healthy subjects. Arch Gen Psychiatry 1988; 45:177–185.

30. Buttinger K, Hollander E, Walsh BT. M-CPP challenges in eating disorder patients. Proceedings of the American Psychiatric Association Annual Meeting, New York, 1990.

31. Hollander E, Stein DJ, DeCaria CM, Cohen L, Saoud J,B, Skodol AE, Kellman D, Rosnick L, Oldham J. Serotonergic sensitivity in borderline personality disorder: preliminary findings. Am J Psychiatry 1994; 151:277–280.

32. DeCaria CM, Stein DJ, Cohen L, Simeon D, Hwang M, Hollander E. Psychobiology of pathological gambling. Presented at First International Obsessive-Compulsive Disorder Congress, Capri, Italy, March 1993.

33. Stein DJ, Hollander E, Cohen L, Simeon D, Aronowitz B. Serotonergic responsivity in trichotillomania: neuroendocrine effects of m-chlorophenylpiperazine. Biological Psychiatry 1995; 37:414–416.

34. Coccaro EF, Siever LJ, Klar HM, Maurer G, Cochrane K, Cooper TB, Mohs RC, Davis KL. Serotonergic studies in affective and personality disorder patients: correlations with behavioral aggression and impulsivity. Arch Gen Psychiatry 1989; 46:587–599.

35. Insel TR. Toward a neuroanatomy of obsessive-compulsive disorder. Arch Gen Psychiatry 1992; 49:739–744.

36. Behar D, Rapoport JL, Berg CJ, Denckla MB, Mann L, Cox C, Fedio P, Zahn T, Wolfman MG. Computerized tomography and neuropsychological test measures in adolescents with obsessive-compulsive disorder. Am J Psychiatry 1984; 41:363–369.

37. Luxenberg JS, Swedo SE, Flament MF, et al. Neuroanatomical abnormalities in obsessive compulsive disorder detected with quantitative x-ray computed tomography. Am J Psychiatry 1988; 145:1089–1093.

38. Stein DJ, Hollander E, Chan S, De Caria CM, Hilal S, Liebowitz MR, Klein DF. Computed tomography and neurological soft signs in obsessive-compulsive disorder. Psychiatry Res: Neuroimaging 1993; 50:143–150.

39. Garber JH, Ananth JV, Chiu LC, Griswold VJ, Oldendorf WH. Nuclear magnetic resonance study of obsessive compulsive disorder. Am J Psychiatry 1989; 146:1001–1005.

40. Robinson D, Wu H, Munne RA, Ashtari M, Alvir JMJ, Lerner G, Koreen A, Cole K, Bogerts B. Reduced caudate nucleus volume in obsessive-compulsive disorder. Arch Gen Psychiatry 1995; 52:393–398.

41. Baxter LR, Phelps ME, Mazziotta JC, Guze BH, Schwartz JM, Seline CE.

Local cerebral glucose metabolic rates in obsessive-compulsive disorder: a comparison with rates in unipolar depression and in normal controls. Arch Gen Psychiatry 1987; 44:211–218.

42. Baxter LR Jr, Schwartz JM, Mazziotta JC, et al. Cerebral glucose metabolic rates in nondepressed patients with obsessive compulsive disorder. Am J Psychiatry 1988; 145:1560–1563.

43. Nordahl TE, Benkelfat C, Semple WE, Bross M, King AC, Cohen RM. Cerebral glucose metabolic rates in obsessive-compulsive disorder. Neuropsychopharmacology 1989; 2:23–28.

44. Swedo SE, Schapiro MB, Brady CL, et al. Cerebral glucose metabolism in childhood-onset obsessive compulsive disorder. Arch Gen Psychiatry 1989; 46:518–523.

45. Martinot JL, Allilaire JF, Mazoyer BM, Hantouche E, Huret JD, Legaut-Demare F, Deslauriers AG, Hardy P, Pappata S, Baron JC, Syrota A. Obsessive-compulsive disorder: a clinical, neuropsychological and positron emission tomography study. Acta Psychiatr Scand 1990; 82:233–242.

46. Rubin RT, Villaneuva-Meyer J, Anath J, Trajmar PG, Mena I. Regional xenon 133 cerebral blood flow and cerebral technetium Tc 99m-HMPAO uptake in unmedicated patients with obsessive-compulsive disorder and matched normal control subjects: determination by high-resolution single-photon emission computed tomography. Arch Gen Psychiatry 1992; 49:695–702.

47. Machlin SR, Harris GJ, Pearlson GD, Hoehn-Saric R, Jeffrey P, Camargo EE. Elevated medialfrontal cerebral blood flow in obsessive-compulsive patients: a SPECT study. Am J Psychiatry 1991; 148:1240–1242.

48. Hollander E, Prohovnik I, Stein DJ. Increased cerebral blood flow during m-CPP exacerbation of obsessive-compulsive disorder. J Neuropsychiatry Clin Neurosci 1995; 7:485–490.

49. Baxter LR Jr., Schwartz JM, Bergman KS, Szuba MP, Guze BH, Mazziotta JC, Alazraki A, Selin CE, Ferng H-K, Munford P, Phelps ME. Caudate glucose metabolic rate changes with both drug and behavior therapy for obsessive-compulsive disorder. Arch Gen Psychiatry 1992; 49:681–689.

50. Swedo SE, Pietrini P, Leonard HL, Schapiro MB, Rettew DC, Goldberger El, Rapoport SI, Rapoport JL, Grady CL. Cerebral glucose metabolism in childhood-onset obsessive-compulsive disorder: revisualization during pharmacotherapy. Arch Gen Psychiatry 1992; 49:690–694.

51. Hoehn-Saric R, Pearlson GD, Harris CJ, Machlin SR, Camargo EE. Effects of fluoxetine on regional cerebral blood flow in obsessive-compulsive patients. Am J Psychiatry 1991; 48:1243–1245.

52. Hollander E, Carrasco JL, Mullen LS, Trungold S, De Caria CM, Towey J. Left hemisphere activation in depersonalization disorder: a case report. Biological Psychiatry 1992; 31:1157–1162.

53. Goyer PF, Andreason PJ, Semple WE, Clayton AH, King AC, Schultz SC, Cohen RM. PET and personality disorders. Biological Psychiatry 1991; 29:43A–185A.

54. Hyde TM, Stacey ME, Coppola R, Handel SF, Rickler KC, Weinberger DR. Cerebral morphometric abnormalities in Tourette's syndrome: a quantitative study of monozygotic twins. Neurology 1995; 45:1176–1182.
55. Peterson BS, Riddle MA, Cohen DJ, Katz LD, Smith JC, Hardin MT, Leckman JF. Reduced basal ganglia volumes in Tourette's syndrome using three-dimensional reconstruction techniques from magnetic resonance images. Neurology 1993; 43:941–949.
56. Peterson BS, Gore JC, Riddle MA, Cohen DJ, Leckman JF. Abnormal magnetic resonance imaging T2 relaxation time asymmetries in Tourette's syndrome. Psychiatry Res 1994; 55:205–221.
57. Braun AR, Stoetter B, Randolph C, Hsiao JK, Vladar K, Gernet J, Carson RE, Herscovitch P, Chase TN. The functional anatomy of Tourette's syndrome: an FDG-PET study. I. Regional changes in cerebral flucose metabolism differentiating patients and controls. Neuropsychopharmacology 1993; 9:277–291.
58. Swedo SE, Rapoport JL, Leonard HL, Schapiro MB, Rapoport SI, Grady CL. Regional cerebral glucose metabolism of women with trichotillomania. Arch Gen Psychiatry 1991; 48:828–833.
59. Tupper DE. Soft Neurological Signs. Orlando, FL: Grune and Stratton, 1987.
60. Quitkin F, Rifkin A, Klein DF. Neurological soft signs in schizophrenia and character disorders. Arch Gen Psychiatry 1976; 33:845–853.
61. Hollander E, Schiffman E, Cohen B, Rivera-Stein M, Rosen W, Gorman JM, Fyer A, Papp L, Liebowitz MR. Signs of central nervous system dysfunction in obsessive-compulsive disorder. Arch Gen Psychiatry 1990; 47:27–32.
62. Aronowitz B, Hollander E, Mannuzza S, Davis J, Chapman T, Fyer AJ. Soft signs and familial transmission of obsessive-compulsive disorder. Poster presented at the 145th annual meeting of American Psychiatric Association, Washington, DC, May 2–7, 1992.
63. Hollander E, Stein DJ, DeCaria CM, Saoud J,B, Klein DF, Liebowitz MR. A pilot study of biological predictors of treatment outcome in obsessive-compulsive disorder. Biological Psychiatry 1993; 33:747–749.
64. Hollander E, DeCaria C, Aronowitz B, Klein DF, Liebowitz MR, Shaffer D. A pilot follow-up study of childhood soft signs and the development of adult psychopathology. J Neuropsychiatry Clin Neurosci 1991; 3(2):186–189.
65. Hollander E, et al. Neurological soft signs in social phobia. Neuropsychiatry Neuropsychol Behav Neurol 1996; 9:182–185.
66. Stein DJ, Hollander E, Cohen L, Frenkel M, Saoud J, DeCaria C, Aronowitz B, Levin A, Liebowitz MR. Neuropsychiatric impairment in impulsive personality disorders. Psychiatry Res 1993; 48:257–266.
67. Stein D, Hollander E, Simeon D, Cohen L, Islam MN, Aronowitz B. Neurological soft signs in female trichotillomania patients, obsessive-compulsive disorder patients, and healthy control subjects. J Neuropsychiatry Clin Neurosci 1994; 6:184–187.

68. Head EK, Bolton D, Hymas N. Deficits in cognitive shifting ability in patients with obsessive-compulsive disorders. Biological Psychiatry 1989; 25:929–937.

69. Flor-Henry P, Yeudall LT, Koles ZJ, Howarth BG. Neuropsychological and power spectral EEG investigations of the obsessive-compulsive syndrome. Biological Psychiatry 1979; 14(1):119–130.

70. Boone KB, Ananth J, Philpott L, Kaur A, Djenderedjian A. Neuropsychological Characteristics of nondepressed adults with obsessive-compulsive disorder. Neuropsychiatry Neuropsychol Behav Neurol 1991; 4:96–109.

71. Christensen KJ, Kim SW, Dysken MW, Hoover DM. Neuropsychological performance in obsessive-compulsive disorder. Biological Psychiatry 1992; 31:4–18.

72. Zielinski CM, Taylor MA, Juzwin KR. Neuropsychological deficits in obsessive-compulsive disorder. Neuropsychiatry Neuropsychol Behav Neurol 1991; 4:110–126.

73. Hollander E, Liebowitz MR, Rosen WG. Neuropsychiatric and neuropsychological studies in obsessive-compulsive disorder. In: Zohar J, Insel T, Rasmussen S, eds. The Psychobiology of Obsessive-Compulsive Disorder. New York: Springer-Verlag, 1991:126–145.

74. Cohen LJ, Hollander E, DeCaria CM, Stein DJ, Simeon D, Liebowitz MR, Aronowitz BA. Specificity of neuropsychological impairment in obsessive-compulsive disorder: a comparison with social phobic and normal controls. J Neuropsychiatry Clin Neurosci 1996; 8:82–85.

75. Moffitt TE, Henry B. Neuropsychological studies of juvenile delinquency and violence: a review. In: Milner J, ed. The Neuropsychology of Aggression. Norwell, MA: Kluwer Academic, 1991.

76. Rugle L, Melamed L. Neuropsychological assessment of attention problems in pathological gamblers. J Nerv Ment Dis 1993; 181:107–112.

77. Bornstein RA, Yang V. Neuropsychological performance in medicated and unmedicated patients with Tourette's disorder. Am J Psychiatry 1991; 148:468–471.

78. Martin A, Pigott TA, Lalonde FM, Dalton I, Dubbert B, Murphy DL. Lack of evidence for Huntington's disease-like cognitive dysfunction in obsessive-compulsive disorder. Biol Psychiatry 1993; 33:345–353.

79. Freeman C, trimble M, Deakin JF et al. Fluvoxamine versus clomipramine in the treatment of obsessive-compulsive disorder: A multi-center, random, double-blind, parallel group comparison. J Clin Psychiatry 1994; 55:301–305.

80. Greist JH, Jefferson JW, Kobak KA, Katzelnick KJ, Serlin RC. Efficacy and tolerability of serotonin transport inhibitors in obsessive-compulsive disorder: A meta-analysis. Arch Gen Psychiatry 1995; 52:53–59.

81. Hollander E, Liebowitz MR, Winchel R, Klumker A, Klein DF. Treatment of body dysmorphic disorder with serotonin reuptake blockers. Am J Psychiatry. 1989; 146:768–770.

82. Hollander E, Cohen LJ, Simeon D. Body dysmorphic disorder. Psychiatric Ann 1993; 23:359–364.

83. Stein DJ, Hollander E, Anthony DT, Schneier FR, Fallon BA, Liebowitz MR, Klein DF. Serotonergic medications for sexual obsessions, sexual addictions, and paraphilias. J Clin Psychiatry 1992; 53:267–271.

84. Messiha FS. Fluoxetine: a spectrum of clinical applications and postulates of underlying mechanisms. Neurosci Biobehav Rev 1993; 17:385–396.

85. Swedo SE, Leonard JL, Rapoport JL, Lenane MC, Goldberger EL, Cheslow DL. A double-blind comparison of clomipramine and desipramine in the treatment of trichotillomania (hair pulling). N Engl J Med 1989; 321:497–501.

86. Fallon BA, Rasmussen SA, Liebowitz MR. Hypochondriasis. In: Hollander E, ed. Obsessive-Compulsive Related Disorders. Washington, DC: American Psychiatric Press, 1993.

87. Hollander E, Liebowitz MR, DeCaria CM, Fairbanks F, Fallon B, Klein DF. Treatment of depersonalization with serotonin reuptake blockers. J Clin Psychopharmocol 1990; 10:200–203.

88. Coccaro EF, Astill JL, Herbert JL, Schut AG. Fluoxetine treatment of impulsive aggression in DSM-III-R personality disorder patients. J Clin Psychopharmacol 1990; 10:373–375.

89. Phillips KA, McElroy S, Keck PE, Pope HG, Hudson JI. Body dysmorphic disorder: 30 cases of imagined ugliness. Am J Psychiatry 1993; 150:302–308.

90. Kaye WH, Weltzin TE, Hsu LKG. Is anorexia nervosa related to obsessive-compulsive disorder and/or altered serotonin activity? Presented at First International Obsessive-Compulsive Disorder Congress, Capri, Italy, March 1993.

91. Hollander E, Cohen LJ, DeCaria C, Stein DJ, Trungold-Apter S, Islam N. Fluoxetine and depersonalization syndrome (letter). Psychosomatics 1992; 33:361.

92. Zohar J, Insel TR, Berman KF, Foa EB, Hill JL, Weinberger DR. Anxiety and cerebral blood flow during behavioral challenge: dissociation of central from peripheral and subjective measures. Arch Gen Psychiatry 1988; 45:167–172.

93. Hollander E, DeCaria C, Gully R, Nitescu A, Suckow RF, Gorman JM, Klein DF, Liebowitz MR. Effects of chronic fluoxetine treatment on behavioral and neuroendocrine response to meta-chlorophenylpiperazine in obsessive-compulsive disorder. Psychiatry Res 1991; 36:1–17.

94. Pollard CA, Ibe IO, Krojanker DN, Kitchen AD, Bronson SS, Flunn TM. Clomipramine treatment of trichotillomania: a follow-up report on four cases. J Clin Psychiatry 1991; 52:128–139.

95. Stein DJ, Hollander E. Low-dose pimozide augmentation of serotonin reuptake blockers in the treatment of trichotillomania. J Clin Psychiatry 1992; 53:123–126.

96. Hollander E, Frenkel M, DeCaria CM, Trungold S, Stein DJ. Treatment of

pathological gambling with clomipramine (letter). Am J Psychiatry 1992; 149:710–711.

97. Shapiro AK, Shapiro ES. Treatment of tic disorders with haloperidol. In: Cohen DJ, Bruun RD, Leckman JF, eds. Tourette's Syndrome and Tic Disorders: Clinical Understanding and Treatment. New York: Wiley, 1988:267–280.

98. Yaryura-Tobias JA, Neziroglu FA. Obsessive-Compulsive Disorders: Pathogenesis, Diagnosis, and Treatment. New York: Marcel Dekker, 1983.

99. Josephson SC, Brondolo E. Cognitive-behavioral approaches to obsessive-compulsive disorders. In: Obsessive-Compulsive Related Disorders. Hollander E, ed. Washington, DC: American Psychiatric Press, 1993.

100. Foa E, Steketee G. Obsessive-compulsive disorder. In: Lindemann C, ed. Handbood of Phobia Therapy: Rapid Symptom Relief in Anxiety Disorders. Northvale, NJ: Jason Aronson, 1989.

101. Neziroglu FA, Yaryura-Tobias JA. Exposure, response prevention and cognitive therapy in the treatment of body dysmorphic disorder. Behav Therapy 1993; 24:431–438.

102. Azrin NH, Nunn RG, Frantz SE. Treatment of hairpulling: a comparative study of habit reversal negative practice training. J Behav Therapy Exper Psychiatry 1980; 11:13–20.

103. Cohen L, Hollander E, Badaracco MA. What the eyes can't see: diagnosis and treatment of somatic obsessions and delusions. Harvard Rev Psychiatry 1994; 2:160–165.

104. Simeon D, Hollander E, Stein D, Cohen L, Aronowitz B. Body dysmorphic disorder in the DSM IV field trial for obsessive compulsive disorder. Am J Psychiatry 1995; 152:1207–1209.

105. McElroy S, Phillips KA, Keck PE, Judson KI, Harrison GP. Body dysmorphic disorder: does it have a psychotic subtype? J Clin Psychiatry 1993; 54:389–395.

106. Fernando N. Monosymptomatic hypochondriasis treated with a tricyclic antidepressant. Br J Psychiatry 1988; 152:851–852.

107. Cotterill JA. Dermatologic non-disease: a common and potentially fatal disturbance of cutaneous body image. Br J Dermatol 1981; 104:611–619.

108. Thomas CS. Dysmorphophobia: a question of definition. Br J Psychiatry 1984; 144:513–516.

109. Vitello B, DeLeon J. Dysmorphia misdiagnosed as obsessive-compulsive disorder. Psychosomatics 1990; 31:220–222.

110. Tamburrino MB, Kaufman R, Hertzer J. Eating disorder history in women with obsessive-compulsive disorder. J Am Med Wom Assoc 1994; 49:24–26.

111. Fahy TA, Osacar A, Marks I. History of eating disorders in female patients with obsessive-compulsive disorder. Int J Eating Disord 1993; 14:439–443.

112. Rubenstein CS, Pigott TA, l'Heureux F, Hill JL, Murphy DL. Preliminary investigation of the lifetime prevalence of anorexia and bulimia nervosa

in patients with obsessive compulsive disorder. J Clin Psychiatry 1992; 53:309–314.

113. Kaye WH, Weltzin TE, Hsu LKG, Bulik CM, McConaha C, Sobkiewics T. Patients with anorexia nervosa have elevated scores on the Yale-Brown Obsessive-Compulsive Scale. Int J Eating Disord 1992; 12:57–62.

114. Fahy TA. Obsessive-compulsive symptoms in eating disorders. Behav Res Ther 1991; 29:113–116.

115. Kaye WH, Weltzin TE, Hsu LKG, Bulik CM. An open trial of fluoxetine in patients with anorexia nervosa. J Clin Psychiatry 1991; 52:464–471.

116. Stein DJ, Hollander E. The obsessive-compulsive disorder spectrum. J Clin Psychiatry 1995; 56:265–266.

117. Swedo SE. Trichotillomania. Psychiatric Ann 1993; 23:402–407.

118. Christensen GA, Mackenzie TB, Mitchell JE. Characteristics of 60 adult chronic hairpullers. Am J Psychiatry 1991; 148:365–370.

119. Cohen LJ, Stein D, Spadaccini E, Rosen J, Aronowitz B. Clinical profile, comorbidity, and treatment history in 123 hairpullers: a survey study. J Clin Psychiatry 1995; 56:319–326.

120. Swedo SE, Leonard HL. Trichotillomania: an obsessive-compulsive disorder? Psychiatric Clin N Am 1992; 15:777–790.

121. Swedo SE. Trichotillomania. In: Hollander E, ed. Obsessive-Compulsive Related Disorders. Washington, DC: American Psychiatric Press, 1993:93–111.

122. Christenson GA, Chernoff Clementz E, Clementz BA. Personality and clinical characteristics in patients with trichotillomania. J Clin Psychiatry 1992; 53:407–413.

123. Swedo SE, Rapoport JL. Annotation: Trichotillomania. J Child Psychol Psychiatry 1991; 32:401–409.

124. Dawber R. Self-induced hair loss. Sem Dermatol 1985; 4:53–57.

125. Bhatia MS, Singhal PK, Rastogi V, Dhar NK, Nigam VR, Taneja SB. Clinical profile of trichotillomania. J Indian Med Assoc 1991; 89:137–139.

126. Stanley MA, Swann AC, Bowers TC, Davis ML, Taylor DJ. A comparison of clinical features in trichotillomania and obsessive-compulsive disorder. Behav Res Ther 1992; 30:39–44.

127. Reeve EA, Bernstein GA, Christensen GA. Clinical characteristics and psychiatric comorbidity in children with trichotillomania. J Am Acad Child Adolesc Psychiatry 1992; 31:132–138.

128. Christensen GA, MacKenzie TB. Trichotillomania, body dysmorphic disorder, and obsessive-compulsive disorder (letter). J Clin Psychiatry 1995; 56:5.

129. lenane mC, Swedo SE, Rapoport JL, Leonard H, Sceery W, Guroff JJ. Rates of obsessive-compulsive disorder in first degree relatives of patients with trichotillomania: a research note. J Child Psychol Psychiatry 1991; 3:925–933.

130. Winchel RM, Jones JS, Stanley B, Molcho A, Stanley M. Clinical characteristics of trichotillomania and its response to fluoxetine. J Clin Psychiatry 1992; 53:302–308.

131. Koran LM, Ringold A, Hewlett W. Fluoxetine for trichotillomania: an open clinical trial. Psychopharmacol Bull 1992; 28:145–149.
132. Christensen GA, Mackenzie TB, Mitchell JE, Callies AL. A placebo-controlled, double-blind crossover study of fluoxetine in trichotillomania. Am J Psychiatry 1991; 148:1566–1571.
133. Christensen GA, Popkin MK, Mackenzie TB, Realmuto GM. Lithium treatment of chronic hair pulling. J Clin Psychiatry 1991; 52:116–120.
134. Friman PC, Finney JW, Christophersen ER. Behavioral treatment of trichotillomania: an evaluative review. Behav Therapy 1984; 15:249–265.
135. Kafka MP. Successful treatment of paraphilic coercive disorder (a rapist) with fluoxetine hydrochloride. Br J Psychiatry 1991; 158:844–847.
136. Anthony DT, Hollander E. Sexual compulsions. In: Hollander E, ed. Obsessive-Compulsive Related Disorders. Washington, DC: American Psychiatric Press, 1993.
137. Emmanuel NP, Lydiard RB, Ballenger JC. Fluoxetine treatment of voyeurism (letter). Am J Psychiatry 1991; 148:950.
138. Bianchi MD. Fluoxetine treatment of exhibition (letter). Am J Psychiatry 1990; 147:1089–1090.
139. Tucker DM, Vannatta K, Rothlind J. Arousal and activation systems and primitive adaptive controls on cognitive priming. In: Stein NL, Leventhal B, Trabasso T, eds. Psychological and Biological Aspects of Emotions. Hillsdale, NJ: Erlbaum, 1990.
140. Davison K. Episodic depersonalization: observations on seven patients. Br J Psychiatry 1964; 110:505–513.
141. Greenberg DB, Hochberg FH, Murray GB. The theme of death in complex partial seizures. Am J Psychiatry 1984; 141:1587–1589.
142. Nuller YL. Depersonalization—symptoms, meaning, therapy. Acta Psychiatr Scand 1982; 66:451–458.
143. Simeon D, Hollander E. Depersonalization disorder. Psychiatric Ann 1993; 23:382–388.
144. Fichtner CG, Horevitz RP, Braun BG. Fluoxetine in depersonalization disorder. Am J Psychiatry 1992; 149:1750–1751.
145. Walsh R. Depersonalization: definition and treatment (letter). Am J Psychiatry 1975; 146:402.
146. Black DW, Wojcieszek J. Depersonalization syndrome induced by fluoxetine (letter). Psychosomatics 1991; 32:468–469.
147. Kellner R, Slocumb JC, Wiggins RJ, et al. The relationships of hypochondriacal fears and beliefs to anxiety and depression. Psychiatr Med 1986; 4:15–24.
148. Noyes R, Reich J, Clancy J, et al. Reduction in hypochondriasis with treatment of panic disorder. Am J Psychiatry 1986; 149:631–635.
149. Craske MG, Rapee RM, Jackel L, et al. Qualitative dimensions of worry in DSM-III-R generalized anxiety disorders subjects and non-anxious controls. Behav Res Ther 1989; 27:397–402.
150. Sako V, Bouman TK. Cognitive behavioral approaches in the treatment of

hypochondriasis: six single case cross-over studies. Behav Res Ther 1992; 30:301–306.

151. Fallon BA, Liebowitz MR, Schneier F, et al. An open trial of fluoxetine for hypochondriasis. In: New Research Program and Abstracts, 144th Annual Meeting of the American Psychiatric Association, New Orleans, LA, NR188, 1991:183.

152. Roy A, Adinoff B, Roehrich L, et al. Pathological gambling: a psychobiological study. Arch Gen Psychiatry 1988; 45:369–373.

153. Moskowitz JA. Lithium and lady luck: use of lithium carbonate in compulsive gambling. NY State J Med 1980; 80:785–788.

154. Leonard HL, Lenane MC, Swedo SE, Rettew DC, Gershon ES, Rapoport JL. Tics and Tourettes's disorder: a 2- to 7-year follow-up of 554 obsessive-compulsive children. Am J Psychiatry 1992; 149:1244–1251.

155. Leckman JF. Tourette's syndrome. In: Hollander E, ed. Obsessive-Compulsive Related Disorders. Washington, DC: American Psychiatric Press, 1993:113–138.

156. Chase TN, Geoffrey V, Gilllespie M, et al. Structural and functional studies of Gilles de la Tourette's syndrome. Rev Neurol (Paris) 1986; 142:851–855.

157. Riddle MA, Hardin MT, King RA et al. Fluoxetine treatment of children and adolescents with Tourette's and obsessive compulsive disorders. J Am Acad Child Adolesc Psychiatry 1990; 29:45–48.

158. McDougle CG, Goodman WK, Leckman JF, Price LH. The psychopharmacology of obsessive compulsive disorder: implications for treatment and pathogenesis. Psychiatr Clin North Am 1993; 16:749–66.

159. Rasmussen SA. Commentary: obsessive-compulsive spectrum disorders. J Clin Psychiatry 1994; 55:89–91.

4

The Neuropsychiatry of OCD

Lisa J. Cohen

Beth Israel Medical Center/
Albert Einstein College of Medicine
New York, New York

Eric Hollander

The Mount Sinai School of Medicine
New York, New York

Dan J. Stein

University of Stellenbosch
Tygerberg, South Africa

Over the past 15 years, there have been remarkable advances in our understanding of the neurological undepinnings of obsessive-compulsive disorder (OCD), with associated treatment advances for this once treatment-refractory disorder. While much work on OCD has centered on the serotonergic model, the neuropsychiatry of OCD has also received increasing attention. Neuropsychiatric investigations have included functional and structural imaging studies, neurological soft-sign exams, electrophysiological studies, and neuropsychological assessment.

Underlying neuroanatomical abnormalities were first suggested by a long-noted association between OCD and neurological disorders. Precipitation of OCD has been reported following numerous neurological disorders, including seizure disorders (1–3), head trauma (4), diabetes insipidus (5), von Economo's (6) and herpes simplex (7) encephalitis, and multiple sclerosis (8). More specifically, a number of neurological disorders associated with basal ganglia disease have been linked with

OCD. These include Sydenham's chorea (9,10), postencephalitic parkinsonism (11), Huntington's disease (12,13), Tourette's syndrome (14,15), and disease of the globus pallidus (16) and head of the caudate (17,18).

NEUROANATOMICAL ABNORMALITIES

Functional and structural neuropathology in OCD patients has been assessed with CT, MRI, PET, SPECT, and rCBF methodologies. Relatively consistent findings have pointed to abnormal activation of an orbital frontal–basal ganglia–thalamic loop (19).

Structural abnormalities have been assessed with CT scan and MRI. Increased ventricle-brain ratios (VBR) in OCD patients relative to controls have been demonstrated in some CT studies but not others. Whereas Behar et al. (20) found greater VBR in adolescent OCD patients relative to controls, Insel et al. (17) found no difference in VBR in adult OCD patients and controls and Luxenberg et al. (18) found no difference in lateral ventrical or third ventrical size in adult OCDs and controls. Likewise, findings of decreased caudate volume on CT are also inconsistent. Luxenberg and colleagues (18) found smaller caudate nucleus volume in OCDs relative to controls whereas Stein et al. (21) reported no difference. Interestingly, Stein et al. (21) found increased VBR in OCD patients with high neurological soft signs compared to both nonpatient controls and OCD patients with low soft signs, suggesting that structural abnormalities may reflect subgroups within OCD patients.

While both CT (17,20) and MRI (22) studies fail to reveal gross pathology of the frontal lobes, abnormalities in frontal tissue (increased T1 signal) have been demonstrated on MRI in 32 OCD patients relative to 14 controls (22). MRI studies, which allow greater precision than CT studies, have also produced contradictory results with regard to caudate volume. Two studies (23,24) demonstrated no difference in caudate volume between OCDs and controls, while another study (25) found increased caudate volume on the right but not left side in OCDs compared to controls.

Robinson et al. (26) assessed the volume of the prefrontal cortex, caudate nucleus, and lateral and third ventricles on MRI in 26 OCD patients and 26 healthy controls. OCD patients demonstrated lower bilateral caudate volume than controls but insignificant differences in ventrical and prefrontal volume. Caudate volume was also associated with level of education, possibly reflecting the plasticity of brain structure. This raises intriguing questions about the mutual influence of structural and functional abnormalities. Future research could assess the longitudinal course of structural abnormalities in OCD as well as possible treatment effects.

In contrast to structural abnormalities, functional abnormalities in the frontal cortex and basal ganglia have been well documented in OCD patients relative to normal controls. On positron emission tomography (PET), increased glucose metabolism was demonstrated in orbitofrontal cortex (27–30), although one study (31) found decreased glucose metabolism. Frontal abnormalities on PET have been related to OCD severity (30) and lowered performance on a frontal-type neuropsychological task (Stroop) (31). Moreover, single-photon emission computed tomography (SPECT) has documented increased blood flow (HMPAO uptake) in frontal cortex (32,33).

Functional abnormalities in the caudate have presented a less consistent picture. PET studies have shown increased (27,28), decreased (31), and unchanged activity in the caudate (29,30). Decreased blood flow in the head of the caudate has been shown on SPECT (32).

In one study with [137]-Xe rCBF, the partial 5-HT agonist mCPP increased OCD symptoms and cortical blood flow, especially in frontal areas. Increase in frontal blood flow correlated with an increase in OC symptoms (34).

Normalization of functional abnormalities following successful treatment of OCD adds further support to the notion of frontal-basal ganglia abnormalities in OCD. Following fluoxetine treatment, reduction both in medial frontal HMPAO uptake on SPECT and in OCD symptoms was documented (35). Baxter et al. (36) demonstrated decreased metabolic activity on PET compared to baseline in the right caudate nucleus following 10-week trials of either fluoxetine or behavior therapy. In another study (37), following 1 year of treatment with either clomipramine or fluoxetine, decreased orbital frontal activity on PET was correlated with treatment response.

In addition, lateralization of neuroanatomical abnormalities has been suggested by several studies showing unilateral findings in both frontal cortex and caudate nucleus, although findings are equivocal as to predominance of left- vs. right-sided pathology (28,38,39).

Finally, psychosurgical findings offer further support of the frontal–basal ganglia–thalamic loop in OCD. Cingulotomy for treatment of a focal seizure originating in the right anterior cingulate gyrus significantly reduced associated OC symptomatology (1). Likewise, leucotomy, thalamotomy, and anterior capsulotomy have been reported to attenuate OCD symptoms (40,41) by interrupting the frontal-thalamic axis.

NEUROLOGICAL SOFT SIGNS

Neurological soft signs provide another measure of neurobehavioral impairment. These are nonlocalizing signs of deviant performance on a motor or sensory task that cannot be attributed to any direct brain lesion

(42). Soft-sign examination assesses fine motor coordination, involuntary and mirror movements, and sensory performance. Elevated soft signs have been found in certain types of schizophrenia and impulsive character subtypes (43), adolescent anxiety disorders (44), attention disorder with hyperactivity (45), and minimal brain dysfunction (46). The fact that several common psychiatric disorders, including subtypes of schizophrenia and affect disorders (43), are not associated with soft signs suggests that soft signs are a relatively specific finding.

In a comparison of 41 adult OCD patients and 20 normal controls matched for age, sex, and handedness, abnormalities were demonstrated in fine motor coordination, involuntary and mirror movements, and visual constructional function (cube drawing) (47). In an expanded sample with 50 OCD patients and 31 normal controls, OCD patients demonstrated greater total and right- and left-sided soft signs (48).

Interestingly, the number of abnormal neurological soft signs in OCD patients was positively correlated with measures of visual-spatial impairment but negatively correlated with measures of executive function (Trailmaking A and B). Moreover, measures of visual-spatial impairment were inversely correlated with Trails A and B (48). This offers further support of the notion that neurological impairment characterizes specific subgroups of OCD patients.

Moreover, increased soft signs in OCD patients was associated with greater symptomatology (47), increased ventricular size on CT (21), greater familial transmission of soft signs (49), and reduced response to serotonin reuptake inhibitors (50).

Finally, a follow-up study of children with high soft signs at age 7 demonstrated a disproportionate rate of OCD, anxiety, affective disorders, and symptoms in adulthood (51).

ELECTROPHYSIOLOGY

Findings from electrophysiological studies have complemented other domains of neuropsychiatric investigation. Electrophysiological studies have demonstrated temporal-lobe EEG abnormalities in some studies (52–54), with less pronounced results in others (20,55). Findings of lateralized abnormalities were consistent with left-hemisphere dysfunction (56,57). Sleep EEGs have been found to differ from normal controls but to be similar to those of depressed patients (1,58). Studies of evoked potentials to visual, auditory, and somatosensory stimuli have shown findings consistent with hyperarousal and overfocused attention (56,57,59–61), although abnormalities may be most evident on complex cognitive tasks (60,62).

NEUROPSYCHOLOGICAL DYSFUNCTION

A growing body of literature on neuropsychological dysfunction in OCD suggests impairments in visual-spatial and visuoconstructional ability (17,63) and frontal-lobe-related executive functions (ability to form, maintain, and switch cognitive sets) (64,65). Findings are inconclusive in regard to attention and memory (20,54,63), although evidence of deficits in visual memory is relatively strong (66).

Nonetheless, numerous methodological problems suggest that results should be interpreted cautiously. Small sample size, insufficient control for the effects of medication use, anxiety, depression, inpatient vs. outpatient status as well as the lack of patient control groups and even in some studies the use of historical norms rather than a nonpatient control group are all inherent problems. Tests are rarely organized into function clusters, decreasing the convergent validity for findings of select functional impairments.

EXECUTIVE DYSFUNCTION

The possibility of executive dysfunction in OCD is of interest given the consistent evidence of abnormal activity in the frontal cortex. Head and colleagues (65) found impairment in 15 drug-free outpatient OCDs relative to matched controls on the Modified Wisconsin Card Sort and on a word-fluency test. Behar et al. (20) studied 16 OCD adolescents relative to matched controls and found impairment on the Money Road Map, which involves discerning and following unstated rules during maze learning. They considered this reflective of executive dysfunction although both tasks have visual-spatial components. Martinot et al. (31) studied 14 nondepressed OCD inpatients, most on medication, and found them impaired on tests of memory and attention that have been associated with executive functions (Rey-Oestereith copy and recall, Trailmaking B, and Stroop). Poor performance on Stroop, which demands focused attention with inhibition of attention to distracting stimuli, was inversely correlated to absolute metabolic values for the prefrontal cortex on PET activity. Verbal fluency was positively correlated with prefrontal metabolic activity.

Flor-Henry et al. (54) administered the Halstead Reitan battery to 11 OCD inpatients and found impairment relative to controls on subtest measures considered sensitive to anterior vs. posterior dysfunction. Christensen et al. (67) found marginally significant differences between 18 nondepressed OCD patients and 18 age-, education-, and gender-matched controls on measures of executive functions (Category Test,

Wisconsin Card Sort, Controlled Word Association, Porteus Maze Test, Word Fluency Test) only when two outliers were removed. Aronowitz et al. (68) found impairment on Trailmaking A, B, and B-A but not on Stroop in 31 OCD patients compared to 21 age- and sex-matched controls.

On the other hand, Zielinski et al. (66) found no differences between 21 OCD patients (some on medication) and controls on measures of executive function. Boone et al. (69) also failed to replicate findings of executive dysfunction with a study of 20 nondepressed OCD patients and 16 controls. Unfortunately, most measures of executive function are associated with presumed hypofunction of the frontal lobes, secondary to lesions of various etiologies, and thus may not be sensitive to hyperfrontality, which may be more characteristic of OCD (27–29).

VISUAL-SPATIAL DYSFUNCTION

Evidence of visual-spatial dysfunction is more conclusive. Higher verbal IQ scores relative to performance IQ scores have been found in OCD (17,69). Boone et al. (69) found impairment on the Hooper Visual Organization Test and on percent retention of the Rey-Oestereith Complex Figure. The latter also implicates visual memory and executive functions. Head et al. (65) found deficits in WAIS-R Block Design, a measure of visual-constructional ability, and the Money Road Test, which also may involve executive functions. Christensen et al. (67) found impairment on recent nonverbal memory tasks and on WAIS Block Design. Zeilinski et al. (66) found impairment in OCD patients relative to controls in tests that measure visual-spatial recall, recognition (false positives on Recurring Figures Test), and sequencing (Corsi's Block Tapping Test). Aronowitz et al. (68) found impairment of visual-constructional and visual memory functions (Benton Visual Retention Test).

ATTENTION AND MEMORY

Findings for attentional and memory deficits in OCD have been inconsistent. Memory impairments have been suggested to account for obsessive checking (70). Zielinski et al. (66) found impaired visual memory but no impairments on the California Verbal Learning Test except on the number of intrusions during immediate recall. WAIS Digit Span, a test of auditory immediate memory, has been found to differentiate patients from controls in some studies (31,54) but not in others (68,69,71). Digit span, however, is also sensitive to attentional deficits.

Attentional problems were interpreted by Martinot et al. (31) when they found impaired performance on Digit Span, a cancelation task, Stroop, and Trailmaking B. These subjects were inpatients and rated higher on trait anxiety. Thus, attentional problems in OCD may be related to level of anxiety. Zielinski et al. (66) found no difference between OCD patients and controls on the Continuous Performance Test, a measure of sustained attention, and found no correlation between anxiety measures and neuropsychological measures. Behar et al. (20) found no differences between adolescent OCD patients and controls on Reaction Time and Two-Flash measures of attention. Thus, the findings on attentional impairment are inconclusive and bear further investigation.

MOTOR-COORDINATION IMPAIRMENT

Impaired coordination of motor programming is possible, considering the broad evidence of basal ganglia involvement. Tests of tactual recognition (e.g., the Tactual Performance Test) have shown impairment (54,67), although more simple tests of motor coordination (e.g., the Purdue Pegboard Test) showed no difference (67).

LATERALIZATION OF NEUROPSYCHIATRIC DYSFUNCTION

There is some indication of lateralization of neuropsychiatric dysfunction in OCD. The strong evidence of impairment in visual-constructional relative to verbal impairment is indicative of right-hemisphere relative to left-hemisphere dysfunction. However, visual-spatial impairment has also been linked to basal ganglia dysfunction (72,73). Wexler et al. (74) documented a lack of normal right-sided dominance in simple line bisection and body turning tasks, suggesting a disruption in normal cerebral laterality. A number of electrophysiological studies (54,56,57) suggest left-hemisphere overactivity or overresponsiveness. Although decreased right-ear advantage, suggesting decreased left-hemisphere function, has been documented (58,75), this has also been associated with decreased awareness of emotion-related words, which is suggestive of decreased right-hemisphere function (75). Brain-imaging findings have been mixed, as there are indications of abnormalities in left, right, or bilateral activity in the caudate, orbitofrontal, and thalamic regions (27,28,37,38).

Thus, although this must be stated with caution, the above findings might support a putative hypothesis of OCD reflecting left-hemisphere hyperfunction with concomitant right-hemisphere hypo-function.

RELATIONSHIP OF NEUROPSYCHIATRIC FINDINGS TO THE SEROTONERGIC MODEL

Recent advances in the study of OCD have stemmed largely from the serendipitous finding of the efficacy of clomipramine. The serotonergic model of OCD gains support from several lines of evidence, including a preferential response to a range of serotonin reuptake inhibitors (SRIs) (76–78), symptom exacerbation and blunted prolactin response following challenge with the partial 5-HT agonist m-CPP in a subgroup of OCD patients (79), and elevated levels of 5-HIAA at baseline in OCD patients who respond to SSRIs (80).

Integrating neuropsychiatric and 5-HT lines of investigation, there is rich innervation of 5-HT fibers in the neuroanatomical areas implicated in OCD, e.g., the basal ganglia and the frontal cortex. Two major tracts of 5-HT neurons originate in the raphe nucleus, one of which originates in the median raphe nucleus and projects to the hippocampus, entorhinal cortex, hypothalamus, amygdala, and parts of the temporal lobes and may be implicated in affective and anxiety disorders (81). The other tract originates in the dorsal raphe nucleus and projects to the striatal, thalamic, and prefrontal areas (81), and thus might be implicated in OCD (Grove et al., unpublished observations).

Despite the convergence of several lines of investigation, the approximately 40% of patients who are refractory to a single SSRI trial suggest a more complicated picture. Heterogeneity within OCD patients has been suggested; more specifically, the existence of discrete subgroups, reflecting either 5-HT dysregulation or overall neurological damage, has been hypothesized (82). Evidence for a dissociation between neurologically and neurochemically impaired patients comes from the relationship of neurological soft signs to decreased responsiveness to SSRI treatment (50), increased ventricle size on CT scan (21), and greater visual-spatial but not executive (frontal) neuropsychological dysfunction (48). Nonetheless, an increase in soft signs may also reflect greater OCD severity, which in turn results in more pervasive neurological impairment.

In sum, neuropsychiatric investigations in OCD have yielded a surprisingly convergent body of literature, broadening our understanding of this very common and debilitating disease. Additional studies might further address the question of heterogeneity, potentially contributing to advances in the treatment of refractory OCD.

REFERENCES

1. Levin BE, Duchowny MS. Association of childhood obsessive compulsive disorder and cingulate epilepsy. Biol Psychiatry 1991; 30:1049–1055.
2. Brickner RM, Rosen AA, Munro R. Physiological aspects of the obsessive state. Psychosom Med 1940; 2:369–383.
3. Bear DM, Fedio P. Quantitative analysis of interictal behavior in temporal lobe epilepsy. Arch Neurol 1977; 34:454–467.
4. McKeon J, McGuffin P, Robinson P. Obsessive-compulsive neurosis following head injury: a report of four cases. Br J Psychiatry 1984; 144:190–192.
5. Barton R. Diabetes insipidus and obsessional neurosis. Am J Psychiatry 1976; 133:235–236.
6. Johnson J, Lucey PA. Encephalitis lethargica, a contemporary cause of catatonic stupor, a report of two cases. Br J Psychiatry 1987; 151:550–552.
7. Khanna S. Neuropsychiatry of obsessive-compulsive disorder: organic basis and organic etiologies. Presented at the First International Obsessive-Compulsive Disorder Conference, Capri, Italy, 1993.
8. George MS, Kellner CH, Fossey MD. Obsessive-compulsive symptoms in a patient with multiple sclerosis. J Nerv Ment Dis 1989; 177:304–305.
9. Chapman AH, Pilkey L, Gibbons MJ. A psychosomatic study of eight children with Sydenham's chorea. Pediatrics 1958; 21:582–595.
10. Swedo SE, Rapoport JL, Cheslow DL, et al. High prevalence of obsessive compulsive symptoms in patients with Sydenham's chorea. Am J Psychiatry 1989; 146:246–249.
11. Schilder P. The organic background of obsessions and compulsions. Am J Psychiatry.
12. Cummings JL, Cunningham D. Obsessive-compulsive disorder in Huntington's disease. Biol Psychiatry 1992; 31:263–270.
13. Dewhurst K, Oliver J, Trick KLK, McKnight AL. Neuropsychiatric aspects of Huntington's diseases. Confinia Neurologica 1969; 31:258–268.
14. Pauls DL, Towbin KE, Leckman JF, et al. Gilles de la Tourette's syndrome and obsessive compulsive disorder: evidence supporting a genetic relationship. Arch Gen Psychiatry 1986; 43:1180–1182.
15. Hollander E, Liebowitz MR, DeCaria C. Conceptual and methodological issues in studies of obsessive-compulsive and Tourette's disorder. Psychiatric Dev 1989; 4:267–296.
16. Laplane D, Levasseur M, Pillon B, Dubois B, Baulac M, Mazoyer B, Tran Dinh S, Sette G, Danze F, Baron JC. Obsessive-compulsive and other behavioural changes with bilateral basal ganglia lesions. Brain 1989; 112(3):699–725.
17. Insel TR, Donnelly ER, Lalakea ML, Alterman IS, Murphy DL. Neurological and neuropsychological studies of patients with obsessive-compulsive disorder. Biol Psychiatry 1983; 18:741–751.
18. Luxenberg JS, Swedo SE, Flament MF, et al. Neuroanatomical abnormali-

ties in obsessive compulsive disorder detected with quantitative x-ray computed tomography. Am J Psychiatry 1988; 145:1089–1093.

19. Insel TR. Toward a neuroanatomy of obsessive-compulsive disorder. Arch Gen Psychiatry 1992; 49:739–744.

20. Behar D, Rapoport JL, Berg CJ, Denckla MB, Mann L, Cox C, Fedio P, Zahn T, Wolfman MG. Computerized tomography and neuropsychological test measures in adolescents with obsessive-compulsive disorder. Am J Psychiatry 1984; 41:363–369.

21. Stein DJ, Hollander E, Chan S, DeCaria CM, Hilal S, Liebowitz MR, Klein DF. Computed tomography and neurological soft signs in obsessive-compulsive disorder. Psychiatry Res Neuroimaging 1993; 50:143–150.

22. Garber JH, Ananth JV, Chiu LC, Griswold VJ, Oldendorf WH. Nuclear magnetic resonance study of obsessive compulsive disorder. Am J Psychiatry 1989; 146:1001–1005.

23. Kellner CH, Jolley RR, Holgate RC, Austin L, Lydiard RB, Laraia M, Ballenger JC. Brain MRI in obsessive-compulsive disorder. Psychiatry Res 1991; 36:45–49.

24. Aylward EH, Schwartz J, Machlin S, Pearlson G. Bicaudate ratio as a measure of caudate volume on MR images. Am J Neuroradiol 1991; 12:1217–1222.

25. Scarone S, Colombo C, Livian S, Ambruzzese M, Ronchi P, Locatelli M, Scotti G, Smeraldi E. Increased right caudate nucleus size in obsessive-compulsive disorder: detection with magnetic resonance imaging. Psychiatry Res Neuroimaging 1992; 45:115–121.

26. Robinson D, Wu H, Munne RA, Ashtari M, Alvir JMJ, Lerner G, Koreen A, Cole K, Bogerts B. Reduced caudate nucleus volume in obsessive-compulsive disorder. Arch Gen Psychiatry 1995; 52:393–398.

27. Baxter LT, Phelps ME, Mazziotta JC, Guze BH, Schwartz JM, Seline CE. Local cerebral glucose metabolic rates in obsessive-compulsive disorder: a comparison with rates in unipolar depression and in normal controls. Arch Gen Psychiatry 1987; 44:211–218.

28. Baxter LR Jr, Schwartz JM, Mazziotta JC, et al. Cerebral glucose metabolic rates in nondepressed patients with obsessive compulsive disorder. Am J Psychiatry 1988; 145:1560–1563.

29. Nordahl TE, Benkelfat C, Semple WE, Bross M, King AC, Cohen RM. Cerebral glucose metabolic rates in obsessive-compulsive disorder. Neuropsychopharmacology 1989; 2:23–28.

30. Swedo SE, Schapiro MB, Brady CL, et al. Cerebral glucose metabolism in childhood-onset obsessive compulsive disorder. Arch Gen Psychiatry 1989; 46:518–523.

31. Martinot JL, Allilaire JF, Mazoyer BM, Hantouche E, Huret JD, Legaut-Demare F, Deslauriers AG, Hardy P, Pappata S, Baron JC, Syrota A. Obsessive-compulsive disorder: a clinical, neuropsychological and positron emission tomography study. Acta Psychiatr Scand 1990; 82:233–242.

32. Rubin RT, Villaneuva-Meyer J, Anath J, Trajmar PG, Mena I. Regional xenon 133 cerebral blood flow and cerebral technetium Tc 99m-HMPAO up-

take in unmedicated patients with obsessive-compulsive disorder and matched normal control subjects: determination by high-resolution single-photon emission computed tomography. Arch Gen Psychiatry 1992; 49:695–702.

33. Machlin SR, Harris GJ, Pearlson GD, Hoehn-Saric R, Jeffrey P, Camargo EE. Elevated medialfrontal cerebral blood flow in obsessive-compulsive patients: a SPECT study. Am J Psychiatry 1991; 148:1240–1242.

34. Hollander E, Prohovnik I, Stein DJ. Increased blood flow during m-CPP exacerbation of obsessive-compulsive disorder. J Neuropsychiatry Clin Neurosci 1995; 7:485–490.

35. Hoehn-Saric R, Pearlson GD, Harris CJ, Machlin SR, Camargo EE. Effects of fluoxetine on regional cerebral blood flow in obsessive-compulsive patients. Am J Psychiatry 1991; 48:1243–1245.

36. Baxter LR Jr, Schwartz JM, Bergman KS, Szuba MP, Guze BH, Mazziotta JC, Alazraki Selin CE, Ferng H-K, Munford P, Phelps ME. Caudate glucose metabolic rate changes with both drug and behavior therapy for obsessive-compulsive disorder. Arch Gen Psychiatry 1992; 49:681–689.

37. Swedo SE, Pietrini P, Leonard HL, Schapiro MB, Rettew DC, Goldberger El, Rapoport SI, Rapoport JL, Grady CL. Cerebral glucose metabolism in childhood-onset obsessive-compulsive disorder: revisualization during pharmacotherapy. Arch Gen Psychiatry 1992; 49:690–694.

38. Calabrese G, Colombo C, Bonfanti A, Scotti G. Caudate nucleus abnormalities in obsessive-compulsive disorder: measurements of MRI signal intensity. Psychiatry Res 1993; 50(2):89–92.

39. Flor HP. Le syndrome obsessionel-compulsif: reflet d'un defaut de regulation frontocaudee de l'hemisphere gauche? Encephale 1990; 16:325–329.

40. Jenike MA, Baer L, Ballantine T, Martuzza RL, Tynes S, Giriunas I, Buttolph L, Cassem NH. Cingulotomy for refractory obsessive-compulsive disorder: a long term follow up of 33 patients. Arch Gen Psychiatry 1991; 48:548–555.

41. Martuzza RL, Chiccoa EA, Jenike MA. Stereotactic radiofrequency thermal cingulotomy for obsessive compulsive disorder. J Neuropsychiatry Clin Neurosci 1990; 2:331–336.

42. Tupper DE, ed. Soft Neurological Signs. New York: Grune & Stratton, 1987.

43. Shaffer D, Schonfeld I, O'Connor PA, Stokman C, Frautman P, Shofer S, Ng S. Neurological soft signs: their relationship to psychiatric disorder and intelligence in childhood and adolescence. Arch Gen Psychiatry 1985; 42:342–351.

44. Mikkelson EJ, Brown GL, Minichiello MD, et al. Neurologic status in hyperactive, enuretic, encopretic and normal boys. J Am Acad Psychiatry 1982; 21:75–81.

45. Nichols PL. Minimal brain dysfunction and soft signs: the collaborative perinatal project. In: Tupper DE, ed. Soft Neurological Signs. New York: Grune & Stratton, 1987:179–199.

46. Quitkin F, Rifkin A, Klein DF. Neurological soft signs in schizophrenia and character disorders. Arch Gen Psychiatry 1976; 33:845–853.

47. Hollander E, Schiffman E, Cohen B, Rivera-Stein M, Rosen W, Gorman JM, Fyer A, Papp L, Liebowitz MR. Signs of central nervous system dysfunction in obsessive-compulsive disorder. Arch Gen Psychiatry 1990; 47:27–32.
48. Hollander E, Cohen L, DeCaria C. Neuropsychiatric studies of OCD. Proceedings of the First Annual International Obsessive-Compulsive Disorder Conference, Capri, Italy, 1993.
49. Aronowitz B, Hollander E, Mannuzza S, Davis J, Chapman T, Fyer AJ. Soft signs and familial transmission of obsessive-compulsive disorder. Poster presented at the 145th annual meeting of American Psychiatric Association, Washington, DC, May 2–7, 1992.
50. Hollander E, DeCaria CM, Saoud JB, Klein DF, Liebowitz MR. Neurological soft signs in obsessive compulsive disorder. Arch Gen Psychiatry 1991; 48:278–279.
51. Hollander E, DeCaria C, Aronowitz B, Klein DF, Liebowitz MR, Shaffer D. A pilot follow-up study of childhood soft signs and the development of adult psychopathology. Clin Res Reports 1991; 3(2):186–189.
52. Jenike MA, Brotman AW. The EEG in obsessive-compulsive disorder. J Clin Psychiatry 1984; 45:122–124.
53. Bingley T, Persson A. EEG studies on patients with chronic obsessive-compulsive neurosis before and after psychosurgery (stereotaxic bilateral anterior capsulotomy). Electroencephalogr Clin Neurophysiol 1978; 44:691–696.
54. Flor-Henry P, Yeudall LT, Koles ZJ, Howarth BG. Neuropsychological and power spectral EEG investigations of the obsessive-compulsive syndrome. Biol Psychiatry 1979; 14:119–130.
55. Insel TR, Gillen JC, Moore A, Mendelson WB, Loewenstein RJ, Murphy DL. Sleep in obsessive-compulsive disorder. Arch Gen Psychiatry 1982; 39:1372–1377.
56. Towey J, Bruder G, Hollander E, et al. Endogenous event-related potentials and selective attention in obsessive-compulsive disorder. Biol Psychiatry 1990; 28:92–98.
57. Shagass C, Roemer RA, Straumanis JJ, Josiassen RC. Distinctive somatosensory evoked potential features in obsessive compulsive disorder. Biol Psychiatry 1984; 19:1507–1524.
58. Rapoport J, Elkins R, Langer D, et al. Childhood obsessive-compulsive disorder. Am J Psychiatry 1981; 138:1545–1554.
59. Shagass C, Roemer RA, Straumanis JJ, Josiassen RC. Evoked potentials in obsessive-compulsive disorder. Adv Biol Psychiatry 1984; 15:69–75.
60. Ciesielski H, Beech HR, Gordon PK. Some electrophysiological observations in obsessional states. Br J Psychiatry 1981; 138:479–484.
61. Beech HR, Ciesielski KT, Gordon PK. Further observations of evoked potentials in obsessional patients. Br J Psychiatry 1983; 142:605–609.
62. Khanna S, Mukundan CR, Channabasavanna SM. Middle latency evoked potentials in obsessive compulsive disorder. Biol Psychiatry 1989; 25:980–983.

63. Diamond BM, Albrecht W, Borison RL. Neuropsychology of obsessive compulsive disorders. Forty-Third Annual Convention and Scientific Program, Society of Biological Psychiatry, Montreal, Canada, May 4–8, 1988.

64. Harvey NS. Impaired cognitive set switching in obsessive compulsive neurosis. IRCS Med Sci 1986; 14:936–937.

65. Head EK, Bolton D, Hymas N. Deficit in cognitive shifting ability in patients with obsessive compulsive disorders. Biol Psychiatry 1989; 25:929–937.

66. Zielinski CM, Taylor MA, Juzwin KR. Neuropsychological deficits in obsessive-compulsive disorder. Neuropsychiatry, Neuropsychol Behav Neurol 1991; 4:110–126.

67. Christensen KF, Kim SW, Dysken MW, Hoover KM. Neuropsychological performance in obsessive-compulsive disorder. Biol Psychiatry 1992; 31:4–18.

68. Aronowitz B, Hollander E, DeCaria C, et al. Neuropsychology of obsessive-compulsive disorder: preliminary findings. Neuropsychiatry, Neuropsychol Behav Neurol 1994; 7:81–86.

69. Boone KB, Ananth J, Philpott L, Kaur A, Djenderedjian AL. Neuropsychological characteristics of nondepressed adults with obsessive-compulsive disorder. Neuropsychiatry, Neuropsychol Behav Neurol 1991; 4:96–109.

70. Rachman S, Hodgson R. Obsessions and Compulsions. Englewood Cliffs, NJ: Prentice-Hall, 1980.

71. Hollander E, Liebowitz MR, Rosen WG. Neuropsychiatric and neuropsychological studies in obsessive-compulsive disorder. In: Zohar J, Insel T, eds. The Psychobiology of Obsessive-Compulsive Disorder. New York: Springer-Verlag, 1991:126–145.

72. Pirozzolo F, Hansch E, Mortimer J, Webster D, Kukowski M. Dementia in Parkinson's disease: a neurological analysis. Brain Cogn 1982; 1:71–83.

73. Boler F, Passafiume D, Keefe NC, Rogers K, Morrow L, Kim Y. Visuospatial impairment in Parkinson's disease: role of perceptual and motor factors. Arch Neurol 1984; 41:485–490.

74. Wexler BE, Yazgan Y, Barr LC, Goodman WK. Abnormalities of cerebral laterality in OCD. Annual Meeting of the American Psychiatric Association, Philadelphia, May 21–16, 1994.

75. Wexler BE, Goodman WK. Cerebral laterality, perception of emotion, and treatment response in obsessive-compulsive disorder. Biol Psychiatry 1991; 29:900–908.

76. The Clomipramine Collaborative Study Group. Clomipramine in the treatment of patients with obsessive-compulsive disorder. Arch Gen Psychiatry 1991; 48:730–738.

77. Perse TL, Griest JH, Jefferson JW, Rosenfeld R, Dar R. Fluvoxamine treatment of obsessive-compulsive disorder. Am J Psychiatry 1987; 12:1543–1548.

78. Turner SM, Jacob RG, Geidel DC, Himmelhoch J. Fluoxetine treatment of obsessive-compulsive disorder. J Clin Psychopharmacology 1985; 5(4):207–212.

79. Hollander E, DeCaria CM, Nitescu A, et al. Serotonergic function in obses-

sive-compulsive disorder: behavioral and neuroendocrine responses to oral m-chlorylpiperazine and fenfluramine in patients and healthy volunteers. Arch Gen Psychiatry 1992; 49:21–28.

80. Thoren R, Asberg M, Bertilsson L, Mellstrom B, Syoquist F, Trachman L. Clomipramine treatment of obsessive-compulsive disorder. II. Biochemical aspects. Arch Gen Psychiatry 1980; 37:1289–1294.

81. Azmitia, EC. The CNS serotonergic system: Progression toward a collaborative organization. In: Meltzer H, ed. Psychopharmacology: The Third Generation of Progress. New York: Raven Press, 1987:61–73.

82. Stein DJ, Hollander E, Cohen L. Neuropsychiatry of obsessive compulsive disorder. In: Hollander E, Zohar J, Marazzati D, Olivier B, eds. Current Concepts in Obsessive Compulsive Disorder. New York: Wiley, 1994:167–182.

5

The Neurochemistry of OCD

Dan J. Stein
University of Stellenbosch
Tygerberg, South Africa

Daphne Simeon and Eric Hollander
The Mount Sinai School of Medicine
New York, New York

INTRODUCTION

The first indication that obsessive-compulsive disorder (OCD) was mediated by a specific neurochemical system was the discovery that clomipramine, a predominantly serotonergic tricyclic antidepressant, was useful in its treatment (1). Subsequent research using pharmacotherapeutic dissection, neurochemical assays, and pharmacological challenges has confirmed that serotonin plays an important role in OCD. However, significant challenges remain in understanding the neurochemistry of OCD—not only in elucidating the specific mechanisms of serotonergic mediation of OCD, but also in determining the role of other neurchemical systems in the disorder. In this chapter we review current research in this area.

THERAPEUTIC DISSECTION

A number of studies have found that serotonin reuptake inhibitors (SRIs) are significantly more effective than noradrenergic reuptake inhibitors in the treatment of OCD (2–4). Indeed, each of the serotonin-specific reuptake inhibitors so far studied in OCD has proven to be an effective treatment (4–7). The selective efficacy of the SRIs in OCD, as well as the relatively long time and high doses that are sometimes necessary for a response, differentiates the disorder from other mood and anxiety disorders, and supports a serotonin hypothesis for OCD.

Nevertheless, several qualifying statements need to be made. First, the mechanism by which the SRIs produce therepeutic efficacy remains unresolved by therapeutic dissection studies. This may be via the action of serotonin on other systems. Second, only 50–60% of patients may respond to the SRIs, and even these patients may not have complete resolution of symptoms (4–7). Patients who do not respond to the SRIs presumably have different neurochemical dysfunctions. Third, medications other than SRIs are sometimes effective in the treatment of OCD. These include a range of antidepressants and anxiolytics (8–10). Fourth, meta-analytical studies show a tendency for the less selective SRIs to be correspondengly more effective than more selective agents in OCD, suggesting that action at sites other than serotonin receptors may also be important (11,12).

McDougle and colleagues (13; Chapter 9, this volume) have found that dopamine blockers are particularly useful in the augmentation of SRIs in OCD patients who have comorbid tics. This finding is consistent with evidence of dopamine dysfunction in tic disorders, and suggests that dopamine may also play an important role in at least a subgroup of OCD patients. Indeed, preclinical research indicates that administration of dopamine agonists produces repetitive behaviors, and clinical research shows a strong association between OCD and tic disorders such as Tourette's syndrome (14).

NEUROCHEMICAL ASSAYS

An early study of clomipramine in adults with OCD indicated that responders had higher levels of the serotonin metabolite 5-hydroxyindole-acetic acid (5-HIAA) in cerebrospinal fluid, and that there was a significant correlation between a decrease in CSF 5-HIAA during treatment and symptomatic improvement (15). Similarly, in children and adolescents with OCD, responders to clomipramine had higher pretreatment platelet serotonin (5-HT) levels and greater decreases in platelet 5-HT concentrations during treatment (16). Indeed, CSF 5-HIAA may be higher in a subgroup of patients with OCD than in normal controls (17). This finding is particularly interesting in light of the well-known association between serotonin hypofunction, as reflected in decreased CSF 5-HIAA, and increased impulsive-aggression (18). Taken together, this work may lead to the postulation that increased serotonergic activity characterizes compulsivity, while serotonin hypofunction reflects impulsivity.

Nevertheless, CSF and platelet findings have not provided unequivocal support for such a hypothesis. Recent CSF studies of adults (19) and children and adolescents (20) with OCD have failed to replicate, or have only partially replicated, earlier work. Interestingly, Leckman and colleagues (21) noted that two patients with violent obsessions had decreased levels of CSF 5-HIAA. Not only is there often a phenomenological overlap in OCD and impulsive-aggressive symptomatology, but the underlying serotonergic bases of these behaviors are likely to be complex and intersecting (22,23).

CSF studies have, moreover, also been used to assess neurochemical systems other than neurotransmitters in OCD. A number of authors have suggested that neuropeptides such as vasopressin or oxytocin may be involved in OCD (19,24). In preclinical paradigms, intracerebroventricular injection of these neuropeptides induces grooming. They also appear to affect cognitive functions (attention and memory) that may be important in OCD (19,24). Despite the equivocal response of OCD to systemic oxytocin, it is possible, then, that brain arginine, vasopressin, oxytocin, or other stress-responsive neuropeptides may have a role in mediating OCD symptoms.

Nevertheless, findings have again been partly inconsistent. Vasopressin arginine concentration was significantly and negatively correlated with obsessive-compulsive symptoms in children and adolescents with OCD (20), and somatostatin was raised in this group compared to conduct-disorder controls (25). During treatment, there was a fall in AVP and corticotropin-releasing factor, and a rise in oxytocin (26). In adults with OCD, however, there was a positive correlation between AVP and OCD severity (19), as well as raised corticotropin-releasing factor (19) and somatostatin (27) compared to controls. Another group did not find elevated AVP in adults with OCD, but did find raised oxytocin levels in patients without a personal or family history of tics (24). Further studies are clearly warranted to investigate a possible role for various neuropeptides in OCD and to determine whether distinct findings are present in discrete OCD subtypes.

PHARMACOLOGICAL CHALLENGES

CSF and platelet studies often provide only a static picture of neurotransmitter function, and they entail a variety of methodological problems. Dynamic studies using specific pharmacological challenges have increasingly been used to provide an additional window on neurotransmitter dysfunction in OCD.

Perhaps the most interesting work has been that undertaken with m-chlorophenylpiperazine (m-CPP), a serotonin agonist. A number of studies have found that m-CPP administration is followed rapidly by an increase in obsessive-compulsive symptoms, and that there is greater blunting of cortisol (28) or prolactin (29) after m-CPP in OCD than in healthy controls.

One hypothesis is that m-CPP, which is also a 5-HT-2 receptor antagonist, exacerbates an underlying serotonin hypofunction, thus increasing symptoms. However, administration of metergoline, a 5-HT-2 antagonist, to OCD patients does not increase symptoms. An alternative hypothesis states that in OCD certain parts of the brain are characterized by serotonin hyperresponsivity (so agonist properties of m-CPP result in behavioral exacerbation), while other brain areas are characterized by serotonin hyporesponsivity (resulting in increased neuroendocrine blunting).

In the experience of Hollander and colleagues (29), only about 50–60% of OCD patients seem to experience exacerbation of symptoms after m-CPP administration—about the same percentage as respond to SRIs. It is notable that after treatment with SRIs, m-CPP no longer results in symptom exacerbation and neuroendocrine function is normalized (30,31). Increased neuroendocrine blunting predicts worse treatment response, suggesting, perhaps, that it is those patients who have greater functional reserve in the serotonin system that respond to SRIs (32).

A number of qualifications again need to be made. m-CPP does not act exclusively on the serotonin system but binds to a variety of receptors. Furthermore, one study found that m-CPP given intravenously resulted in symptom exacerbation, but not m-CPP given orally (33). Another study found no symptom exacerbation after intravenous m-CPP, and neuroendocrine blunting only in females (34). Administration of the serotonin agonist MK-212 resulted in a relatively blunted neuroendocrine response in OCD patients but did not increase OCD symptoms (35). m-CPP differs from MK-212 in that it also has 5-HT-1D agonist effects, which may account for these behaviorial differences. Clearly, further research on serotonin agonists, with better control for methodological differences between previous studies, needs to be undertaken.

Other serotonergic agents have been used in pharmacological challenge research. Research on fenfluramine, a serotonin releaser and reuptake blocker, has resulted in mixed findings, with neuroendocrine blunting in some studies but not in others (29). The 5-HT-1A agonists buspirone and ipsapirone did not differentially affect prolactin response in OCD patients and controls (36,37). Furthermore, after long-term treatment with fluoxetine, although there was blunting of neuroendocrine responses to buspirone, this did not correlate with decrease in symptoms (38). The serotonin precursor tryptophan did not lead to neuroendocrine blunting prior to treatment, and may even have been associated with enhanced responses (34,39). Tryptophan depletion during SRI treatment resulted in increased depressive symptoms but not in increased OCD symptoms (40). However, administration during SRI treatment of metergoline (41), a 5-HT-1/5-HT-2 antagonist, or of ritanserin (42), a 5-HT-2A/2C antagonist, resulted in OCD exacerbation. Similarly, treatment of schizophrenia with clozapine, a neuroleptic with 5-HT-2 antagonism, may result in increased OCD symptoms (43).

In general, then, there may be a shift from pretreatment exacerbation of OCD by serotonin agonists to posttreatment exacerbation of OCD by serotonin antagonists. Perhaps there is a compensatory increase in postsynaptic serotonin function prior to treatment, with equilibration of serotonin function by SRIs. The range of different results are not, however, neatly explicable by any one hypothesis. The complexity of the serotonin system makes necessary further research with more specific ligands to attempt to elucidate the role of different receptor subtypes in OCD.

What about neurochemical systems other than serotonin in OCD? It is notable that a range of agents such as lactate (44) and yohimbine (45) do not exacerbate OCD—differentiating OCD symptoms from anxiety and panic symptoms. Similarly, studies of the hypothalamic-pituitary-adrenal (HPA) axis in OCD have been inconsistent, perhaps differentiating OCD from depression (46). Nevertheless, pharmacological challenge studies do demonstrate some evidence for a role for the noradrenergic, dopaminergic, cholinergic, and opioid systems in OCD.

Intravenous administration of the noradrenergic α_2-agonist clonidine induced a transient reduction in OCD symptoms (47). Nevertheless, neuroendocrine findings in OCD patients after clonidine have been inconsistent (47–49). Growth-hormone response to the acetylcholinesterase inhibitor pyridostigmine was significantly elevated in OCD patients compared with controls (50). Dopamine agonists may increase OCD-like symptoms, but have not done so when administered as a pharmacological challenge (51–56). The opioid antagonist naloxone may also increase OCD symptoms in some patients (57). Clearly, then, further research on the relationship between serotonin and these other systems in OCD is required.

DISCUSSION

A crucial question concerns the relationship between neurochemical function and what is known about the neuroanatomical underpinnings of OCD. As discussed in Chapter 4 of this volume, dysfunction in prefrontal–basal ganglia–thalamic circuits has received much attention in OCD research. Indeed, there is evidence that serotonergic fibers project to the head of the caudate and to prefrontal circuits (58). We administered m-CPP to patients and then did regional cerebral blood flow (rCBF) analyses (59). In those patients in whom there was an exacerbation of OCD symptoms, there was a significant increase in cortical perfusion.

This finding once again raises the question of the relationship between compulsivity and impulsivity. Certainly increased impulsivity is often seen in association with frontal dysfunction, suggesting that compulsivity is characterized by hyperfrontality and impulsivity by hypofrontality. On the other hand, increased frontal activity in OCD may be a compensatory phenomenon—an attempt to decrease dysfunctional output from the basal ganglia. This increased activity may include upregulation of serotonin function. After successful pharmacotherapy, there might be both equilibration of serotonin function and normalization of frontal activity.

An appropriately complex analysis of neurochemical dysfunction in OCD must take into account interactions between serotonin and other brain systems. We found that, compared to controls, OCD patients showed blunted pHVA responses to fenfluramine administration. This finding is consistent with dysregulation of serotonin–dopamine interactions in OCD (60). As suggested earlier, however, a good deal of further research, perhaps using multiple pharmacological challenges, is necessary to further investigate the interactions of neurochemical systems in OCD.

While we have learned a good deal about the neurochemistry of OCD in the last decade or so, much more work remains to be done to understand this complex disorder. While neurochemical assays have methodological limitations, additional work, particularly on postmortem specimens, will prove helpful in determining variation in serotonergic function in different parts of the brain in OCD. Additional studies using more specific pharmacological challenges, and combining pharmacological challenges with functional neuroimaging, will also further advance our understanding of OCD.

REFERENCES

1. Fernandez-Cordoba E, Lopez-Ibor Alino J. La monoclorimipramina en enfermos psiquiatricos resistentes a otros tratamientos. Acta Luso-Esp Neurol Psiquiatr Ciene Afines 1967; 26:119–147.
2. Thoren P, Asberg M, Cronholm B, et al. Clomipramine treatment of obsessive compulsive disorder. I. A controlled clinical trial. Arch Gen Psychiatry 1980; 37:1281–1285.
3. Zohar J, Insel TR. Obsessive-compulsive disorder: psychobiological approaches to diagnosis, treatment, and pathophysiology. Biol Psychiatry 1987; 22:667–687.
4. Goodman WK, Price LH, Delgado PL, et al. Specificity of serotonin reuptake inhibitors in the treatment of obsessive-compulsive disorder: comparison of fluvoxamine and desipramine. Arch Gen Psychiatry 1990; 47:577–585.
5. Tollefson GD, Rampey AH, Potvin JH, et al. A multicenter investigation of fixed-dose fluoxetine in the treatment of obsessive-compulsive disorder. Arch Gen Psychiatry 1994; 51:559–567.
6. Montgomery SA, McIntyre A, Osterheider M, et al. A double-blind, placebo-controlled study of fluoxetine in patients with DSM-III-R obsessive-compulsive disorder. Eur Neuropsychopharmacol 1993; 3:143–152.
7. Chouinard G, Goodman W, Greist J, et al. Results of a double-blind placebo controlled trial of a new serotonin reuptake inhibitor, sertraline, in the treatment of obsessive-compulsive disorder. Psychopharmacol Bull 1990; 26:279–284.
8. Fogelson DL, Bystritsky A. Imipramine in the treatment of obsessive-compulsive disorder with and without major depression. Ann Clin Psychiatry 1991; 3:233–237.
9. Hewlett WA, Vinogradov S, Agras WS. Clomipramine, clonazepam, and clonidine treatment of obsessive-compulsive disorder. J Clin Psychopharmacol 1992; 12:420–430.
10. Vallejo J, Olivares J, Marcos T, et al. Clomipramine versus phenelzine in obsessive-compulsive disorder: a controlled clinical trial. Br J Psychiatry 1992; 161:665–670.
11. Jenike MA, Hyman S, Baer L, et al. A controlled trial of fluvoxamine in obsessive-compulsive disorder: Implications for a serotonergic theory. Am J Psychiatry 1990; 147:1209–1215.
12. Stein DJ, Spadaccini E, Hollander E. Meta-analysis of pharmacotherapy trials for obsessive compulsive disorder. Int Clin Psychopharm 1995; 10:11–18.
13. McDougle CJ, Goodman WK, Leckman JF, et al. Haloperidol addition in fluvoxamine-refractory obsessive-compulsive disorder: a double-blind pla-

cebo-controlled study in patients with and without tics. Arch Gen Psychiatry 1994; 51:302–308.

14. Goodman WK, McDougle CJ, Price LH, et al. Beyond the serotonin hypothesis: a role for dopamine in some forms of obsessive compulsive disorder? J Clin Psychiatry 1990; S51:36–43.

15. Thoren P, Asberg M, Bertilsson L, et al. Clomipramine treatment of obsessive-compulsive disorder. II. Biochemical aspects. Arch Gen Psychiatry 1980; 37:1289–1294.

16. Flament MF, Rapoport JL, Murphy DL, et al. Biochemical changes during clomipramine treatment of childhood obsessive-compulsive disorder. Arch Gen Psychiatry 1987; 44:219–225.

17. Insel TR, Mueller EA, Alterman I, et al. Obsessive-compulsive disorder and serotonin: is there a connection? Biol Psychiatry 1985; 20:1174–1188.

18. Stein DJ, Hollander E, Liebowitz MR. Neurobiology of impulsivity and impulse control disorders. J Neuropsych Clin Neurosci 1993; 5:9–17.

19. Altemus M, Pigott T, Kalogeras K, et al. Abnormalities in the regulation of vasopressin and corticotrophin releasing factor secretion in obsessive-compulsive disorder. Arch Gen Psychiatry 1992; 49:9–20.

20. Swedo SE, Leonard HL, Kruesi MJP, et al. Cerebrospinal fluid neurochemistry in children and adolescents with obsessive-compulsive disorder. Arch Gen Psychiatry 1992; 49:29–36.

21. Leckman JF, Goodman WK, Riddle MA, et al. Low CSF 5HIAA and obsessions of violence: Report of two cases. Psychiatry Res 1990; 33:95–99.

22. Stein DJ, Hollander E, Simeon D, et al. Impulsivity scores in patients with obsessive-compulsive disorder. J Nerv Ment Dis 1994; 182:239–240.

23. Stein DJ, Hollander E. Impulsive aggression and obsessive-compulsive disorder. Psychiatric Ann 1993; 23:389–395.

24. Leckman JF, Goodman WK, North WG, et al. The role of central oxytocin in obsessive compulsive disorder and related normal behavior. Psychoneuroendocrinology 1994; 19:723–749.

25. Kruesi MJP, Swedo S, Leonard H, et al. CSF somatostatin in childhood psychiatric disorders: A preliminary investigation. Psychiatry Res 1990; 33:277–284.

26. Altemus M, Swedo SE, Leonard HL, et al. Changes in cerebrospinal fluid neurochemistry during treatment of obsessive-compulsive disorder with clomipramine. Arch Gen Psychiatry 1994; 51:794–803.

27. Altemus M, Pigott T, L'Heureux F, et al. CSF somatostatin in obsessive-compulsive disorder. Am J Psychiatry 1993; 150:460–464.

28. Zohar J, Mueller EA, Insel TR, et al. Serotonergic responsivity in obsessive-compulsive disorder: comparison of patients and healthy controls. Arch Gen Psychiatry 1987; 44:946–951.

29. Hollander E, DeCaria C, Nitescu A, et al. Serotonergic function in obsessive compulsive disorder: behavioral and neuroendocrine responses to oral m-CPP and fenfluramine in patients and healthy volunteers. Arch Gen Psychiatry 1992; 49:21–28.

30. Zohar J, Insel TR, Zohar-Kadouch RC, et al. Serotonergic responsivity in obsessive-compulsive disorder: effects of chronic clomipramine treatment. Arch Gen Psychiatry 1988; 45:167–172.
31. Hollander E, DeCaria C, Gully R, et al. Effects of chronic fluoxetine treatment on behavioral and neuroendocrine responses to meta-chlorophenylpiperazine in obsessive-compulsive disorder. Psychiatry Res 1991; 36:1–17.
32. Hollander E, Stein DJ, DeCaria CM, et al. A pilot study of biological predictors of treatment outcome in obsessive-compulsive disorder. Biol Psychiatry 1993; 33:747–749.
33. Pigott TA, Hill JL, Grady TA, et al. A comparison of the behavioral effects of oral versus intravenous mCPP administration in OCD patients and the effect of metergoline prior to iv mcpp. Biol Psychiatry 1992; 33:3–14.
34. Charney DS, Goodman WK, Price LH, et al. Serotonin function in obsessive-compulsive disorder. Arch Gen Psychiatry 1988; 45:177–185.
35. Bastani B, Nash JF, Meltzer HY. Prolactin and cortisol responses to MK-212, a serotonin agonist, in obsessive-compulsive disorder. Arch Gen Psychiatry 1990; 47:833–839.
36. Lucey JV, Butcher G, Clare AW, et al. Buspirone-induced prolactin responses in obsessive-compulsive disorder (OCD): is OCD a 5HT2 receptor disorder. Int Clin Psychopharmacol 1992; 7:45–49.
37. Lesch KP, Hoh A, Disselkamp-Tietze J, et al. 5-hydroxytryptamine1A receptor responsivity in obsessive compulsive disorder: comparison of patients and controls. Arch Gen Psychiatry 1991; 48:540–547.
38. Lesch KP, Hoh A, Schulte HM, et al. Long-term fluoxetine treatment decreases 5-HT1a receptor responsivity in obsessive compulsive disorder. Psychopharmacology 1991; 105:415–420.
39. Fineberg NA, Cowen PJ, Kirk JW, et al. Neuroendocrine responses to intravenous L-tryptophan in obsessive compulsive disorder. J Affect Disord 1994; 32:97–104.
40. Barr LC, Goodman WK, McDougle CJ, et al. Tryptophan depletion in patients with obsessive-compulsive disorder who respond to SRIs. Arch Gen Psychiatry 1994; 51:309–317.
41. Benkelfat C, Murphy DL, Zohar J, et al. Clomipramine in obsessive-compulsive disorder: further evidence for a serotonergic mechanism of action. Arch Gen Psychiatry 1989; 46:23–28.
42. Ergovesi S, Ronchi P, Smeraldi E. 5-HT2 receptor and fluvoxamine effect in obsessive compulsive disorder. Hum Psychopharmacol Clin Exp 1992; 7:287–289.
43. Hwang MY, Stein DJ, Simeon D, Hollander E. Clozapine, obsessive symptoms, and serotonergic mechanisms. Am J Psychiatry 1993; 150:1435.
44. Gorman JM, Liebowitz MR, Fyer AJ, et al. Lactate infusions in obsessive-compulsive disorder. Am J Psychiatry 1985; 142:864–866.
45. Rasmussen SA, Goodman WK, Woods SW, et al. Effects of yohimbine in obsessive-compulsive disorder. Psychopharmacology 1987; 93:308–313.
46. Bailly D, Servant D, Dewailly D, et al. Corticotropin releasing factor stimu-

lation test in obsessive compulsive disorder. Biol Psychiatry 1994; 35:143–146.

47. Hollander E, DeCaria C, Nitescu A, et al. Noradrenergic function in obsessive-compulsive disorder: behavioral and neuroendocrine responses to clonidine and comparison to healthy controls. Psychiatry Res 1991; 37:161–177.

48. Siever LJ, Insel TR, Jimerson DC, et al. Growth hormone response to clonidine in obsessive-compulsive patients. Br J Psychiatry 1983; 142:184–187.

49. Lee MA, Cameron OG, Gurguis GNM, et al. Alpha-2 adrenoceptor status in obsessive-compulsive disorder. Biol Psychiatry 1990; 27:1083–1093.

50. Lucey JV, Clare AW, Dinan TG. Elevated growth hormone responses to pyridostigmine in obsessive-compulsive disorder: evidence of cholinergic supersensitivity. Am J Psychiatry 1993; 150:961–962.

51. Frye PE, Arnold LE. Persistent amphetamine-induced compulsive rituals: response to pyridoxine (B6). Biol Psychiatry 1981; 16:583–587.

52. Insel TR, Hamilton J, Guttmacher L, et al. d-Amphetamine in obsessive compulsive disorder. Psychopharmacology 1983; 80:231–235.

53. Koizumi H. Obsessive compulsive symptoms following stimulants. Biol Psychiatry 1985; 20:1332–1337.

54. Borcherding BG, Keysor CS, Rapoport JL, et al. Motor/vocal tics and compulsive behaviors on stimulant drugs: is there a common vulnerability? Psychiatry Res 1990; 33:83–94.

55. Joffe RT, Swinson RP, Levitt AJ. Acute psychostimulant challenge in primary obsessive-compulsive disorder. J Clin Psychopharmacol 1991; 11:237–241.

56. Rosse RB, Fay-McCarthy M, Collins JP, et al. Transient compulsive foraging behavior associated with crack cocaine use. Am J Psychiatry 1993; 150:155–156.

57. Insel TR, Pickar D. Naloxone administration in obsessive-compulsive disorder: report of two cases. Am J Psychiatry 1983; 140:1219–1220.

58. Parent A. Serotonergic innervation of the basal ganglia. J Comp Neurol 1990; 299:1–16.

59. Hollander E, Prohovnik I, Stein DJ. Obsessions and cerebral blood flow during pharmacological challenge with m-CPP. J Neuropsychiatry Clin Neurosci 1995; 7:485–490.

60. Hollander E, Stein DJ, Saoud JB, et al. Effects of fenfluramine on plasma pHVA in OCD. Psychiatry Res 1992; 42:185–188.

6

Veterinary Models of OCD

N. H. Dodman, A. Moon-Fanelli, and P. A. Mertens
Tufts University School of Veterinary Medicine
North Grafton, Massachusetts

S. Pflueger
Tufts University School of Medicine
Boston and Baystate Medical Center
Springfield, Massachusetts

Dan J. Stein
University of Stellenbosch
Tygerberg, South Africa

Until 1991, when Goldberger and Rapoport (1) reported that dogs with acral lick dermatitis responded to treatment with the antiobsessional agent clomipramine, there was no evidence to support a spontaneously occurring animal model of obsessive-compulsive disorder (OCD). Indeed, the term (obsessive) compulsive behavior was virtually unheard of in veterinary medicine. Now, a few years later, acral lick dermatitis is being considered a possible model for human OCD, and the term "compulsive behavior" has been introduced into veterinary medicine to cover a multitude of repetitive behaviors and behavioral syndromes previously referred to as displacement behaviors or stereotypies (2). What is the difference, then, between a compulsive behavior and a stereotypy? The term stereotypy is normally reserved for simple movement disorders such as tremors, tics, and perseverations (3,4). Compulsive behaviors, however, are more complicated and are often preceded by a recurring thought that drives the behavior. As more complicated forms of stereo-typy, such as stereotyped operant behavior, are appreciated in animals and the concept of OCD in humans broadens to include other repetitive behaviors such as trichotillomania, the distinction between the two types of behavior becomes even less evident (5,6). In addition, tic disorders and some forms of OCD are comorbid, implying that there may be underlying mechanisms in common (7,8).

Recently, evidence has emerged that OCD and stereotypies may originate in similar brain regions and involve similar neurotransmitters, with serotonin and dopamine featuring prominently in both conditions (6,9,10). The basal ganglia are probably one of the primary repositories for innate behaviors that underlie displacement behaviors, stereotypy, and OCD (9,11,12). Certain of these innate behavioral patterns may be expressed as a consequence of anxiety resulting from stress (frustration or conflict) and be performed repetitively and inappropriately (13,14). The type of repetitive behavior that is liberated seems to be a function of the species, breed, age, sex, and the level of arousal. From a neuroethological perspective, it should be possible to predict the likely expression of compulsive behaviors in various species of domestic animals. Each behavior may involve slightly different neural circuitry and thus may respond differently to pharmacological treatment.

Figure 1 is a schematic showing putative interactions of the various neurotransmitters in the propagation of compulsive behavior. Stress is known to release ACTH and β-endorphin, and endorphin release is thought to propagate repetitive behaviors via a dopaminergic mechanism (15–18). In addition, stress has been shown to release norepinephrine, which in turn activates serotonin (19,20). Serotonin has an inhibitory influence on dopaminergic pathways and should reduce repetitive behaviors (21). Serotonin reuptake inhibitors are the most widely efficacious group of compounds used to treat animals affected with various compulsive behaviors (22–25).

The following discussion focuses on veterinary models of OCD, including dogs, cats, birds, horses, and farm and zoo animals that exhibit repetitive (compulsive) behaviors. The models that have been studied most extensively are described in detail; others will be alluded to or tabulated. The classification of behaviors referred to is along neuroethological lines. Each species has particular sets of fixed action patterns that have evolved to ensure optimal survival of that species. It appears that the various species-typical compulsive behaviors arise from these hard-wired adaptive behaviors and originate when genetic and environmental circumstances favor their expression. Genetic factors may include not only the propensity for species-typical behavior but also the susceptibility for a compulsive behavioral response to chronic or acute stress.

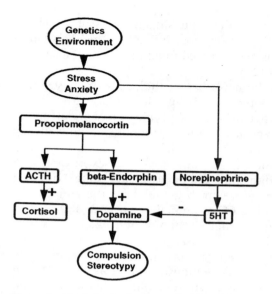

Figure 1   Hypothetical schematic illustrating the interaction of key neurotransmitters in compulsive behavior.

NEUROETHOLOGICAL VIEW OF COMPULSIVE BEHAVIOR IN ANIMALS

Because of the parallels between OCD and animal stereotypies, a number of authors have proposed neuroethological models to explain the origin of OCD in humans (1,10,13). A key component of this hypothesis is that certain behavioral "subroutines" related to grooming and other behaviors necessary for survival have been programmed into the human brain by natural selection. Rapoport suggests that compulsive activity results from the malfunction of higher brain centers so that patterns of adaptive behavior are replayed repeatedly. A neuroethological approach lends credence to the validity of pursuing animal models to facilitate analysis of this condition (26).

The hypothesis that OCD manifests as a disturbance of genetically encoded behaviors necessary for survival stems from classic ethological theories of fixed action patterns. Early ethologists recognized that adaptive behavior could be subdivided into distinct motor patterns, called fixed action patterns, that were expressed in a coordinated fashion (27–29). These fixed action patterns were defined as innate and adaptive behavioral sequences consisting of "stereotyped" movements that are very similar in all members of a species. The fundamental "form constant movements" do not have to be learned by the animal, and provide, like morphological characteristics, distinguishing features of a species. The genetic basis for these behaviors is substantiated by the observation that such fixed action patterns are observed in all members of a species, even those raised in isolation (29).

While all behavior has a heritable basis, ethologists emphasize that for some behaviors only the potentiality is inherited. Many animals are preprogrammed to learn particular species-specific behaviors at preordained times in their lives. Exposure to the appropriate stimulus during this critical period will result in the expression of the normal species-typical behavior. Thus, variation in the developmental expression of a fixed action pattern occurs, with some innate behaviors being expressed in full form at birth and others developing gradually as the animal matures. Furthermore, the response of an animal to eliciting stimuli (releasers) may vary depending on internal stimuli and external events. Depending on the animal's level of arousal, the expression of a fixed action pattern may range from mere intention movements to completely executed actions. Ethological studies demonstrate that aspects of fixed action patterns may be modified by environmental events to fine-tune the animal's behavior. Learning thus may provide the final motor components that are most adaptive to an individual's environment. For this reason, even though behaviors associated with survival have long been considered innate, or "hard-wired," variability in expression occurs.

Fixed action patterns usually proceed without any indication of insight into the species-preserving function of the activity on the part of the animal. This is supported by the inappropriate repetitive behaviors exhibited by some animals when placed in a chronically stressful environment. Under such circumstances, the observed behavior patterns are not activated from their normal source but are stimulated by the conflicting (stressful) situation in which the animal finds itself. Animals in a conflictive situation, in which two or more "drives" are simultaneously activated, may exhibit behaviors that appear to be irrelevant to any of the tendencies in conflict. These misdirected behaviors are referred to as displacement behaviors. As an example, deer engage in sham feeding when the tendency to remain conflicts with a tendency to flee (30). Continued conflict/stress may, in some instances, result in the repetitive performance of fixed action patterns in inappropriate contexts—so-called stereotypies or compulsive behaviors.

OCD AND STEREOTYPY: ARE THEY SYNONYMOUS?

Abnormal repetitive behaviors typically involve motor patterns associated with predation, feeding, grooming, social behavior, sexual behavior, agonistic behavior, and locomotion. Historically, all such dysfunctional behaviors displayed by animals have been categorized as stereotypies whereas similar patterns exhibited by humans have been referred to as compulsions. Recently, the terms *stereotypy* and *compulsion* have come to be used interchangeably in veterinary medicine. While this broad-spectrum interpretation of ritualistic behavior in animals has heuristic value, it remains to be demonstrated whether OCD in humans and stereotypies in animals are homologous. Careful comparison of compulsive behavior exhibited by humans and stereotypies in animals reveals numerous similarities (Table 1).

Development and Characteristics of Stereotypies

The origin of repetitive locomotor movements displayed by captive animals has been attributed to displacement behaviors that subsequently may evolve into stereotypy (31). The development of stereotypic behavior is usually ascribed to exposure to suboptimal environmental conditions in which animals are faced with unresolvable conflicts (31,32). Environments are particularly stressful if the stressor is unpredictable or uncontrollable, or inhibits the expression of instinctive behaviors necessary to satisfy normal physiological and psychological needs (33). If situations of conflict/stress continue, the prevailing displacement behaviors may become ingrained. Under these circumstances, when the source of conflict is removed, the behaviors may continue to be performed repetitively and pointlessly without a stimulus. At this point, the threshold is lowered such that the behavior appears to be expressed almost in vacuo. Prolonged conflict is thought to induce central pathophysiological changes that promote the development of stereotypies/compulsive behavior (34). It is almost as if the neural circuitry becomes "well-worn." It has also been suggested that such behaviors may have an inhibitory effect on sympathetic nervous activity (35). A number of studies have associated the performance of stereotypies with reducing distress, anxiety, or aggression (36,37). By way of comparison, humans with OCD frequently report that engaging in their compulsions relieves the anxiety associated with their obsessions.

Stereotypic behavior historically has not been considered a heritable disorder but rather a motoric pattern that has become established in response to a suboptimal environment or conflict-producing experience (31). There are several problems with this simplistic view: 1) if stereotypies are nothing more than a by-product of exposure to suboptimal environments, that would not account for the species-specificity of the motor patterns elicited; 2) it does not explain the observed individual

Table 1   Comparison of Compulsive Behavior in Humans and Stereotypies in Animals

Characteristics/ pharmacological response	Human OCD	Animal stereotypy
Genetic/familial	Evidence for heritable component	Evidence for heritable component
Onset	Childhood/adolescence, but may present at any age	Often young, many start around puberty but may present at any age
Obsessions/ compulsions	Obsession leading to compulsive behavior or obsessions/compulsions alone	Obsessions unknown; compulsive behavior
Phenomenology	Hard-wired survival behaviors performed repetitively	Species/breed-typical behaviors performed repetitively
Magnitude	Time-consuming (more than 1 hr/day); interferes with normal functioning; physical injury	Time-consuming (more than 1 hr/day); interferes with normal functioning; physical injury
Complexity	Complex	Simple or complex
Function of behavior	To relieve mounting tension	Unknown (but physically restraining an animal from performing the ritualized behavior causes anxiety)
Response to SSRI	Many forms respond to this treatment over time	Many forms respond to this treatment over time
Response to opioid blockade	Some OC spectrum conditions respond	Some respond
Response to dopamine blockade	Some OC spectrum conditions respond	Some respond
Associated with brain disorder	Seizures	Some types associated with partial seizures

differences in the tendency to express repetitive behaviors in response to stress; 3) it does not account for the spontaneous onset of stereotypic behavior in seemingly non-stressful environments; and 4) it does not address the familial nature of such abnormal behavior. Whatever the origin, once a stereotypic behavior has become established, it is difficult to extinguish even after the animal is returned to a more suitable environment. It has been our experience that at this stage the stereotypy takes on characteristics that conform closely to DSM-IV criteria for OCD (4).

Relevant Characteristics of OCD

OCD is a complex, chronic, high-frequency psychiatric illness. It manifests itself through obsessions or compulsions that are perceived, at least initially, as ego-dystonic (4). The compulsions are often performed in response to an obsession or according to certain rules. The ritualized aspect of the compulsion is typically stereotyped. Young children and adults may exhibit identical symptoms, which suggests that biological preprogramming may be involved (9,38,39). One diagnostic feature of OCD is the manifestation of recurrent behaviors or thoughts severe enough to interfere significantly with an individual's normal activities. These rituals may sometimes result in physical injury, and impede normal social interactions. Over time, obsessive-compulsive symptoms may wax and wane, and the compulsions may even take on a different form. Affected persons may show a progression of symptoms that correlate with behaviors that might be considered specifically adaptive for their age group. For example, children may exhibit purely ritualized actions, whereas washing is typical of adolescence and ruminations are common in adults (38). In one-third to one-half of all OCD patients, the onset of the condition occurs in early childhood or adolescence (9).

Compulsive behavior in people and repetitive behavior in animals are not necessarily attributable to an identifiable stressor, although in all species, once the behavior is firmly established, stress and other psychological factors may exacerbate the signs (14,31,32,40). In this way, stress/anxiety may function as a nonspecific releaser. In addition, the ontogeny is similar, being sudden or gradual in both. Puberty is a particularly sensitive period for the onset of repetitive behavior in animals as it is in people. When viewed from this perspective, repetitive behavior in animals and compulsive behavior in humans are similar.

Etiology of Stereotypies and OCD

Phylogenetically, stereotypic behavior seems ubiquitous and thus perhaps too general to be considered equivalent to OCD. Nevertheless, not all members of a species exhibit stereotypic behavior when confronted with stress. Why should one animal express ritualized, repetitive behaviors in response to suboptimal conditions whereas another, in a seemingly identical environment, does not? Individual differences in physiological tolerance for stress and the ability to devise appropriate coping mechanisms may predispose certain individuals to develop compulsive responses (32). Such predispositions may be influenced by genetic factors and early experience (41). Animals with anxious or hyperactive temperaments would be expected to have a lower threshold for developing repetitive behaviors.

Early adverse experiences can have long-term effects on an individual's ability to cope with stress (42). For animals sensitized early in life, repetitive behaviors may subsequently be exhibited when there is little or no discernible stress. For example, an association between premature weaning and "wool-sucking" and other aberrant oral behaviors has been suggested in cats (43). Also, forced early weaning in foals can lead to stall-walking as a displacement behavior and this may predispose to anxiety-driven compulsive stall-walking later in life (44).

Not all behaviors that have been classified as stereotypies or obsessive-compulsive are induced by past or present exposure to stressful experiences. Compulsive behaviors resulting from head injuries, complicated birth, or bacterial and viral infections point to a primary biological etiology in some cases (9,26,45,46). Neurological disorders in humans that have been found to occur concurrently with OCD include epilepsy, Sydenham's chorea, postencephalitic Parkinson's disease, and toxic lesions of the basal ganglia (26). A similar association between repetitive behaviors and neurological disorders has been found in some animals (47–49). The comorbidity of OCD and other neurologically based disorders implies that physical as well as psychological factors can release the behaviors that comprise the enumerated obsessive-compulsive spectrum of disorders.

Genetic Factors of Compulsive Behaviors

Data from twin and family studies indicate that some forms of OCD may have a heritable component (8,50,51). Rapoport (9) reported that 20% of OCD probands have a first-degree relative with OCD, and noted that fathers and sons rarely exhibit identical symptoms. This implies that their behaviors have a biological basis and are not learned or modeled. However, whereas the specific motor patterns expressed may be genetically encoded with few degrees of freedom, obsessive-compulsive behavior itself may not be completely hard-wired. In most cases, the phenotypic expression of symptoms is thought to result from an interplay of genetic and environmental influences (50,51).

A number of studies have been conducted to investigate the proposed genetic underpinnings of OCD. In a recent review (50), Rasmussen summarizes the existing data from twin and family studies. The majority of studies, although not all, support the hypothesis that OCD is familial. The greatest risk for relatives was found for patients at the extreme of the severity spectrum, and rates were higher for relatives when probands showed an early age of onset. Several family studies indicate that subthreshold OCD conditions may be transmitted in families with OCD (52,53). Data from twin studies support the hypothesis that OCD is part of a broader inherited spectrum of neurotic anxiety (51). If certain families within a species are more vulnerable to developing OCD in response to exposure to various types of stress, then perhaps what is heritable is the propensity to react to stress by developing compulsive behavior. Some individuals who are genetically predisposed to OCD may never experience a sufficiently stressful environment to cause the expression of compulsive behaviors. Others may wax and wane in the severity of their condition depending on their level of exposure to and tolerance for stress. Genetic relationships have also been suggested for some forms of OCD and Tourette's disorder/chronic tics and trichotillomania (8,54–57). Veterinary models developed from research in progress support a broad-spectrum interpretation and conform to genetic data presented for the human condition (vide infra).

Pharmacological Treatment of Stereotypies and OCD

Stereotypies in animals and OCD in humans both respond positively to treatment with selective serotonin reuptake inhibitors (SSRIs) (1,23,24,58–60). The response to SSRIs, however, is not consistent and often incomplete (59,61). Enhanced improvement may be obtained when behavioral modification techniques are implemented simultaneously with pharmacological treatment (61). Pharmacological criteria alone are not diagnostic for OCD because SSRIs have a broad spectrum of effects and are efficacious in the treatment of a wide variety of other disorders, including depression, anxiety, and aggression (62). In addition, repetitive behaviors in animals and some forms of OCD in humans may respond to treatment with other medications, such as opioid agonists and dopamine antagonists (25,59,63–66).

CANINE COMPULSIVE BEHAVIOR

Innate behaviors that have been important for the survival of canids include grooming, predatory behavior, ingestive behavior, sexual activity, communication, aggression, and locomotion. Abnormal expression of a variety of these normal species-typical behaviors occurs in some domestic dogs and can become so severe that owners must seek professional help for their canine companions (Table 2). Grooming behaviors expressed to excess in domestic dogs include excessive licking of body parts, particularly the extremities of the limbs; nail-biting; and foot-

Table 2 Canine Compulsive Behavior—Most Promising Models for OCD Research

Condition	Description	Presumed derivation	Familial/genetic status	Age of onset	Temperament of affected individuals	Precipitating events/ circumstances	Comorbidity	Pharmacological responsiveness
Lick granuloma	Repetitively licking distal extremities of limbs	Grooming behavior	Possible genetic underpinnings (affects large breeds)	Variable (usually mature dogs)	Tend to be highly strung, anxious, or hyperactive	Separation/ isolation	Separation anxiety, noise phobia	SSRIs, opioid antagonists
Flank-sucking	Mouthing the flank regions	Ingestive behavior (nursing)	Probably genetic, mainly in Dobermans	Puberty or young adulthood	High-strung, anxious	Stress	Lick granuloma	Opioid antagonists
Tail-chasing	Continuously running in tight circles, attempting to grasp tail	Predatory behavior	Probably genetic, occurs mainly in Bull Terriers and German Shepherds (or crosses)	Puberty or young adulthood	Hyperactive, anxious	Estrus, changing environment, postsurgery, other stresses, excitement	Compulsive behavior toward objects, aggression, partial seizures, hyperactivity	SSRIs, anticonvulsants
Compulsive object playing	Dogs spend many hours a day engrossed in oral activities directed toward objects e.g., tennis ball, log, or chew toy	Predatory behavior	Suspected genetic underpinnings; occurs mainly in known predatory breeds, e.g., Bull Terrier, Retriever	Prepubertal; puberty	High-strung, anxious	Stress	Tail-chasing, flank-sucking, hyperactivity	SSRIs

chewing. Common repetitive movements considered components of the predatory sequence include snapping at imaginary flies, shadow-chasing, tail-chasing, and compulsive behavior with objects, expressed as excessive retrieving, chasing, and carrying. Repetitive chewing and sucking on objects or self (flank-sucking) may represent displaced nursing behavior to the point of compulsion. Polydipsia, polyphagia, and pica occur in dogs and may reflect displaced ingestive behavior. Repetitive digging or floor-scratching and stereotypic pacing are all locomotor activities that some dogs perform to excess. Compulsive digging and floor- or dirt-scratching could be categorized as displaced behaviors relating to food caching or denning activity. Since locomotor activity is intrinsic to most behaviors necessary for survival, it is not surprising that some dogs exposed to prolonged conflict resort to pacing or other motoric components of adaptive behavior. Such behaviors may be associated with escape or territorial patrolling. Finally, rhythmic barking or howling may also constitute a problem for dog owners. Under normal circumstances, a bark serves a social function by eliciting attention or acting as a warning signal or threat. Depending on the context, howls function to strengthen social bonds, reaffirm social status, announce territorial occupancy, or serve as individual identification that may lead to reunification with the group. Compulsive barking or howling with no eliciting stimulus represents an adaptive response that has misfired. Working from the premise that stereotypic manifestations of these species-typical behaviors might be considered canine equivalents of OCD, it is logical to extend animal models beyond those for grooming behaviors.

Genetic Variability Underlying Breed Differences in Predatory Behavior

For carnivores, obtaining food involves three systems of behavior: 1) investigatory behavior for locating prey that employs various sensory systems, all of which have been accentuated in some breeds of dogs; 2) agonistic behavior to stalk, herd, chase, and kill the prey; and 3) ingestive behavior (67).

Although predatory behavior is displayed by all canids, the extent of expression of specific motor sequences has been highly modified by artificial selection. Reviewing the variety of breeds, it becomes apparent that, through artificial selection, man has been able to produce different breeds of dogs suited to various "occupations" by selecting for specific elements of the predatory sequence. Enhancement of specific sensory systems essential to the investigatory phase of predation has been selected for in breeds such as sight hounds and scent hounds. Breeds that differ qualitatively in expression of specific agonistic motor components are also abundant. Behavioral studies with different breeds of domestic dogs illustrate this concept (68,69). The Siberian Husky, for example, is described as behaviorally representative of the domestic canid's progenitor, the wolf. This breed exhibits the full range of appetitive and consummatory sequences characteristic of the predatory behavior of the wild ancestral form. Border Collies, a breed of livestock-conducting dogs, display the appetitive, searching, and stalking behaviors, but do not follow through with the full range of consummatory behaviors. Retrievers and Setters go so far as to locate and retrieve prey, but the predatory sequence is attenuated. Livestock-guarding dogs exhibit virtually no aspects of the predatory sequence. Thus, it is evident that through artificial selection for specific aspects of the predatory sequence, the phenotype can be limited to some components but not others, such that the genetic systems involved can be expressed in different combinations or separately.

Clinical data we have accrued suggests that breeds that are "genetically predisposed" to a specific aspect of the predatory sequence may preferentially exhibit that behavior in a ritualized, repetitive manner when exposed to prolonged conflict. Many sheepherding breeds have a predilection for ball-chasing, stereotypic pacing, and fence-running. German Shepherds are particularly prone to these behaviors and to tail-chasing. Hunting breeds may preferentially display a compulsive tendency to retrieve and carry objects. One Retriever that was diagnosed as suffering from separation anxiety began to retrieve and cache shoes repetitively in the absence of its owner. However, these breeds do not necessarily manifest specific components of the predatory sequence as compulsive behavior. Another Labrador Retriever that was initially an insatiable retriever of objects developed compulsive self-grooming—specifically, acral lick dermatitis—when a change in family lifestyle resulted in decreased interaction between the dog and its owner. Thus, a change in circumstance that might not readily be recognized by the owner as constituting a stressor may correspond with the onset of a displacement activity with repetitive features. The observation that the resulting behaviors resemble species-specific fixed action patterns and may preferentially reflect breed-specific behavioral characteristics supports the hypothesis that conflict/anxiety/stress may unleash primitive behavior in an inappropriate context.

Compulsive Predatory Behavior in Bull Terriers

Ancestors of the Bull Terrier breed include the Bulldog and the English white terrier. Bulldogs were selected for a tendency to attack the nose of a bull and hang on rather than employing the slash attack from the rear preferred by wolves and many other breeds of dogs. Terrier breeds have been selected for the tendency to attack prey and continue attacking regardless of any injury suffered. During the 1800s, these predatory techniques were valued in Bull Terriers, a breed that was originally developed for killing rats, baiting bear and badger, and fighting dogs in a pit. Thus, these dogs were selected for the full predatory sequence, with a special emphasis on having the tenacity to "bring down" and "hold on" to prey. For this breed, the tendency to be overinvolved with a task formed the basis for selection. Coincidentally, breeders may also have been selecting for a comparatively hyperactive temperament.

From our clinical and research experience, compulsive behaviors reflecting predatory tendencies have constituted the primary complaints from Bull Terrier owners (70). Considering the breed's genetic background, it is not surprising that they would be predisposed to express aspects of predatory behavior out of context. Typical compulsive behaviors include tail-chasing, repetitive and ritualized behavior with objects, and iterative ingestion of inedible material. While many owners consider tail-chasing and compulsive behavior with objects to be normal idiosyncrasies of the breed, for some affected dogs the compulsion can be debilitating. Within the breed, these behaviors are expressed on a continuum ranging from mild and not too disturbing in some dogs to extreme and very disruptive in others. Based on DSM-IV criteria, we consider these activities to constitute a model for OCD when 1) they consume more than 3–8 hours of the animal's time per day, 2) physical injury results as a consequence of the repetitive nature of the behavior, and 3) the behavior significantly interferes with the dog's normal functioning and social relationship with the owner (4). Frustration or conflict may result if moderate or severely affected dogs are prevented from performing the compulsion.

Compulsive Behavior with Objects

Survey and clinical data collected for over 180 Bull Terriers at the Tufts Behavior Clinic indicate that approximately 25% of this sample population displayed compulsive behavior toward such objects as toys, logs, or food dishes (70). This percentage most likely represents an overestimate for the entire breed population since family data were collected from probands, their relatives, and other affected animals presenting at the clinic. Based on the previously described criteria, this preliminary figure includes subthreshold as well as threshold dogs. The behaviors exhibited consist of stereotyped, repetitive, and excessive chasing, carrying, and/ or chewing of inedible items. When provided with a suitable substrate, these dogs will spend from 3 hours per day to almost all waking hours engaged in compulsive activity directed toward the object. For threshold individuals, the compulsion can be so severe that the dog loses weight, suffers exhaustion, and incurs physical injury. While some can be temporarily distracted from the activity, most resume almost immediately when permitted. If the compulsion is prevented, dogs may appear anxious, resort to another repetitive behavior such as tail-chasing, or exhibit aggression. Dogs that are singularly focused on an object may reject their owner, preferentially engaging in the repetitive behavior. Frequently, one specific object elicits the compulsive response. A dog that exhibits compulsive behavior toward a tennis ball or log is often, although not always, normal with respect to its interaction with most other objects. When owners refuse to participate in play in an attempt to decrease the frequency of the undesired behavior, some dogs have been reported to develop their own repetitive activities, such as releasing a ball at the top of stairs or a hill and repeatedly chasing and retrieving the object. They persist to the point of exhaustion and perform this behavior to the exclusion of most other normal activities. Apart from their compulsive behavior with a particular object, many of these dogs are normal in most other respects.

Our preliminary data indicate that the onset of compulsive activity frequently, although not exclusively, precedes or coincides with the approach of sexual maturation. Additionally, the data suggest that hyperactive or anxious dogs may be more susceptible to physiological, psychological, or environmental stress, which may exacerbate if not precipitate the compulsions. A moderate to significant decrease in the frequency and intensity of compulsive behavior directed toward objects has been observed in four of seven affected dogs following treatment with SSRIs (70). The three remaining dogs were not allowed access to the objects that had previously elicited the compulsive behavior so the effect of treatment for these animals remains unknown. These three animals were concurrently being treated for tail-chasing.

Repetitive behavior with objects appears to stem from primitive predatory behaviors that have been emancipated from their original context. Although the exact mode of transmission has yet to be determined, our pilot data suggest that genetic factors are important for the tendency to develop compulsions toward objects (71). A heritable component is suspected since the behavior appears to run in particular family lines and only some animals are affected within a given sibship. Compulsive behavior directed toward objects has been expressed by dogs that have not had an opportunity to learn this behavior from other dogs and have not been subjected to substandard environments that might result in excessive activity of this sort.

Tail-Chasing

While tail-chasing and compulsive behavior with objects phenomeno-logically appear to be distinct, careful inspection of the behaviors suggests that they both contain predatory features. Therefore, the preceding comments regarding the predatory nature of compulsive behavior with objects also apply to tail-chasing.

The phenotypic presentation of tail-chasing behavior in Bull Terriers represents a continuum, from some dogs that engage in slow to moderately rapid rotation while fixated on the tail to others that engage in rapid spinning bouts during which the dog seems unfocused and dissociated from its surroundings. For some, it seems that spinning occurs spontaneously although it may be attributed to increased arousal, anticipation, or excitement. For others, a glimpse of their tail is enough to trigger the behavior. They fixate on the tail, begin to "stalk" it slowly, and progress to feverish whirling in tight circles in an attempt to grab their tail. This behavior may culminate in self-mutilation caused by grabbing and biting the tail. The frequency and severity of expression range from mild and desultory to near-constant spinning that severely interferes with the dog's health and normal functioning. Dogs in this latter seriously affected group, in particular, will continue to spin beyond the point of exhaustion, and they seem to lack self-control and appear extremely anxious. The behavior is similar to the repetitive, ritualized behaviors observed in humans suffering from OCD in the sense that the animal is compelled to repeat the same motion continuously and has little ability to stop. Some owners of mildly to moderately affected dogs report that the animal will chase its tail in a location out of view of the owner if it has been reprimanded repeatedly for tail-chasing.

Tail-chasing occurs equally in males and females. However, in our experience, males often appear more severely affected and more difficult to treat. The onset of tail-chasing typically occurs between 6 months to 2 years of age, although it may present at any time. The behavior seems to be more common in hyperactive or anxious dogs. Furthermore, the development of tail-chasing is frequently associated with exposure to environmental or psychological stress, including ownership changes, anesthesia, estrus, and parturition; in some cases, however, there is no known stressful trigger. The development of tail-chasing differs between individual dogs, varying from a gradual to a sudden onset. When the behavior is displayed occasionally by young puppies, owners often disregard it as play, but the behavior may escalate as the dog ages and tail-chasing can become a singular focus. In some dogs the frequency of tail-chasing, as well as the duration of bouts, may decrease with age.

Tail-chasing is the sole compulsion in some dogs, but others exhibit tail-chasing and compulsions with objects simultaneously. Occasionally, a dog will switch from one compulsion to another. For example, if the primary compulsive response focuses on objects, the dog may switch to tail-chasing, particularly if the desired object is removed. The association of this compulsive behavior with anxious or hyperactive temperaments, its occurrence following exposure to stress, typically pubertal age of onset (although variable), and the waxing, waning, and mutating nature of the compulsions all mirror the human condition of OCD. Additional support for classifying tail-chasing as a manifestation of compulsive disorder is provided by the partial or complete cessation of the behavior in response to SSRIs such as clomipramine and fluoxetine (70).

Tail-chasing behavior has been variably diagnosed as a seizure-related phenomenon or an opioid-mediated stereotypy (47,49,72,73). Electroencephalographic abnormalities and abnormal brain geometry have been reported in tail-chasing Bull Terriers (47,48). The association of compulsive behavior with seizure activity is not entirely surprising, as some humans diagnosed with OCD also exhibit a concurrent seizure disorder (59).

Both tail-chasing and spinning are most likely varying levels of expression of the same phenotype since breeding of mild tail-chasers can result in severe spinners, and juveniles that occasionally chase their tails may subsequently express severe spinning. Our preliminary data indicate that tail-chasing in Bull Terriers occurs in certain pedigrees and segregates within sibships (71). In this particular population, it is most likely transmitted as a polygenic disorder. Data from critical test crosses will be necessary to develop a definitive genetic model indicating the exact mode of inheritance.

Compulsive Behavior of Dogs Related to Grooming

Ethology and Neurophysiology of Grooming Behavior

Self-grooming serves several functions: cleaning the body surface, thermoregulation, parasite control, and self-comforting behavior (74–76). In social species, allogrooming facilitates social integration by functioning as a bonding signal and appeasement gesture. Grooming may be performed as a displacement activity, occurring after an animal has been exposed to novel, stressful, or conflicting stimuli. The activity of grooming is thought to have a de-arousing effect after exposure to a stressor, and consequently may function as a coping mechanism (76,77).

A variety of neural pathways have been implicated in grooming behavior. Hypothalamic stimulation experiments suggest that grooming is a preprogrammed and innate behavior (78). Similar brain regions may be involved in the pathophysiology of OCD (79,80). The mechanism of self-grooming in response to arousing external stimuli is thought to involve an ACTH-oxytocin-dopamine pathway (81,82).

Acral Lick Dermatitis

Canine acral lick dermatitis (ALD) (synonym: lick granuloma) is a psychogenic disorder of dogs characterized by continuous licking and chewing of the distal extremities of the limbs (83–85). The condition can arise at any age and does not appear to affect either sex preferentially (86,87). Affected dogs usually present with localized alopecia, skin ulcers, and granulomatous lesions in the areas of the dorsum of the carpus or tarsus (58,83,84,88,89). Medical conditions such as pyodermatitis, allergies, foreign bodies, and neoplasia sometimes initiate the licking; however, even after the primary cause has been eliminated, a susceptible dog may continue to lick. Once the dog has engaged in indiscriminate grooming of the legs and paws for an extended period of time, local histopathological processes increase the dog's urge to groom (90).

Social isolation, confinement, and other stressors are thought to be associated with the onset of this condition and may also increase the intensity and frequency of the behavior (9,83–86). Once the licking behavior has been established, it may be performed at any time, even in the owner's presence. Dogs that have been punished for this behavior may actively avoid their owners to engage in bouts of self-directed licking. At the Tufts University Behavior Clinic, approximately 70% of the dogs diagnosed with ALD have comorbid fear or anxiety-based conditions, such as thunderstorm phobia or separation anxiety.

ALD occurs predominantly in large breeds of dogs. Doberman Pinschers, Labrador Retrievers, and Great Danes are overrepresented in the population of affected dogs, and the condition may occur more frequently within individual families (9,58,91). Preliminary data collected from a family of affected Dobermans suggest that ALD may be transmitted as a simple dominant Mendelian segregant; however, the precise mode of inheritance cannot be definitely ascertained until more data have been collected (92).

A variety of treatment modalities, including physical restraint, topical therapy and opioid antagonists have been used with varying degrees of success (25,58,84–86,88,93–97). Goldberger and Rapoport's study of 37 dogs with ALD demonstrated that clomipramine is an effective treatment for this otherwise refractory condition (1). Twenty-five percent of dogs with ALD treated at the Tufts University Behavior Clinic over a 6-month period exhibited 100% improvement following approximately 3 months of treatment with clomipramine 2 mg/kg administered orally. The success rates for the remaining cases varied from an overall improvement of 80% (55% of the dogs) to 60% (10% of the dogs) to 50% (10% of the dogs).

To substantiate the role of serotonin in ALD, Rapoport (9,98) attempted to replicate the results of previous studies in which metachlorophenylpiperazine (m-CPP), a 5-HT receptor agonist, was administered to human patients with OCD and anxiety disorders. Administration of m-CPP to human patients is associated with an increase in anxiety and OC behavior (99,100). Rapoport's m-CPP challenge in dogs with ALD did not produce analogous results, since the dogs became somnolent and did not respond with increased anxiety or obsessive-compulsive behavior (9). Because the sedation noted in these dogs may have been dose-related, we repeated the study in five ALD dogs using lower doses of m-CPP (0.25–0.5 mg/kg) that did not cause somnolence. Preliminary analysis of the results of this trial did not indicate an increased frequency or intensity of compulsive licking in treated dogs, although the dogs did respond to auditory stimuli with an increased startle response.

FELINE COMPULSIVE BEHAVIOR

Innate behaviors that are particularly relevant to cats in terms of survival include predation, ingestive behavior, self-grooming, scent marking, and sexual and territorial defensive behaviors. Abnormal repetitive behaviors related to ingestive behavior, grooming, and, possibly, territorial defensive behavior include wool-sucking/texture-related eating disorder, psychogenic alopecia, compulsive lip- and nose-licking, compulsive paw-licking, compulsive hair-playing, and, possibly, feline hyperesthesia syndrome and tail-biting (Table 3). Hoarding, which occurs in Munchkin cats, may be more closely related to predation. The most common repetitive behavior problem of domestic cats, anxiety-related urine marking, has some compulsive elements but is not generally regarded as true compulsive behavior. Interestingly, however, the latter condition is often refractory to behavior-modification therapy and environmental manipulation, but a subset of these cats can be controlled by treatment with anxiety-reducing medication, such as buspirone and benzodiazepines, as well as antidepressant drugs, including SSRIs (24,101).

Compulsive Behavior Related to Feeding: Wool-Sucking/Texture-Related Eating Disorder

Wool-sucking, in which cats nurse compulsively on woolen or acrylic substrates or their own hair, is a compulsive behavior that occurs most

Table 3 Feline Compulsive Behavior—Most Promising Models for OCD Research

Condition	Description	Presumed derivation	Familial/genetic basis	Age of onset	Temperament of affected individuals	Precipitating events/circumstances	Pharmacological responsiveness
Wool-sucking	Nursing behavior directed toward woolen/acrylic substrates, sometimes progresses to frank ingestive behavior	Nursing/ingestive behavior	Oriental breeds	Post-weaning	High-strung	Confinement	SSRIs
Psychogenic alopecia	Compulsive self-grooming, often involving limbs and abdomen	Grooming behavior	Some breed specificity, e.g., Singapora and Ocicat	Variable	Anxious/fearful	Stress or conflict	SSRIs, opioid antagonists, dopamine antagonists
Lip- and nose-licking	Repetitive licking of upper lip and nostril causing ulceration/granuloma	Grooming behavior	Any breed	Variable	Not determined	Anxiety (?)	Not known
Compulsive paw-licking	Repeatedly dabbling paw in water bowl then licking paw	Grooming behavior	American Shorthair and British Shorthair	Variable	Not determined	Confinement (?)	SSRIs
Hoarding	Hoarding unusual objects	Prey retrieval (?)	Munchkin	Adolescence	Not determined	Not known	Dopamine antagonists (?)

commonly in Oriental breeds, especially Siamese, although it is also seen in other purebred and mixed-breed cats. It appears to be particularly common in more active breeds. The condition resembles a displaced nursing behavior, and may be the feline equivalent of thumb-sucking. Because of the breed predilection, wool-sucking is thought to have genetic underpinnings, possibly related to the comparatively anxious temperament of affected breeds and perhaps to early weaning.

Some cats exhibiting wool-sucking behavior show a developmental progression to aberrant ingestive behavior, characterized by a predilection for woolen, acrylic, cotton, or plastic substrates. This eating compulsion can sometimes be redirected onto more acceptable substrates, such as high-fiber food. Alternatively, SSRIs reduce the frequency of the behavior in many affected cats (92). Cats treated in this way show a gradual decrease in the frequency of the behaviors over several weeks, and may progress to an estimated 90–95% level of improvement. This time course mirrors the response of many human OCD patients treated with SSRIs.

Compulsive Behavior Related to Grooming

Psychogenic Alopecia

From an ethological perspective, self-grooming serves a variety of functions in the cat, including basic cleaning, removing parasites, and providing comfort when the animal experiences duress. Normally cats spend a great deal of each day self-grooming (102). In susceptible animals exposed to environmental stressors, however, grooming behavior may become excessive and inappropriate, leading to depilation and alopecia. A cat presented to one of the authors (NHD) began grooming excessively when another cat was introduced into the home. This cat initially responded to treatment with an opioid antagonist, naltrexone. An opioid antagonist was selected for treatment because endogenous opioids are known to be involved in propagation of self-scratching (103). Interestingly, compulsive face-picking (neurotic excoriations) in humans has also been found to respond to treatment with an opioid antagonist (104). Dopamine antagonists have also been reported as effective treatments for psychogenic alopecia in cats, raising the possibility that compulsive self-directed grooming may involve opioid-mediated activation of a dopamine-facilitated behavior (63). Recently, most cats with psychogenic alopecia presented at our clinic have been treated with SSRIs. The results have been encouraging, with the majority of cases responding similarly, in both time course and degree, to other compulsive behaviors in people and animals (92).

Some evidence is beginning to emerge that feline psychogenic alopecia has a heritable component. One strain of Singapora cats exhibits compulsive self-grooming that appears to be inherited as a recessive trait (105). Phenomenological similarities exist between feline psychogenic alopecia and human trichotillomania. Trichotillomania, classified as an impulse-control disorder, is now considered by some to be an obsessive-compulsive spectrum disorder, which has many similarities to classical OCD—including, as in cats with psychogenic alopecia, a positive response to treatment with SSRIs (5,106,107). In addition, opioid antagonists and dopamine antagonists are beneficial adjuvants to other forms of therapy in both conditions (64).

Compulsive Hair-Playing

Certain members of a new cat breed, the Ojos Azules, exhibit an unusual variation of hair-pulling behavior in that the object of their attention is human hair. Affected cats begin by rubbing against the owner's face, then burrowing in—and finally frantically pulling on—the scalp hair. The behavior is sufficiently problematic that cats showing this trait are usually banished from the family's sleeping quarters. Domestic cats engage in allogrooming with offspring and other feline members of the household. Such behavior promotes bonding and may serve as a conciliatory gesture and aid in the distribution of pheromones. When the behavior is redirected toward their owners as opposed to conspecifics, the activity may represent an aberrant form of social grooming.

The behavior appears to be transmitted as a single-gene disorder, although the preliminary pedigree data do not permit definitive assessment of the inheritance pattern (Figure 2).

Compulsive Lip- and Nose-Licking

One of the most fundamental forms of feline grooming behavior is licking of the lips or nose. These are two distinct actions, which rarely overlap (102). Because of the abrasiveness of the cat's tongue, repetitive licking of the lips or nose seen in some cats may result in irritation and ulceration of these areas. Treatment of these conditions has been largely unsuccessful to date, perhaps because the resulting lesions have been viewed as dermatological problems. Some components of a dermatological problem termed the eosinophilic granuloma complex are now thought to have genetic and psychogenic factors (108). One aspect of this complex, which presents as an indolent ulcer of the upper lip, or lip granuloma, and which is three times more common in females than males, seems to be a particularly likely candidate for a compulsive behavioral etiology (109). Working from first principles, a logical approach

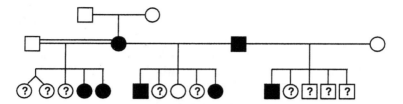

Figure 2 Pedigree of repetitive hair-playing in cats (solid symbols).

to treatment would be to address possible environmental causes of anxiety and to treat with either an opioid antagonist, a dopamine antagonist, or an SSRI.

Compulsive Paw-Licking

A colony of American short-haired cats in Springfield, Massachusetts, exhibits an unusual form of repetitive grooming behavior (105). Affected cats dabble their paws in the water bowl, often knocking it over, and then proceed to lick their paws for a while before repeating the behavioral sequence. This deviation from normal cleaning/grooming behavior can be so troublesome that water bowls for these cats must be anchored or designed to prevent spillage. The behavior appears to be inherited rather than learned (Figure 3), and preliminary results indicate that it responds to treatment with SSRIs (105). The same trait was observed in a colony of British shorthairs. Very young children exhibit a similar compulsive behavior, finger-licking, which may be analogous (110).

Feline Hyperesthesia Syndrome

This complicated behavioral condition has some features that appear stereotypic or compulsive and others that appear frankly neurological. Affected cats—almost always Siamese or Siamese crosses—exhibit dilated pupils, rippling skin, and bouts of frenetic self-directed grooming (111). Agitation is obvious during an attack, which may last from a few seconds to half a minute. An apparent sensitivity to touch, which can trigger attacks, accounts for the name of this syndrome, which is usually associated with heightened affect and aggression. It has been suggested that the signs are manifestations of mental problems associated with an unstable personality, frustrations of various kinds, environmental pressures, and possibly even minimal brain damage (112). Partial seizures have been suggested as being associated with this condition, and some cats have shown improvement when treated with phenobarbital (113). The association between seizure activity and OCD has been reported in some human patients with OCD; a similar pathophysiological mechanism may be operating in cats with feline hyperesthesia syndrome (45). We have successfully treated affected cats with SSRIs, which seem to have the effect of leveling mood, as well as directly inhibiting the self-directed attacks (92).

Compulsions Possibly Related to Territorial Defense Behavior

A curious condition occurs in some cats, which, in a state of heightened affect and agitation, attack and bite their own tails. This self-injurious behavior may be a manifestation of feline hyperesthesia syndrome (described above) or may be a separate condition. Affected cats are usually housecats confined to the home, and some manifest the behavior when territorial challenges are presented by outside cats. The resulting situation appears to be one of anxiety and frustrated conflict. Because affected cats tend to be more dominant than deferent in terms of their underlying temperament, it is possible that the self-directed attacks may be dominance-driven redirected behavior. The condition is reminiscent of the floating-limb syndrome that affects solitary housed primates (114). Affected primates attack one of their own hind feet, which they hold poised in midair behind their head. The result is an unresolvable dominance struggle between the monkey and its own appendage. Like the monkeys, in the process of delivering the self-directed attacks some cats may inflict significant self-injury. The feline condition responds to treatment with opioid antagonists and SSRIs and may be a feline form of OCD in which intraspecific aggression is the misdirected underlying natural behavior (92).

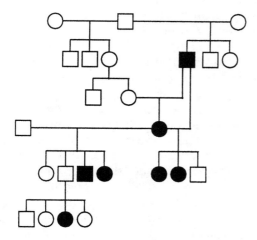

Figure 3   Pedigree of paw-licking in cats (solid symbols).

Compulsive Behavior Related to Predation: Hoarding

A unique form of hoarding behavior has recently been observed in a large kindred of Munchkin cats, a breed characterized by unusually short legs. These cats are attracted to unusual objects, such as key rings, pens, or jewelry. When confronted with an object of interest, the cat will immediately pick up the item in its mouth and carry it to a preferred hiding place. The objects are usually taken to a single consistent location and are not subsequently removed for play. Although the behavior may be reminiscent of a mother cat's moving her litter to another nest site or the retrieval of a wandering kitten, the behavior is seen in both sexes. Prey retrieval is another possible underlying behavior. Hoarding does not appear to be a learned behavior since the trait does not usually manifest itself until adolescence, long after kittens have left their birthplace for new homes.

Hoarding behavior in laboratory animals appears to require intact dopamine function in the CNS. After disruption by lesions of the dopamine system, it can be restored by the administration of L-dopa (21). The need to save unneeded objects is a relatively common symptom of OCD in humans.

AVIAN COMPULSIVE BEHAVIOR

Preening in birds serves a hygienic and thermoregulatory function. However, birds also groom one another (allopreening), particularly avian species such as parrots that are highly social and form persistent pair bonds (115). Allopreening has evolved into a ritualized communicative signal primarily to solidify social bonds and to function as an appeasement display to inhibit attacks by conspecifics (115). Feather-picking is a common behavior problem in captive avian species. The condition is characterized by excessive preening, which inhibits the normal growth of feathers. The birds usually chew on feathers that seem "different" from others, for example, feathers that are currently growing and clipped feathers. Occasionally bleeding occurs when vascularized feathers (blood feathers) are affected. When engaging in extensive chewing, the birds tend to pull these feathers with their beak, grab them with their feet, and hold and "examine" them for a period of time until they eventually lose interest and drop the feather. The loss of feathers occurs most commonly in circumscribed areas under the wings, on the abdomen, and surrounding the tail. In extreme cases, preening may result in self-mutilative behavior, such as skin-chewing and -tearing.

Although organic diseases (bacterial and viral infection, parasites, autoimmune factors, toxic elements, lesions, malnutrition, and endocrine imbalances) have been implicated as causes of feather-picking, en-

vironmental factors are known to play a significant role in its development. Proposed stressors that correlate with the onset of feather-picking
include isolation or inadequate interaction with the owners, reproduc-
tive frustration (lack of mates or wrong choice of cage mates), inadequate housing or management, and malnutrition (116–119).

In our experience, it appears that some breeds, e.g., the Cockatoo
and the African Gray, are affected more frequently. A genetic predispo-
sition for feather-picking has been suggested, but remains to be demonstrated (117,120–122).

Treatment of feather-picking birds has included therapy of underlying medical conditions, hooded (Elizabethan) collars, beak-grinding and
-notching, application of foul-tasting sprays, and environmental enrich-
ment. For nonmedical etiologies, the condition is refractory to such treatments. Pharmacological treatment of feather-picking aimed at achieving
sedation, using diazepam or phenobarbital, has met with little success
(117,121). Recent studies indicate that feather-picking may respond to
SSRIs (122,123). Preliminary results from our clinical studies on the use of
fluoxetine in 25 birds strongly support this contention, indicating an overall improvement ranging from 60 to 100% (124). Relapses do occur, particularly as the feathers begin to grow back, and we recommend increasing
the dosage to get the birds through this period. An association with anxious temperaments is also indicated—approximately 30% of all birds enrolled in our study show clinical signs of separation anxiety manifested by
excessive vocalization whenever the owner leaves the room.

Phenomenological similarities between feather-picking/self-mutila-
tion in birds and some forms of human OCD, including trichotillomania
and self-mutilation, are striking (10). Due to the differences between
human and avian anatomy and physiology, a direct comparison of human OCD and this avian compulsion seems inadequate at first. It should
be noted, however, that although the configuration of the avian and
mammalian brain differs, their structure and function have been shown
to be comparable (123). Because of the phenomenological and pharmacological similarities between some forms of human OCD and avian
feather-picking and self-mutilation, the latter may provide a suitable
model for the study of at least some aspects of OCD.

EQUINE COMPULSIVE BEHAVIOR

Horses are social animals that in their natural environment live in
groups or bands (102). In this situation, 60–70% of their day is normally
occupied by grazing (102). As they graze, they walk slowly from place
to place but, as potential prey animals, they are ready to flee quickly
when alarmed. When not feeding, horses may rest or engage in various

aspects of their social repertoire, which include, for example, both affiliative and sexual behavior. Mutual grooming is one feature of affiliative behaviors that is typical for horses. Aggression, also part of the social repertoire, is necessary to maintain a stable hierarchy within the herd, genetic soundness, and "survival of the fittest."

Preventing a horse, or any other animal, from performing its natural behaviors by confinement and social isolation could be viewed as a form of social stress. This, coupled with the common but unnatural twice-daily feeding regimen imposed by horse owners, might be responsible for the high percentage of equine compulsive behaviors, the so-called stall vices. A recent study (125) indicated that about 15% of all stabled horses show some form of compulsive behavior. The compulsive behaviors expressed reflect aberrations of normal species-typical behaviors. Motor patterns reflecting aspects of feeding behavior, locomotion, and sexual behaviors are particularly prevalent.

Compulsions Related to Feeding Behavior

Feeding comprises several different behavioral components that blend together to create the process by which food is ingested. These components include prehension, mastication, and deglutition. Repetitive behaviors related to prehension include lip-flapping, wood-nibbling, and cribbing, whereas compulsions related to mastication and deglutition include tongueing and aerophagia (Table 4).

Cribbing is one of the most common equine compulsions, affecting 1 to 3% of the equine population. Affected horses anchor their upper incisor teeth on a ledge or surface, lean back, tense their neck muscles, and retract their larynx, and may engulf a bolus of air (aerophagia). There is some evidence that cribbing is familial, although environmental factors and learning are thought to play a role in its development (126). Affected horses appear more anxious and vigilant than noncribbing counterparts, and have been described as hyperkinetic (66). To date, there is no reliable treatment for cribbing, although various physical methods of preventing the behavior have been tried, ranging from anticribbing collars to electrical aversion therapy, and even surgery to remove the large ventral neck muscles (128). Research indicates that cribbing is opioid-mediated and that opioid antagonists are almost completely effective in preventing the behavior (66). Dopaminergic mechanisms may be secondarily involved because morphine, which precipitates compulsive walking, digging, and cribbing in horses, appears to produce these behavioral effects through dopaminergic activation (18). Serotonin may have a modulating influence because SSRIs produce a

Table 4 Equine Compulsive Behavior—Most Promising Models for OCD Research

Condition	Description	Presumed derivation	Familial/ genetic status	Age of onset	Temperament of affected individuals	Precipitating events/ circumstances	Pharmacological responsiveness
Lip-flapping	Lips are drawn apart and smacked together repeatedly	Ingestive behavior	Unknown	Variable	Not determined	Confinement	Unknown
Wood-nibbling	Prehensive movements with incisor teeth directed toward wooden surfaces	Ingestive behavior	Unknown	Variable	Not determined	Confinement	Unknown
Cribbing	Horse grasps ledge or surface with incisor teeth, leans back, tenses neck muscles; sometimes associated with aerophagia	Ingestive behavior	Suggested familial basis	Young	More active/ anxious than counterparts	Inactivity, boredom (presumed), imitation	Opioid antagonists, dopmaine antagonists, SSRIs
Tongueing	Tongue moves in a front-to-back motion	Ingestive behavior	Unknown	Variable	Not determined	Unknown	Unknown

decrement in the behavior (128). One working hypothesis linking these neurotransmitters is that anxiety and stress increase opioid production, which in turn activates neostriatal dopamine pathways to induce the behavior (66) (Figure 1). Because highly palatable rations increase central endorphin release, it was anticipated that cribbing frequency would increase in affected horses following ingestion of palatable food, and this has been confirmed (129,130). What was not anticipated was that the mean peripheral β-endorphin level of cribbing horses was little more than half that of controls (130). Plasma β-endorphin levels have been found to be low in human subjects with OCD and some subgroups of pathological gamblers (131,132).

Compulsions Related to Locomotion

The most common locomotor compulsions in horses are stall-walking and weaving. Stall-walkers constantly walk the perimeter of their stalls, often leaving a circular track in their bedding material. Weavers move their heads from side to side, moving their weight from one foot to another in a stereotypic fashion. The latter behavior represents an abbreviated form of fence running, a displacement behavior that arises from conflict. Stall-walking, like cribbing, is enhanced by opioid receptor agonists (morphine) and dopamine agonists and attenuated by opioid antagonists (18,133). Weaving is also enhanced by morphine and dopamine agonists and is exacerbated by stress and frustration, but it is refractory to treatment with doses of opioid antagonists that would be effective in the treatment of cribbing (18,66). Both conditions appear to have neurophysiological and behavioral similarities to some forms of OCD in humans.

Compulsions Related to Sexual Behavior

One particularly intriguing equine compulsive behavior appears to be motivated by conflict and sexual arousal (for example, males may be triggered by a mare in estrus). The condition, which has been variously described as equine self-mutilation syndrome, flank-biting, and equine self-directed aggression, appears to share many features with Tourette's syndrome (134). The most striking behavioral manifestation involves a gross head–neck motor tic, with the horse making downward or sideways glancing movements during what appears to be a self-directed attack. Some horses actually bite themselves, hence the term self-directed aggression. Affected horses also strike out with one limb (hemiballismus) during a bout, and may grunt or squeal during what is a fairly stereotyped motor sequence. They also appear to be preoccupied with the walls of their enclosure. There is a suggestion that some horses may have a problem crossing thresholds, as they often buck or rear when confronted with such obstacles. In general, affected horses appear to be frustrated by their environment. They are often hyperactive and appear excited and agitated, especially during a bout. The behavior is exacerbated by stress and attenuated when the horse is engaged in an absorbing activity. It affects males more frequently than females (7 to 1), and is usually first seen in the preadolescent or adolescent horse. An atypical presentation was seen in a geriatric (22-year-old) horse that engaged in the behavior for the first time following head trauma (134). Tourette's syndrome can also arise secondary to trauma (135).

The syndrome appears to have a familial distribution. Although the condition is uncommon, with an incidence of 0.04–0.7% of the equine population, often more than one family member is affected (134). In one family that we studied, a sire and two male sibling progeny were all affected (136). In another family, the grandsire, the sire, and the horse in question were all affected.

Pharmacological studies in affected horses have demonstrated the efficacy of opioid antagonists and dopamine antagonists (acepromazine and haloperidol), α_2-adrenergic agents (detomidine), and the SSRI clomipramine in reducing the intensity and frequency of bouts (136,137). Catecholamine agonists appear to enhance the Tourette-like behavior (137). Progestins and castration ameliorate signs of "equine Tourette's" in some horses (134). The antiandrogen flutamide reduces the severity of clinical signs of Tourette's syndrome in people (138).

REPETITIVE BEHAVIOR IN FARM AND ZOO ANIMALS

Farm Animals

Due to current concerns over animal welfare, stereotypic behavior in farm animals, particularly sows and heifers, has been studied in great detail (31,139). While repetitive behaviors in food-production animals have not been viewed as models for the human condition of OCD, the species-typical patterns of expression and the eliciting factors conform to other potential animal models previously discussed and support a neuroethological approach (Table 5). Stereotypies in farm animals generally involve a disturbance in appetitive and consummatory behaviors, which is to be expected given their herbivorous nature. Oral "vices" observed in cattle and pigs include bar-biting, tongue-rolling, nostril-licking, and chewing. Tongue-rolling is considered a stereotypy when a cow repeatedly rolls its tongue inside or outside of its mouth in an undeviat-

Table 5 Zoo and Farm Animal Compulsive Behavior—Most Promising Models for OCD Research

Condition	Species	Description	Presumed derivation	Age of onset	Precipitating events/ circumstances	Pharmacological responsiveness
Bar-biting	Sow	Biting and chewing on objects	Ingestive	Variable	Confinement; not observed in unrestricted environments	Opioid antagonist
Tongue-rolling	Cow, sow	Rolling tongue, as during feeding	Ingestive	Variable	Confinement; not observed in unrestricted environments	—
Hair-licking	Calf	Excessive self-directed licking	Ingestive/ grooming	Young/ weaning	Early weaning; low-fiber diet; bucket-feeding leading to lack of suckling?	—
Redirected suckling	Calf	Sucking on objects/ other animals' umbilici or preputia	Ingestive	Young/ weaning	Early weaning; low-fiber diet; bucket-feeding leading to lack of suckling?	—

Condition	Species	Description	Presumed derivation	Age of onset	Precipitating events/ circumstances	Pharmacological responsiveness
Masturbation	Monkey	Self-directed sexual act	Sexual behavior	Variable	Confinement; not observed in unrestricted environments	—
Hair-pulling	Monkey/ primate	Self-directed removal of body hair	Grooming	Variable	Confinement; not observed in unrestricted environments	—
Weaving	Bear, elephant, monkey/ primate	Shifting weight from one leg to the other	Locomotor	Variable	Confinement; not observed in unrestricted environments	SSRI
Pacing	Felidae, bear	Walking in a specific pattern	Locomotor	Variable	Confinement; not observed in unrestricted environments	Opioid

—Not determined.

ing fashion. Bar-biting is defined as clamping the jaws around a bar and moving the head back and forth while chewing on the bar (140). The behaviors typically emerge as a reaction of highly aroused animals to a stressful environment (42,141). Factors constituting stress include poor housing conditions, food restriction, confinement, and tethering (140,142,143).

Repetitive behaviors may also be age-specific. Veal calves that are weaned early develop a stereotyped form of tongue-rolling that involves the end of the tongue curving back into the mouth and being sucked on before being extended again. This seems to be displaced suckling behavior and contrasts with the behavior of adult cows, whose tongueing stereotypies include components of the movements involved in pulling up vegetation (37,144).

Stereotypic behavior in sows, which involves oral activities such as chewing, rooting, sham (vacuum) sucking, and drinking, has been observed predominantly in tethered animals. Cronin (145) proposed that stereotypies of tethered sows develop from escape attempts. However, an ethological interpretation would suggest that all these behaviors are associated with appetitive and consummatory behaviors. When an animal is frustrated by a stressful environment, the resulting repetitive behaviors frequently mimic primary survival behaviors that are species-specific.

Stereotypies in farm animals are thought to function as a "coping mechanism" (31,35,36,146). The performance of stereotyped behavior has been correlated with a reduction in physiological signs of stress, including a decrease in cortisol levels and a reduced incidence of abomasal (stomach) ulceration (147–150). The development of stereotypies may be influenced by individual temperamental and physiological differences. Terlouw et al. (151) demonstrated that tethering is not a prerequisite for the development of stereotypies in sows and that individual differences in susceptibility figure prominently. Studying oral stereotypies in calves, Dantzer (152) suggested that these abnormal behaviors occur in individual animals that have a pathological deviation of neurochemical systems within the brain.

Not much is known about the brain centers and neurotransmitters involved in compulsive behavior in farm animals. Presumably the basal ganglia are the repositories for the naturalistic behaviors released as in other species, including humans. What little evidence there is about neurotransmitter involvement points to an opioid-dopamine interaction, but serotonergic agents have yet to be investigated. Opioids are thought to be involved in the propagation of stereotypic bar-biting in tethered sows because treatment with the opioid blocker naloxone has been shown to be effective (149,153).

Zoo Animals

Confinement and isolation seem to be the most important components in the development of displacement activities and stereotypies in wild species maintained in captivity. The behavior patterns of these animals vary, depending on the species affected (Table 5). Primates, for example, indulge in behaviors such as continuous rocking, excessive self-grooming, and continuous masturbation (31,114). One of us (NHD) was consulted recently regarding a female long-tailed macaque whose compulsive masturbation had evolved into rectal probing when a neighboring male macaque was moved from view. Her two offspring, who lived in the same enclosure with her, also evidenced rectal probing, suggesting that learned and environmental influences were operating. Polar bears, leopards, tigers, elephants, and many other species are known to spend a considerable amount of time performing behaviors related to locomotion (pacing, weaving), grooming (in extreme cases, self-mutilation), eating or drinking, and vocalization when confined in a zoo or a comparable environment (42,154–156).

Parallels between compulsive behavior in zoo animals and that in other species suggest that these conditions share similar etiologies and mechanisms. Opioid pathways appear to be involved, at least in some zoo-animal stereotypies, as treatment with the opioid antagonist naltrexone has led to improvement in some cases (157). Serotonergic drugs have not been used extensively for treatment of these animals, but preliminary results are promising. Recently, a polar bear at the Calgary Zoo that paced continuously for 70% of its active (awake) time showed a 30% decrease in pacing over 3 weeks when treated with fluoxetine.

The striking neuroethological similarities between compulsive behaviors of zoo animals and obsessive-compulsive-spectrum/obsessive-compulsive-related behaviors lends support to the putative biobehavioral homology of these apparently diverse conditions. When viewed in an ethological light, it can be seen that zoo-animal compulsions may also serve as valid models for human OCD research (10).

CONCLUSION

The preceding interpretation of repetitive behaviors in animals (stereotypies) and the often more complex compulsive behaviors in humans as variations on a biological theme has heuristic value and is worthy of serious consideration. A neuroethological explanation for the similarities provides the conceptual framework in which the better investigated "stereotypies" of animals and human OCD can be honed to indicate apparent biological homology. The phenomenological and neuropharmacological evidence is particularly compelling in some veterinary models such as ALD, the tail-chasing and repetitive behavior with objects of dogs, psychogenic alopecia of cats, feather-picking in birds, and some of the repetitive behaviors exhibited by captive primates. A neuroethological explanation for these behaviors based on innate behavior patterns encoded in the basal ganglia region of the brain is well founded scientifically and suggests that most compulsive behaviors are fundamental survival behaviors performed to excess and out of context (10,158). Although the same basic brain regions may be involved in animal stereotypy and human OCD, different behaviors appear to involve slightly different neural circuitry and neurotransmitters; however, serotonergic, dopaminergic, and opioidergic pathways appear to feature prominently. This intrinsic diversity has been one of the factors delaying a unifying theory of stereotypies and OCD, and may account for the different pharmacological responsiveness of the individual conditions.

Another obvious difficulty in cross-species comparisons has been the nature of the hard-wired behavior patterns. From anything but a neuroethological perspective, it is difficult to see why there should be any similarities at all between the ring-hoarding Munchkin cat and a person who keeps checking that the taps are turned off. These phenotypic discrepancies are explicable when they are considered as species-specific survival behaviors that have become disassociated from their original context. Other stumbling blocks have been the complexity of the behaviors and their association, or not, with associated cognitive processes. Stereotypies, for example, were thought to be extremely simple repetitive movements that were performed automatically and served no purpose. Now familial, temperamental, and environmental factors predisposing susceptible individuals to stereotypies are receiving more attention. Also, recent neurophysiological and neuropharmacological data indicate that these conditions are more easily explicable as a form of neurophysiological escape from psychological stressors. This situation is reminiscent of human compulsive behaviors that seem to have anxiety-related underpinnings and comorbidity and appear to affect genetically vulnerable individuals.

One hypothetical limitation of animal models is that an obsession per se, which is characteristic of so many human forms of OCD, cannot be demonstrated or measured and, in many cases, may not even occur in animals. This makes study of pure obsessions impossible, but does not preclude meaningful investigation of compulsive components, whether they occur in isolation or are preceded by a presumed obsession. However, some adults and many young children exhibit ritualistic behavior with few, if any, preceding obsessions so recurrent urges are not necessary precursors of compulsive behavior and their absence does not preclude the ability to make an accurate diagnosis or to apply logical and effective treatments. The concept advocated by early ethologists, that animals respond to environmental stimuli without cognition, is currently being contested by some modern animal behaviorists (159–162). It appears that animals do have sentience and the ability to experience themselves as independent agents. In support of this, animals show a range of behavioral problems similar to those encountered in human psychiatry, including depression, eating disorders, separation anxiety, and phobias, and they respond to similar interventions (163). Animals do not have the same behavioral routines and agendas that humans do, and for this reason would not be expected to manifest the same compulsions as those of humans with OCD. Also, animals do not have the same social pressures as humans and are unlikely to feel guilty about performing compulsive behaviors of any sort, grooming or otherwise. Instead, they indulge in their own species-specific behaviors with little or no regard for the social consequences of their actions. Although it has not been scientifically measured, it is possible that animals could experience an "obsession with incompleteness" that compels them to perform the same actions repeatedly. Whether this new view will ever find application in OCD research remains questionable. Unlike humans, companion and domestic animals do not have large frontal lobes and, presumably, do not have such complex emotional features (14).

One advantage of using spontaneously occurring animal models to study OCD is that large, relatively homologous populations of affected individuals can be compared with their symptomless counterparts under similar managemental and environmental conditions. Physiological, pharmacological, and anatomical studies of these populations are eminently feasible, and may shed new light on some currently unresolved issues. Another advantage of using animals in the study of OCD is that genealogical studies would be facilitated since breeding records are available for many species. The short generation time and large litters of some species lend themselves well to breeding experiments and gene-tracking. The use of animal models provides a new perspective on the study of human compulsive disorder and, with this new approach, a better understanding of all aspects of this group of conditions—including genetics, neurophysiology, neuropharmacology and treatment—should be possible.

There do seem to be some very strong analogies, if not homology, between animal repetitive behaviors and human OCD. We believe that with appropriate selection of the correct veterinary models, much can be unraveled to further our understanding of the spectrum of human OCD and related disorders.

REFERENCES

1. Goldberger E, Rapoport J. Canine acral lick dermatitis: Response to the antiobsessional drug clomipramine. J Am Anim Hosp Assoc 1991; 22:179–182.
2. Luescher UA. Conflict, stereotypic and compulsive behavior. Proceedings of American Veterinary Medical Association Annual Meeting, San Francisco, CA, 1994.
3. Frith CD, Done DJ. Stereotyped behavior in madness and in health. In: Cooper SJ, Dourish CT, eds. Neurobiology of Stereotyped Behavior. Oxford: Clarendon Press, 1990:232–259.
4. American Psychiatric Association. Diagnostic and Statistical Manual of Mental Disorders. 4th ed. Washington, DC: American Psychiatric Association, 1994.
5. Stein DJ, Hollander E. The spectrum of obsessive-compulsive-related disorders. In: Hollander E, ed. Obsessive Compulsive–Related Disorders. Washington, DC: American Psychiatric Press, 1993:241–271.
6. Robbins TW, Mittleman G, O'Brien J, Winn P. The neuropsychological significance of stereotypy induced by stimulant drugs. In: Cooper SJ, Dourish CT, eds. Neurobiology of Stereotyped Behavior. Oxford: Clarendon Press, 1990:26–63.
7. Baer L. Factor analysis of symptom subtypes of obsessive compulsive disorder and their relation to personality and tic disorders. J Clin Psychiatry 1994; 55(3):18–23.
8. Pauls DL, Alsobrook H, Goodman W, Rasmussen S, Leckmon JF. A family study of obsessive-compulsive disorder. Am J Psychiatry 1995; 152(1):76–84.
9. Rapoport JL. Recent advances in obsessive-compulsive disorder. Neuropsychopharmacology 1991; 5:1–10.
10. Stein DJ, Shoulberg N, Helton K, Hollander E. The neuroethological approach to obsessive compulsive disorder. Comprehen Psychiatry 1992; 33(4):274–281.
11. Rapoport JL, Wise SP. Obsessive-compulsive disorder: evidence for basal ganglia dysfunction. Psychopharm Bull 1988; 24(3):380–384.
12. Stahl SM. Basal ganglia neuropharmacology and obsessive-compulsive disorder: the obsessive-compulsive disorder hypothesis of basal ganglia dysfunction. Psychopharm Bull 1988; 24(3):370–374.
13. Insel TR. Obsessive-compulsive disorder: new models. Psychopharmacology Bull 1988; 24(3):365–369.
14. Insel TR, Mos J, Berend O. Animal models of obsessive compulsive disorder. In: Hollander E, Zohar J, Marazziti D, Olivier B, eds. Current Insights

in Obsessive Compulsive Disorder. New York: Wiley, 1994:117–135.

15. Axelrod J, Reisine TD. Stress hormones: their interaction and regulation. Science 1984; 224:452–459.

16. Cabib S, Puglisi-Allegra S, Oliverio A. Chronic stress enhances apomorphine-induced stereotyped behavior in mice: involvement of endogenous opioids. Brain Res 1984; 298:138–140.

17. Knott PJ, Hutson PH. Stress-induced stereotypy in the rat: neuropharmacological similarities to Tourette syndrome. In: Friedhoff AJ, Chase TN, eds. Gilles de la Tourette Syndrome. New York: Raven Press, 1982:233–238.

18. Shuster L, Dodman NH, D'Allesandro T, Zuroff S. Reverse tolerance to the stimulant effects of morphine in horses. Equine Vet Sci 1984; 4(5):233–236.

19. De Boer T, Nefkens F, Van Helvoirt A. The alpha 2 adrenoceptor antagonist Org 3770 enhances serotonin transmission in vivo. Eur J Pharmacol 1994; 253:R5–R6.

20. Shibasaki T, Tsumori C, Hotta M, Imaki T, Yamada K, Demura H. The response pattern of noradrenaline release to repeated stress in the hypothalamic paraventricular nucleus differs according to the form of stress in rats. Brain Res 1995; 670:169–172.

21. Goodman WK, McDougle CJ, Price LH, Riddle MA, Pauls DL, Leckman JF. Beyond the serotonergic hypothesis: a role for dopamine in some forms of obsessive-compulsive disorder. J Clin Psychiatry 1990; 51:8(suppl):36–43.

22. Stein DJ, Borchelt P, Hollander E. Pharmacotherapy of naturally occurring anxiety symptoms in dogs. Res Comm Psych Psychiatry Behav 1994; 4:39–48.

23. Overall KL. Use of clomipramine to treat ritualistic stereotypic motor behavior in three dogs. J Am Vet Med Assoc 1994; 205(12):1733–1741.

24. Dodman NH. Pharmacological treatment of behavioral problems in cats. Vet Int 1994; 4:13–20.

25. Dodman NH, Shuster L, White SD, Court MH, Parker D, Dixon R. Use of narcotic antagonists to modify stereotypic self-licking, self-chewing, and scratching behavior in dogs. J Am Vet Med Assoc 1988; 193:815–819.

26. Rapoport JL. The biology of obsessions and compulsions. Scientific American 1989; 83–89.

27. Tinbergen N. The Study of Instinct. London: Oxford University Press, 1951.

28. Lorenz K. Evolution and Modification of Behavior. Chicago: University of Chicago Press, 1966.

29. Eibl-Eibesfeldt I. Ethology: The Biology of Behavior. New York: Holt, Rinehart and Winston, 1970.

30. Muller-Using D. Ubereinige bisher unbeachtete Ubersprunghandlungen bei hoheren saugern. Z Tierpsychol 1952; 9:479–481.

31. Mason GJ. Stereotypies: a critical review. Anim Behav 1991; 41:1015–1037.

32. Dallaire A. Stress and behavior in domestic animals. Ann NY Acad Sci 1993; 697:269–274.

33. Levine S, Coe C., Wiener SG. Psychoendocrinology of stress: a psychobiological perspective. In: Levine S, Brush FR, eds. Psychoendocrinology. New York: Academic Press, 1989.
34. Ridley RM, Baker HF. Stereotypy in monkeys and humans. Psychol Med 1982; 12:61–72.
35. Schouten WGP, Wiepkema PR. Coping styles of tethered sows. Behav Proc 1991; 25:125–132.
36. Cooper JJ, Nicol CJ. The "coping hypothesis" of stereotypic behavior: a reply to Rushen. Anim Behav 1993; 45:616–618.
37. Mason GJ. Forms of stereotypic behavior. In: Lawrence AB, Rushen J, eds. Stereotypic Animal Behavior Fundamentals and Applications to Welfare. Wallingford, England: CAB International, 1993.
38. Rapoport JL. The Boy Who Couldn't Stop Washing: The Experience and Treatment of Obsessive-Compulsive Disorder. New York: EP Dutton, 1989.
39. Swedo S, Rapoport JL, Leonard H, et al. Obsessive compulsive disorder in children and adolescents: clinical phenomenology of 70 consecutive cases. Arch Gen Psychiatry 1989; 46:335–341.
40. Winchel RM. Trichotillomania: presentation and treatment. Psychiatric Ann 1992; 22(2):84–89.
41. Ladewig J, DePassile AM, Rushen J, Schouten W, Terlouw C, von Borell E. Stress and the physiological correlates of stereotypic behavior. In: Lawrence AB, Rushen J, eds. Stereotypic Animal Behavior Fundamentals and Applications to Welfare. Wallingford, England: CAB International, 1993.
42. Luescher UA, McKeown DB, Halip J. Stereotypic or obsessive-compulsive disorders in dogs and cats. In: Marder AR, Voith V, eds. Veterinary Clinics of North America. Small Animal Practice. Vol 21(2). Philadelphia: WB Saunders, 1991:401–413.
43. Hart BL, Hart LA. Canine and Feline Behavioral Therapy. Philadelphia: Lea & Febiger, 1985.
44. Luescher UA, et al. Equine stereotypies (videotape). University of Guelph production, Guelph, Ontario, 1990.
45. Kettle P, Marks I. Neurological factors in obsessive-compulsive disorder. Br J Psychiatry 1986; 149:315–319.
46. Robbins TW, Sahakian BJ. Behavioural and neurochemical determinants of drug-induced stereotypy. In: Clifford-Rose F, ed. Metabolic Disorders of the Nervous System Progress in Neurobiology Series. London: Pittman, 1981:244–291.
47. Dodman NH, Knowles K, Shuster L, Moon-Fanelli A, Tidwell A, Keen CL. Behavioral changes associated with suspected complex partial seizures in Bull Terriers. J Am Vet Med Assoc 1996; 208(5):688–691.
48. Blackshaw JK, Sutton RH, Boyhan MA. Tail chasing or circling behavior in dogs. Canine Practice 1994; 19(3):7–11.
49. Dodman NH, Bronson R, Gliatto J. Tail chasing in a bull terrier. J Am Vet Med Assoc 1993; 202(5):758–760.
50. Rasmussen SA. Genetic studies of obsessive-compulsive disorder. Ann Clin Psychiatry 1993; 5:241–248.

51. Rasmussen SA. Genetic studies of obsessive-compulsive disorder. In: Hollander E, Zohar J, Marazzati D, Olivier B, eds. New York: Wiley, 1994:105–113.
52. Lenane MC, Swedo SE, Leonard H, et al. Psychiatric disorders in first-degree relatives of children and adolescents with obsessive-compulsive disorder. J Am Acad Child Adolesc Psychiatry 1990; 29:407–412.
53. Black DW, Noyes R, Goldstein RB, Blum N. A family study of obsessive-compulsive disorder. Arch Gen Psychiatry 1992; 49:362–368.
54. Robertson MM, Gourdie A. Familial Tourette's syndrome in a large British pedigree—associated psychopathology, severity, and potential for linkage analysis. Br J Psychiatry 1990; 156:515–521.
55. Pauls DL, Leckman JF. The inheritance of Gilles de la Tourette's syndrome and associated behaviors: evidence for autosomal dominant transmission. N Engl J Med 1986; 315:997–999.
56. Pauls DL, Towbin KE, Leckman J, Zahner GEP, Cohen DJ. Gilles de la Tourette's syndrome and obsessive-compulsive disorder. Arch Gen Psychiatry 1986; 43:1180–1182.
57. Lenane MC, Swedo SE, Rapoport JL, Leonard H, Sceery W, Guroff JJ. Rates of obsesesive-compulsive disordser in first degree relatives of patients with trichotillomania: a research note. J Child Psychol Psychiatry 1992; 33(5):925–993.
58. Rapoport JL, Ryland DH, Kriete M. Drug treatment of canine acral lick: an animal model of obsessive compulsive disorder. Arch Gen Psychiatry 1992; 49:517–521.
59. Jenike MA. Pharmacologic treatment of obsessive-compulsive disorders. Psych Clin N Amer 1992; 15(4):895.
60. Hewlett WA, Vinogradov S, Agras WS. Clomipramine, clorazepam and clonidine treatment of obsessive-compulsive disorder. J Clin Psychopharmacol 1992; 12(6):420–429.
61. Montgomery SA. Pharmacological treatment of obsessive compulsive disorder. In: Hollander E, Zohar J, Marazziti D, Olivier B, eds. Current Insights in Obsessive Compulsive Disorder. New York: Wiley, 1994: 215–225.
62. Rasmussen SA. Obsessive compulsive spectrum disorders. J Clin Psychiatry 1994; 55(3):89–91.
63. Willemse T. The effect of dopamine antagonists on psychogenic alopecia in cats. In: Kwotchka KW, White SD, eds. Proceedings of the Second World Congress of Veterinary Dermatology, Montreal, Quebec, Canada, 1992: 51.
64. Stein DJ, Hollander E. Low dose pimozide augmentation of serotonin reuptake blockers in the treatment of trichotillomania. J Clin Psychiatry 1992; 53(4):123–126.
65. Christenson G, Crow SJ, MacKenzie TB, Crosby RD, Mitchell JE. A placebo controlled double blind study of naltrexone for trichotillomania. New Research Abstracts of the American Psychiatric Association Annual Meeting 1994:212.
66. Dodman NH, Shuster L, Court MH, Dixon R. Investigation into the use of

narcotic antagonists in the treatment of a stereotypic behavior pattern (crib-biting) in the horse. Am J Vet Res 1987; 48:311–319.

67. Scott JP, Fuller JL. Dog Behavior: The Genetic Basis. Chicago: University of Chicago Press, 1965.

68. Arons CD. Genetic Variability Within a Species: Differences in Behavior, Development, and Neurochemistry Among Three Types of Domestic Dogs and Their F1 Hybrids. Ph.D. dissertation, University of Connecticut, Storrs, CT, 1989.

69. Coppinger R, Glendinning J, Torop E, Matthay C, Sutherland M, Smith C. Degree of behavioral neoteny differentiates canid polymorphs. Ethology 1987; 75:89–108.

70. Moon-Fanelli A, Dodman NH. Tufts University, Grafton, MA, 1995. Data on file.

71. Moon-Fanelli AA, Dodman NH, Ginsburg BE. Compulsive stereotypy in Bull Terriers: a genetic system gone awry. Proceedings of Animal Behavior Society Meeting, Lincoln, NB, July 8–13, 1995.

72. Pemberton PL. Feline and canine behavior control: progestin therapy. In: Kirk RE, ed. Current Veterinary Therapy. Vol VII. Philadelphia: WB Saunders, 1980:62–71.

73. Brown SA, Crowell-Davis S, Malcolm T, Edwards P. Naloxone-responsive compulsive tail chasing in a dog. J Am Vet Med Assoc 1987; 190:884–886.

74. Bolles RC. Grooming behavior in the rat. J Comprehen Physiol Psychol 1966; 53(3):306–310.

75. Thiessen DD. Body temperature and grooming in the Mongolian gerbil. Ann NY Acad Sci 1988; 525:27–39.

76. Jolles J, Rompa-Barendregt J, Gipsen WH. Novelty and grooming behavior in the rat. Behav Neural Biol 1979; 25:563–572.

77. Spruijt BM, Van Hooff JA, Gipsen WH. The ethology and neurobiology of grooming behaviour. Physiol Rev 1992; 72(3):825–852.

78. Van Erp AMN. Manipulation of neuronal circuitry underlying self-grooming behavior in the rat. Proefschrift ter Verkrijging van de Graad van Doctor aan de Rjiksuniversiteit Leiden, 1993.

79. Yardley CP, Neziroglu F. Compulsions, aggression, and self-mutilation: a hypothalamic disorder? J Orthomolec Psychiatry 1978; 7(2):114–117.

80. Rapoport JL, Swedo SE, Leonard L. Childhood obsessive compulsive disorder. J Clin Psychiatry 1992; 53(4):11–16.

81. Argiolas A, Melis MR, Gessa GL. Yawning and penile errection: central dopamine-oxytocin-adrenocorticotropin connection. Ann NY Acad Sci 1988; 525:330–337.

82. Cools AR, Spruijt BM, Ellenbroeck BA. Role of central dopamine in ACTH-induced grooming behavior in rats. Ann NY Acad Sci 1988; 525:338–349.

83. Voith L. Acral lick dermatitis in the dog. Canine Pract 1986; 14(4):15–22.

84. Muller GH, Kirk RW, Scott DW. Small animal dermatology. 4th ed. Philadelphia: WB Saunders, 1989:750–757.

85. Scott DW, Walton DK. Clinical evaluation of a topical treatment for canine acral lick dermatitis. J Am Hosp Assoc 1984; 20:565–570.

86. White SD. Naltrexone treatment of acral lick dermatitis in dogs. J Am Vet Med Assoc 1990; 196(7):1073–1076.

87. Van Nes JJ. Electrophysiological evidence of sensory nerve dysfunction in 10 dogs with acral lick dermatitis. J Am Vet Med Assoc 1986; 22:157–160.

88. Young MS, Manning TO. Psychogenic dermatosis. Dermatol Rep 1984; 3:1–8.

89. Voith V. Behavioral disorders. In: Davis L, ed. Handbook of Small Animal Therapeutics. New York: Churchill-Livingstone, 1985:519–535.

90. Hart BJ, Powell KL. Antibacterial effects of saliva: role of maternal peri-parturient grooming and in licking wounds. Physiol Behav 1990; 48:383–386.

91. Overall KL. Recognition, diagnosis, and management of obsessive-compulsive disorders. Canine Pract 1992; 17(4):39–42.

92. Dodman NH. Tufts University Veterinary School, Grafton, MA, 1985. Data on file.

93. Doering GG. Acral lick dermatitis: medical management. Canine Pract 1974; 5:21–25.

94. Reid JS. Acropruritic granuloma. In: Kirk RW, ed. Current Veterinary Therapy. Vol V. Philadelphia: WB Saunders, 1974:441–443.

95. Bullock JE. Acupuncture treatment of canine lick granuloma. Calif Vet 1978; 32(4):14–15.

96. Richardson JS, Zaleski WA. Naloxone and self-mutilation. Biological Psychiatry 1983; 18:99–101.

97. Herman BH, Hammock MK, Arthur-Smith A. Naltrexone decreases self-injurious behavior. Ann Neurol 1987; 22:550–552.

98. Murphy DL, Pigott TA. A comparative examination of a role for serotonin in obsessive compulsive disorder, panic disorder, and anxiety. J Clin Psychiatry 1990; 51(4):53–60.

99. Charney DS, Woods SW, Goodman WK, et al. Serotonin function in anxiety. II. Effects of serotonin agonist *m*-CPP in panic disorder patients and healthy subjects. Psychopharmacology 1987; 92:14–24.

100. Murphy DL, Mueller EA, Hill IJL, et al. Comparative anxiogenic, neuro-endocrine, and other physiologic effects of m-chlorophenylpiperazine given intravenously or orally to healthy volunteers. Psychopharmacology 1989; 98:275–282.

101. Hart BL, Eckstein RA, Powell KL, Dodman NH. Effectiveness of buspirone on urine spraying and inappropriate urination in cats. J Am Vet Med Assoc 1993; 203(2):254–258.

102. Houpt KA. Domestic Animal Behavior. 2d ed. Ames, IA: Iowa State University Press, 1991.

103. Stoessl AJ. Dopamine D1 receptor agonist–induced grooming is blocked by the opioid receptor antagonist naloxone. Eur J Pharmacol 1994; 259:301–303.

104. Smith KC, Pittlekow MR. Naltrexone for neurotic excoriations. J Am Acad Dermatol 1989; 20:860–861.

105. Pfluger S. Baystate Medical Center, Springfield, MA, 1995. Personal communication.
106. Winchel RM, Jones SJ, Stanley B, Molcho A, Stanley M. Clinical characteristics of trichotillomania and its response to fluoxetine. J Clin Psychiatry 1992; 53:304–308.
107. Swedo SE. Trichotillomania: an obsessive compulsive spectrum disorder? In: Jenike MA, ed. Obsessional Disorders. Pediatric Clinics of North America. Vol 15. Philadelphia: WB Saunders, 1992:777–790.
108. Song MD. Diagnosing and treating feline eosinophilic granuloma complex. Vet Med 1994; 89:1141–1145.
109. Scott DW. The skin. In: Holzworth J, ed. Diseases of the Cat. Philadelphia: WB Saunders, 1987:619–675.
110. Rettew DC, Swedo SE, Leonard AL, et al. Obsessions and compulsions across time in 79 children and adolescents with obsessive-compulsive disorder. J Am Acad Child Adolesc Psychiatry 1992; 31:1050–1056.
111. Holzworth J. The skin. In: Holzworth J, ed. Diseases of the Cat. Philadelphia: WB Saunders, 1987:654–655.
112. Parker AJ, O'Brien DP, Sawchirk SA. The nervous system. In: Pratt PW, ed. Feline Medicine. Santa Barbara, CA: Am Vet Public, 1983.
113. Summers BA, Barlough JF. Nervous system and disorders. In: Siegal M, ed. The Cornell Book of Cats. New York: Villard Books, 1989:216.
114. Kraemer GW, Clarke AS. The behavioral neurobiology of self-injurious behavior in rhesus monkeys. Prog Neuro-Psychopharmacol Biol Psychiatr 1990; 14:S141–S168.
115. Wilson EO. Sociobiology: The new synthesis. Cambridge, MA: Belknap Press of Harvard University Press, 1975.
116. Fudge A. Avian giardiasis: Diagnosis, disease syndrome, and therapy. Proceedings of the Association of Avian Veterinarians, 1986:155–164.
117. Rosskopf WJ. Feather picking in psittacine birds: a clinician's approach to diagnosis and treatment. Proceedings of the Association of Avian Veterinarians, 1986:265–276.
118. Davis CS. Parrot psychology and behavior problems. Vet Clin N Am 1991; 21(6):1281–1288.
119. Davis C. Behavior modification counseling—an alliance between the veterinarian and behavior consultant. Sem Avian Exotic Med 1995; 4(1):39–42.
120. Keiper RR. Studies of stereotypy function in the canary. Anim Behav 1970; 18:353–357.
121. Rosskopf WJ, Woerpel W. The psittacine mutilation syndrome: management, incidence, possible etiology and therapy. Proceedings of the Association of Avian Veterinarians, 1990:301–304.
122. Ramsay EC, Grindlinger H. Treatment of feather picking with clomipramine. Proceedings of the Association of Avian Veterinarians, 1992:379–382.
123. Johnson CA. Chronic feather picking: a different approach to treatment. Proceedings of the International Conference on Avian Medicine, 1987:125–142.

124. Mertens PA, Dodman NH. Tufts University School of Veterinary Medicine, Grafton, MA, 1995. Data on file.
125. Luescher UA, McKeown DB, Halip J. Reviewing the causes of obsessive-compulsive disorders in horses. Vet Med May 1991:527–530.
126. Vecchiotti GG, Galanti R. Evidence of heredity of cribbing, weaving, and stall walking in thoroughbred horses. Livest Prod Sci 1986; 14:91–95.
127. Hakansson A, Franzen P, Pettersson H. Comparison of two surgical methods for treatment of crib-biting in horses. Equine Vet J 1992; 24:494–496.
128. McDonald S. Pennsylvania Veterinary School, New Bolton, PA, 1992. Personal communication.
129. Dum J, Gramsch C, Herz A. Activation of hypothalami β-endorphin pools by reward induced by highly palatable food. Pharmacol Biochem Behav 1983; 18:443–444.
130. Gillham S, Dodman NH, Shuster L, Kream R, Rand W. The effect of diet on cribbing behavior and plasma β-endorphin in horses. Applied Anim Behav Sci 1994; 41:147–153.
131. Weizman R, Gil-Ad I, Mermesh H, Munitz H, Laron Z. Immunoreactive β-endorphin, cortisol and GH plasma levels in obsessive-compulsive disorder. Clin Neuropharmacol 1990; 13:297–302.
132. Blaszczynski AP, Winter SW, McConaghy N. Plasma endorphin levels in pathological gamblers. J Gambling Behav 1986; 2:3–14.
133. Dodman NH, Shuster L. Tufts University Veterinary School, Grafton and Boston, MA, 1985. Unpublished data on file.
134. Dodman NH, Normile J, Shuster L, Rand W. Equine self-mutilation syndrome (57 cases). J Am Vet Med Assoc 1994; 204(8):1219–1223.
135. Adeloye A, Kouka N, Kuwait R. Gilles de la Tourette's syndrome associated with head injury: a case report. J Natl Med Assoc 1991; 83:1018–1020.
136. Dodman NH, Shuster L, Court MH, Patel J. Use of a narcotic antagonist (nalmefene) to suppress self-mutilative behavior in a stallion. J Am Vet Med Assoc 1988; 192(11):1585–1586.
137. Shuster L, Dodman NH. Pharmacologic study of equine Tourette's disease. Tufts University, 1995. Data on file.
138. Peterson BS, Leckman JF, Scahill L, et al. Steroid hormones and Tourette's syndrome: early experience with antiandrogen therapy. J Clin Psychopharmacol 1994; 14(2):131–135.
139. Laurence AB, Rushen J. Stereotypic animal behavior: fundamentals and applications to welfare. Wallingford, England: CAB International, 1993.
140. Redbo I. The influence of restraint on the occurrence of oral stereotypies in cows. Appl Anim Behav Sci 1992; 35:115–123.
141. Danzer R. Behavioral, physiological and functional aspects of stereotyped behavior: a review and re-interpretation. J Anim Sci 1986; 62:1776–1786.
142. Rushen JP. Stereotypies, aggression and feeding schedules of tethered sows. Appl Anim Behav Sci 1985; 14:137–147.
143. Terlouw EM, Lawrence AB. Long-term effects of food allowance and

housing on development of stereotypies in pigs. Appl Anim Behav Sci 1993; 38:103–125.

144. Fraser AF, Broom DM. Farm Animal Behavior and Welfare. London: Ballieres Tindall, 1990.

145. Cronin GM. The development and significance of abnormal stereotyped behavior in tethered sows. Ph.D. dissertation, Agricultural University of Wageningen, The Netherlands, 1985.

146. Cronin GM, Wiepkema PR, van Ree JM. Endogenous opioids are involved in abnormal stereotyped behaviors of tethered sows. Neuropeptides 1985; 6:527–530.

147. Wiepkema PR. Behavioural aspects of stress. In: Wiepkema PR, Van Adrichem PWM, eds. The Biology of Stress in Farm Animals. Dordrecht: Martinus Nijhoff, 1987:113–134.

148. Redbo J. Stereotypies and cortisol secretion in heifers subjected to tethering. Appl Anim Behav Sci 1993; 38:213–225.

149. Hessing MJC, Hagelso AM, Schouten WGP, Wiepkema PR, van Beek JAM. Individual behavioral and physiological strategies in pigs. Physiol Behav 1993; 55:39–46.

150. Rushen J. The "coping hypothesis" of stereotypic behaviours. Anim Behav 1993; 45:613–615.

151. Terlouw EMC, Lawrence AB, Illius AW. Influences of feeding level and physical restraint on the development of stereotypies in sows. Anim Behav 1991; 42:981–992.

152. Dantzer R. Animal welfare methodology and criteria. Rev Sci Tech Off Int Epiz 1994; 13(1):291–302.

153. Cronin GM, Wiepkema PR, van Ree JM. Endorphins implicated in stereotypies of tethered sows. Experientia 1986; 42:198–199.

154. Berkson G, Mason WA, Saxon SV. Situation and stimulus effects on stereotyped behaviors of chimpanzees. J Comp Physiol Psychol 1963; 56:786–792.

155. Meyer-Holzapfel M. Abnormal behavior in zoo animals. In: Fox MV, ed. Abnormal Behavior in Animals. New York: WB Saunders, 1968:475–480.

156. Wechsler B. Stereotypies and attentiveness to novel stimuli: a test in polar bears. Appl Anim Behav Sci 1992; 33:381–388.

157. Kenny DE. Use of naltrexone for treatment of psychogenically induced dermatoses in five zoo animals. J Am Vet Med Assoc 1994; 205:1021–1023.

158. Wise S. A brief history of the basal ganglia. In: Carroll B, ed. Psychopathology of the Brain. New York: Raven Press, 1991.

159. Griffen DR. The Question of Animal Awareness. New York: Rockefeller University Press, 1976.

160. Griffen DR. Animal Thinking. Cambridge, MA: Harvard University Press, 1984.

161. Ristau CA, ed. The Minds of Other Animals: Essays in Honor of Donald R. Griffin. New Jersey: Lawrence Erlbaum, 1991.

162. Cheney DL, Seyfarth RM. How Monkeys See the World: Inside the Mind of Another Species. Chicago: University of Chicago Press, 1991.
163. Stein DJ, Dodman NH, Borchelt P, Hollander E. Behavioral disorders in veterinary practice: relevance to psychiatry. Comprehen Psychiatry 1994; 35(4):275–285.

7

Serotonin-Reuptake Inhibitors in the Treatment of OCD

Darin Dougherty and Scott L. Rauch

Massachusetts General Hospital
and Harvard Medical School
Boston, Massachusetts

INTRODUCTION

Obsessive-compulsive disorder (OCD) has a lifetime prevalence of 1–3% worldwide (1). A number of available treatments, including behavioral therapy and pharmacological intervention, are effective in ameliorating the symptoms of OCD. Initial medication therapies provide clinically significant improvement in approximately 60% of OCD patients, and a higher percentage may benefit following serial trials of various agents (2,3). Therefore, up to 40% of patients with OCD do not experience significant benefits from initial medication treatment trials (2,3); treatment resistance may be defined as failure to achieve 25% reduction of baseline symptoms.

Serotonin-reuptake inhibitors (SRIs) represent the first-line pharmacological treatment for OCD. In contrast, predominantly noradrenergic reuptake blockers do not show antiobsessional efficacy. Although current theories regarding the mechanism of action of SRIs may prove overly simplistic, it is known that SRIs inhibit presynaptic serotonergic reuptake (4,5). Reuptake blockade extends the period that serotonin remains in the synaptic cleft, and thus presumably increases serotonergic neurotransmission. However, this reuptake inhibition occurs rapidly whereas clinical benefits are not seen for weeks. Therefore, more complex molecular mechanisms, such as changes in second-messenger systems, are hypothesized to actually mediate the therapeutic antiobsessional effects of SRIs (6).

In addition to OCD, SRIs are used in the treatment of a number of other disorders including major depression, panic disorder, social phobia, and eating disorders. Because SRIs are effective treatments for such disorders, some theorists have inferred that dysregulation of the serotonergic system plays a role in their pathophysiology. In fact, SRIs probably do provide their beneficial effects through their interactions with the serotonergic system. Likewise, SRIs can cause side effects via their primary action as inhibitors of serotonin uptake, as well as through interactions with other receptor systems.

In this chapter we review the clinical data pertaining to the use of SRIs for OCD. We present pharmacokinetic, pharmacodynamic, and side-effect information in addition to highlighting possible interactions between SRIs and other common medications. Finally, we offer recommendations regarding the treatment of OCD with SRIs.

CLINICAL ASSESSMENT

Differential Diagnosis and Comorbidity

Although the diagnosis of OCD is often straightforward, heralded by classic symptoms, sometimes OCD presents with atypical features. Conversely, other disorders may present with symptoms reminiscent of OCD: the ruminations of depression, intrusive thoughts or delusions of psychotic disorders, and stereotyped behaviors of organic mental disorders, to name a few. Comprehensive clinical evaluation with careful differential diagnosis is essential before initiating treatment for OCD.

Even with proper diagnosis, psychiatric comorbidity is common in OCD. It is estimated that up to two-thirds of all patients with OCD have lifetime comorbidities (1,7). These comorbid conditions not only serve to cloud the diagnostic picture, but can also influence the selection of optimal treatments. Fortunately, many of the conditions that occur with OCD are likewise responsive to SRIs.

Treatment Response

Once treatment has been initiated for OCD, it is important to monitor the patient's response over time. The degree of symptom resolution, or lack thereof, will direct the clinician regarding dosage adjustment or switching to an alternative treatment. Although it is possible to assess treatment response qualitatively through periodic clinical interviews, we recommend the regular use of validated scales such as the Yale-Brown Obsessive Compulsive Scale (Y-BOCS) to quantify the ongoing severity of OCD symptoms (8,9). Studies of response rates with SRIs show that approximately 60% of patients will experience at least a 25–35% decrease in symptoms (3). Although clinical research protocols typically operationalize responder status in terms of this 25 or 35% reduction in Y-BOCS score, in clinical practice, the benchmark for acceptable response must be determined in collaboration with the patient. Furthermore, although the Y-BOCS score is an excellent gauge of symptomatic improvement, the overall change in quality of life must also be considered. It is important at the outset of treatment to inform patients that 100% reduction of symptoms is rare. Finally, in addition to systematic assessment of efficacy, it is equally important for clinicians to ask about side effects at every visit.

GENERAL DESCRIPTION AND PHARMACOLOGY OF THE SRIs

Description

SRIs include clomipramine (Anafranil), fluoxetine (Prozac), sertraline (Zoloft), paroxetine (Paxil), and fluvoxamine (Luvox). Of these, fluoxetine, sertraline, paroxetine, and fluvoxamine are the newer so-called "selective serotonin-reuptake inhibitors" (SSRIs), characterized by minimal affinity or pharmacological action at receptor sites other than the serotonin transporter. Clomipramine, on the other hand, is a tricyclic antidepressant (TCA). Thus, although clomipramine's serotonin-reuptake-blocking properties are similar to those of the SSRIs, it also has pharmacologically significant affinity for cholinergic and adrenergic receptors, thereby influencing its side-effect profile.

Pharmacology

While all SRIs block reuptake of serotonin presynaptically, there are other pharmacological characteristics that distinguish these agents from one another, including differences in metabolism, half-life, protein binding, and effects on other neurotransmitter systems (see Table 1) (4,10,11). All SRIs undergo hepatic metabolism and renal excretion. SRIs may be divided into those with active and those with inactive metabolites. For clomipramine, fluoxetine, and sertraline, which have active metabolites, the half-life of the daughter compound must be considered when estimating duration of effect after dosing. In general, measuring serum levels of SRIs and/or their metabolites has not been useful in determining effective dosage or predicting clinical response.

Table 1 Pharmacological Profile of SRIs

	Fluoxetine	Paroxetine	Sertraline	Fluvoxa-mine	Clomipramine
Half-life (hrs)	24–72	20	25	15	19–37
Metabolite	Active	Inactive	Active	Inactive	Active
Protein binding (%)	94	95	99	77	97
Uptake inhibition (Ki)[a]					
5-HT (nM)	25	1.1	7.3	6.2	7.4
NE (nM)	500	350	1,400	1,100	96
DA (nM)	4200	2000	230	>10,000	9100

[a] Lower Ki indicates higher affinity for uptake inhibition.
Source: Refs. 4,5,10,11.

Protein binding may influence levels of available drug in at least two ways: 1) if the patient is on other highly protein-bound medicines, competition can produce elevated levels of the SRI and/or the other agent and 2) hypoproteinemia, as seen in chronic medical illness, malnutrition, or advanced age, can lead to higher concentrations of unbound SRI (i.e., the active form). There are subtle differences in the relative affinities of the various SRIs for monoaminergic reuptake sites, and more prominent differences between clomipramine and the SSRIs with respect to anticholinergic and antiadrenergic postsynaptic effects. As elaborated below, these pharamacological distinctions do not appear to have major consequences in terms of differential efficacy, but they do influence side-effect profile.

EFFICACY OF SRIs FOR OCD

Numerous studies demonstrate the efficacy of SRIs in the treatment of OCD (see Table 2) (12–37). Clomipramine has been commercially available the longest, and therefore represents the most studied and arguably the most tried and true of the antiobsessional agents. Numerous trials, including placebo-controlled studies, indicate that clomipramine is an effective antiobsessional treatment, significantly superior to placebo (12–18) and nonserotonergic antidepressant agents (18–25). The SSRIs have also been studied in rigorous fashion, and proven effective as antiobsessional medications (26–34). In addition to the abundant data in adults, there are analogous studies demonstrating the antiobsessional efficacy of SRIs in children and adolescents (see Table 3) (38–44).

Table 2 Controlled Trials of SRI Therapy for OCD in Adult Patients

Studies	Conditions	Results
Clomipramine (CMI) vs. Placebo or Non-SRIs (12–25)		
Karabanow, 1977 (12)	CMI vs. placebo	CMI superior to placebo
Montgomery, 1980 (13)	CMI vs. placebo crossover	CMI superior to placebo
Mavissakalin et al., 1985 (14)	CMI vs. placebo	CMI superior to placebo
Jenike, 1989 (15)	CMI vs. placebo	CMI superior to placebo
Greist et al., 1990 (16)	CMI vs. placebo	73% improved on CMI
		6% improved on placebo
CMI collaborative group, 1991 (17)	CMI vs. placebo	38–44% decrease Sx with CMI
		3–5% decrease Sx with placebo
Thoren et al., 1980 (18)	CMI vs. nort. vs. placebo	CMI, but not nort., superior to placebo
Ananth et al., 1981 (19)	CMI vs. amitriptyline	CMI superior to amitriptyline
Insel et al., 1983 (20)	CMI vs. clorgyline	CMI effective; clorgyline not
Zahn et al., 1984 (21)	CMI vs. clorgyline	CMI superior to clorgyline
Volavka et al., 1985 (22)	CMI vs. imipramine	CMI superior to imipramine
Cui, 1986 (23)	CMI vs. doxepin	78% improve on CMI
		36% improve on doxepin
Lei, 1986 (24)	CMI vs. imipramine crossover	CMI superior to imipramine
Zhao, 1991 (25)	CMI vs. amitriptyline	95% improve on CMI
		56% improve on amitriptyline
SSRIs vs. Placebo or Non-SRIs (26–34)		
Perse et al., 1987 (26)	Fluvoxamine vs. placebo	Fluvoxamine superior to placebo
Goodman et al., 1989 (27)	Fluvoxamine vs. placebo	Fluvoxamine superior to placebo
Jenike, 1990 (28)	Fluvoxamine vs. placebo	Fluvoxamine superior to placebo

Table 2 Continued

Studies	Conditions	Results
Rasmussen et al., in press (29)	Fluvoxamine vs. placebo	Fluvoxamine superior to placebo
Goodman et al., 1990 (30)	Fluvoxamine vs. desipramine	Fluvoxamine superior to desipramine
Chouinard et al., 1990 (31)	Sertraline vs. placebo	Sertraline superior to placebo
Jenike et al., 1990 (32)	Sertraline vs. placebo	Sertraline superior to placebo
Greist et al., 1992 (33)	Sertraline vs. placebo	Sertraline superior to placebo
Tollefson et al., 1994 (34)	Fluoxetine vs. placebo	Fluoxetine superior to placebo
SRIs vs. SRIs (35–37)		
Den Boer et al., 1987 (35)	CMI vs. fluvoxamine	Comparable efficacy
Freeman et al., 1994 (36)	CMI vs. fluvoxamine	Comparable efficacy
Pigott et al., 1990 (37)	CMI vs. fluoxetine	Comparable efficacy

Table 3 Controlled Trials of SRI Therapy for OCD in Children and Adolescents

Study	Conditions	Results
Flament et al., 1985 (38,39)	CMI vs. placebo	CMI superior to placebo
Devaugh-Geiss et al., 1992 (40)	CMI vs. placebo	37% decrease Sx on CMI 8% decrease Sx on placebo
Rapoport et al., 1980 (41)	CMI vs. DMI vs. placebo	No differences
Leonard et al., 1988 (42)	CMI vs. DMI	CMI superior to DMI
Leonard et al., 1991 (43)	CMI substituted with DMI in 50%	89% on DMI relapsed 18% on CMI relapsed
Riddle et al., 1992 (44)	Fluoxetine vs. placebo	Fluoxetine superior to placebo

With respect to relative efficacy among SRIs, few adequately powered head-to-head studies have been performed. Thus far, no published results provide compelling data to support the superiority of any SRI over others in terms of antiobsessional efficacy (35–37). Greist and colleagues (3) performed a meta-analysis of four large multicenter placebo-controlled trials of SRIs for the treatment of OCD. This meta-analysis incorporated data from hundreds of patients treated with clomipramine, fluoxetine, fluvoxamine, or sertraline. All four medications were shown to be superior to placebo for the treatment of OCD. Although the meta-analysis suggests that clomipramine is superior to the three SSRIs in that greater clinical improvement was seen with clomipramine, limitations in the methodology of the meta-analysis have been acknowledged. For instance, the fact that clomipramine had been studied prior to the availability of other SRIs meant that subjects enrolled in clomipramine trials necessarily represented an SRI-naive cohort, whereas a substantial proportion of patients enrolled in subsequent trials of the SSRIs were SRI nonresponders.

ADMINISTRATION OF SRIs FOR OCD

Several administration parameters for SRIs differ when they are used as antiobsessionals versus when they are used as antidepressants. First, SRI trials for OCD may require longer duration; at least 10 weeks is recommended to fairly assess the antiobsessional response to a given agent. Second, the dosages of SRIs recommended in the treatment of OCD often exceed those recommended for depression (45). Guidelines regarding SRI dose ranges for OCD are as follows: 150–250 mg/day for clomipramine, 40–80 mg/day for fluoxetine, 50–200 mg/day for sertraline,

200–300 mg/day for fluvoxamine, and 40–60 mg/day for paroxetine. Although the target doses of these agents may be higher when used for OCD, starting doses should be comparable to or even lower than those used in the treatment of depression. Third, guidelines regarding duration of treatment and antiobsessional medication discontinuation are tentative. Extant data as well as anecdotal collective experience suggest that OCD symptoms typically return following abrupt discontinuation of SRIs (46). Additional studies are necessary to determine optimal strategies for minimizing dose and duration of SRIs in the long-term treatment of OCD. Similarly, insufficient data are available regarding optimal antiobsessional dosages and treatment duration in pediatric populations.

SIDE EFFECTS AND DRUG INTERACTIONS

Side effects

Efficacy must be weighed against side effects when choosing between treatment options for any disorder. Furthermore, the importance of a medication's side-effect profile is magnified when the treatment is likely to be chronic, as is often the case in OCD. All SRIs can cause side effects attributable to their fundamental serotonergic mode of action. In addition, clomipramine, as is typical for TCAs, is most apt to cause anticholinergic and antiadrenergic side effects, whereas SSRIs tend to cause fewer side effects mediated via nonserotonergic receptor systems (see Tables 4 and 5) (4,10,11,47–51).

TCAs such as clomipramine have effects beyond those attributable to their properties as reuptake inhibitors (51). They are known to have a quinidine-like antiarrhythmic effect that slows intracardiac conduction. Although generally an issue only in patients with known cardiac disease, occasional adverse effects may be seen in patients with no documented pre-existing condition. Furthermore, the cardiac conduction effects of TCAs lead to much greater toxicity than seen in SSRIs when

Table 4 Side Effects of Tricyclic Antidepressants (e.g., Clomipramine)

Anticholinergic: dry mouth, blurred vision, constipation, urinary hesitancy
Antiadrenergic: postural hypotension
Cardiac conduction abnormalities (e.g., prolonged QT)
Decreased seizure threshold
Weight gain
Sexual dysfunction

Source: Refs. 47,49–51.

Table 5   Side Effects of SSRIs

Agitation/insomnia
Gastrointestinal distress
Headache
Sexual dysfunction

Source: Refs. 4,10,11,48,49,51.

large doses are taken, as in the context of overdose. This is a critical issue, because suicide attempts can be a factor in OCD as well as in common comorbid disorders, such as major depression. TCAs have anticholinergic effects that can cause tachycardia, blurred vision, fever, constipation, urinary retention, and confusion (10). Orthostatic hypotension may occur as a result of alpha$_1$-adrenergic antagonism (10). Lastly, clomipramine is known to lower seizure threshold (50).

SSRIs are relatively safe compared to TCAs. Few, if any, cases of death have been reported following overdose with SSRIs. Although side effects are generally less severe, one may see agitation or anxiety, nausea, headaches, and sexual dysfunction (4). While any of these side effects can contribute to noncompliance, sexual dysfunction is seen in as many as one-third of patients (48) but may not be readily reported unless the clinician specifically inquires about it. There is little systematic data on the treatment of SSRI-induced sexual dysfunction, but case reports and clinical practice have shown that effective interventions may include switching to another SSRI or adding yohimbine (an alpha$_2$-adrenergic antagonist), amantidine (a dopamine agonist), cyproheptadine (an antihistaminic/antiserotonergic agent), or buspirone (49).

Drug Interactions

Patients being treated for OCD are often taking other medications concurrently. Therefore, potential drug interactions must be considered when selecting an antiobsessional agent. In addition to well-established drug interactions known to occur in conjunction with clomipramine (or other TCAs), individuals may also experience idiosyncratic reactions (see Table 6) (47,49,51–55). Some medications interact with clomipramine by influencing its plasma concentration, while others potentiate clomipramine's side effects via synergy at relevant receptor sites. For instance, the hypotensive effects of clomipramine can be exacerbated by alpha-methyldopa, beta-adrenergic blockers, clonidine, diuretics, and low-potency antipsychotics. Quinidine and other class Ia antiarrhythmics as well as thioridazine, mesoridazine, and pimozide may add to cardiotoxic

Table 6   Tricyclic Antidepressant Drug Interactions

Interaction	Agents
Prolong cardiac conduction time	Type Ia antiarrhythmics
Raise TCA level and prolong QT interval	Phenothiazines
Additive hypotensive effect	Alpha-adrenergic blockers
Increase prothrombin time	Warfarin
Raise TCA levels	Cimetidine, disulfiram, methylphenidate
Lower TCA levels	Oral contraceptives, alcohol, phenytoin

Source: Refs. 47,49,51–55.

effects of TCAs. Numerous common medications that have anticholinergic effects can synergize with TCAs to produce anticholinergic toxicity, including antihistamines, antiparkinsonians, low-potency antipsychotics, over-the-counter sleeping pills, and antispasmodics or antidiarrheals. Conversely, TCAs such as clomipramine can potentiate the effects of warfarin or block the effects of guanethidine.

SSRIs can participate in drug interactions as a consequence of effects on the hepatic cytochrome P450 system (see Table 7) (52–54). As each SSRI is metabolized by one or more isoenzymes of cytochrome P450, they may either inhibit or induce the corresponding enzymatic activity, thereby affecting the metabolism of other drugs. Conversely, other medications can inhibit or induce the P450 system, thereby modulating the metabolism of SRIs. Table 7 outlines known P450 interactions, categorized by the isoenzymes involved (52–54). It is important to realize that there is tremendous individual variation in these P450 effects. In addition, the fact that SSRIs are highly protein-bound can lead to drug interactions that do not involve the cytochrome P450 system per se. For example, SSRIs can compete with warfarin, carbamezapine, and valproate for protein-binding sites, leading to increased levels of these agents, with accompanying adverse effects. In general, these interactions do not represent absolute contraindications to coadministration. Rather, the cognizant pharmacologist need only be attentive regarding necessary adjustments to the dose of SRIs or other medications in this context.

RECOMMENDATIONS AND SPECIFIC TREATMENT GUIDELINES

There are overwhelming data supporting the efficacy of SRIs for OCD, and they are undeniably the first-line pharmacological treatment for OCD. Although most patients with OCD will need chronic treatment with SRIs, gains made via behavioral therapy may facilitate SRI dose

Table 7 Cytochrome P450 Drug Interactions

Enzyme	Fluoxetine	Fluvoxamine	Paroxetine	Sertraline	Drug Interaction
1A2		×			TCAs, theophylline, antipsychotics
2D6	×		×	×	TCAs, antipsychotics, type Ic antiarrhythmics
2C	×	×		×	Phenytoin, diazepam, tolbutamide
3A4	×	×		×	Carbamazepine, alprazolam, terfenadine, astemizole

Source: Refs. 52–54.

reductions or even permit discontinuation of medication altogether. When using SRIs for OCD, start at low doses to minimize side effects, including their potential initial anxiogenic effects. The dosage of SRIs should then be gradually advanced as tolerated to an initial target. For instance, fluoxetine might be advanced from 10 mg per day to 60 mg per day over a 3-week period. As previously noted, response to a given dosage cannot be fairly assessed in less than 10 weeks. Some experts prefer advancing the medication, as tolerated, to a maximum dose within the recommended range. Then, following an additional 10 weeks of treatment, if response is unsatisfactory, augmentation strategies or transition to an alternative SRI can be initiated in the interest of greatest time efficiency. On the other hand, if the response to a maximal tolerated dose is satisfactory, the dose can be gradually reduced after a few weeks, so the minimum effective dosage can be titrated in the context of maintenance therapy.

Despite the pharmacological similarities among the SRIs, patients may prove responsive to one agent while being resistant to another. We recommend that at least three adequate serial trials of SRIs (including two different SSRIs as well as clomipramine) before a patient should be considered SRI-refractory. If a given SRI is well tolerated but ineffective, it may be most prudent to proceed with augmentation before moving on to the next SRI trial. Some clinicians are inclined to forgo augmentation if an SRI alone is completely ineffective, pursuing augmentation only in the face of partial response. Augmentation strategies and non-SRI alternative monotherapies are discussed in Chapters 8 and 9. Interestingly, limited experience with intravenous clomipramine indicates that this alternative route of administration might provide relief in patients refractory to oral SRI therapies (56).

SUMMARY

In summary, SRIs are the first-line pharmacological treatment for OCD. Used correctly, the majority of patients experience clinically significant improvement on these agents, although residual symptoms are common. Several factors should be taken into account when prescribing an SRI. Initial selection from among the available agents should be based on subtle differences in pharmacology, side-effect profile, and known drug interactions. In general, SSRIs tend to be better tolerated than clomipramine; however, along with considerations about drug interactions, treatment decisions should be made on a case-by-case basis. Likewise, although prevailing differences between the SRIs with respect to efficacy have not been proven, individual patients may well show substantial differential responses. Practices pertaining to starting dosage and rate of up-titration can be influenced by a patient's disposition regarding potential side effects and his sense of urgency in seeking symptom relief. As reviewed elsewhere, other pharmacotherapies or behavioral therapy may augment the beneficial effects of SRIs. Thus, although future scientific advances may someday provide superior treatments, SRIs remain the mainstay of pharmacotherapy for OCD.

ACKNOWLEDGMENTS

Research and educational activities at the Massachusetts General Hospital Obsessive Compulsive Disorders Unit are supported in part via the David Judah Research Fund. The authors thank Michael Jenike, M.D., for his mentorship in this domain.

REFERENCES

1. Rasmussen SA, Eisen JL. The epidemiology and differential diagnosis of obsessive compulsive disorder. J Clin Psychiatry 1994; 55(suppl):5–14.
2. Goodman WK, McDougle CJ, Price LH. Pharmacotherapy of obsessive compulsive disorder. J Clin Psychiatry 1992; 53(suppl):29–37.
3. Greist JH, Jefferson JW, Kobak KA, et al. Efficacy and tolerability of serotonin transport inhibitors in obsessive compulsive disorder: a meta-analysis. Arch Gen Psychiatry 1995; 52:53–60.
4. Grimsley SR, Jann MW. Paroxetine, sertraline, and fluvoxamine: new selective serotonin reuptake inhibitors. Clin Pharm 1992; 11:930–957.

5. Preskorn SH. Basic neuropharmacology of SSRIs. In: Preskorn SH, ed. Clinical Pharmacology of Selective Serotonin Reuptake Inhibitors. Oklahoma: Professional Communications, 1996:33–62

6. Hyman SE, Nestler EJ. Initiation and adaptation: a paradigm for understanding psychotropic drug action. Am J Psychiatry 1996; 153:151–162.

7. Karno M, Golding JM, Sorenson SB, et al. The epidemiology of obsessive compulsive disorder in five US communities. Arch Gen Psychiatry 1988; 45:1094–1099.

8. Goodman WK, Price LH, Rasmussen SA, et al. The Yale-Brown Obsessive Compulsive Scale (Y-BOCS). Part I. Development, use, and reliability. Arch Gen Psychiatry 1989; 46:1006–1011.

9. Goodman WK, Price LH, Rasmussen SA, et al. The Yale-Brown Obsessive Compulsive Scale (Y-BOCS). Part II. Validity. Arch Gen Psychiatry 1989; 46:1012–1016.

10. Richelson E. The pharmacology of antidepressants at the synapse: focus on newer compounds. J Clin Psychiatry 1994; 55(suppl):34–39.

11. Tollefson GD. Selective serotonin reuptake inhibitors. In: Schatzberg AF, Nemeroff CB, eds. Textbook of Psychopharmacology. Washington, DC: American Psychiatric Press, 1995:161–182.

12. Karabanow O. Double-blind controlled study in phobias and obsessions. J Int Med Res 1977; 5(suppl):42–48.

13. Montgomery SA. Clomipramine in obsessional neurosis: a placebo-controlled trial. Pharmaceutical Med 1980; 1(2):189–192.

14. Mavissakalian M, Turner SM, Michelson L, et al. Tricyclic antidepressants in obsessive compulsive disorder: antiobsessional or antidepressant agents? Am J Psychiatry 1985; 142:572–576.

15. Jenike MA, Baer L, Summergrad P, et al. Obsessive compulsive disorder: a double-blind placebo-controlled trial of clomipramine in 27 patients. Am J Psychiatry 1989; 146:1328–1330.

16. Greist JH, Jefferson JW, Rosenfeld R, et al. Clomipramine and obsessive compulsive disorder: a placebo-controlled double-blind study of 32 patients. J Clin Psychiatry 1990; 51(7):292–297.

17. Clomipramine Collaborative Group. Clomipramine in the treatment of patients with obsessive compulsive disorder. Arch Gen Psychiatry 1991; 48:730–738.

18. Thoren P, Asberg M, Cronholm B, et al. Clomipramine treatment of obsessive compulsive disorder. I. A controlled clinical trial. Arch Gen Psychiatry 1980; 37:1281–1285.

19. Ananth J, Pecknold JC, van den Steen N, et al. Double-blind comparative study clomipramine and amitriptyline in obsessive neurosis. Prog Neuropsychopharmacol 1981; 5(3):257–262.

20. Insel TR, Murphy DL, Cohen RM, et al. Obsessive compulsive disorder: a double-blind trial of clomipramine and clorgyline. Arch Gen Psychiatry 1983; 40:605–612.

21. Zahn TP, Insel TR, Murphy DL. Psychophysiological changes during phar-

macological treatment of patients with obsessive compulsive disorder. Br J Psychiatry 1984; 145:39–44.

22. Volavka J, Neziroglu F, Yaryura-Tobias JA. Clomipramine and imipramine in obsessive compulsive disorder. Psychiatry Res 1985; 14(1):83–91.

23. Cui YE. A double-blind trial of chlorimipramine and doxepin in obsessive compulsive disorder. Chung Hua Shen Ching Shen Ko Tsa Chih 1986; 19(5):279–281.

24. Lei BS. A crossover treatment of obsessive compulsive neurosis with imipramine and clomipramine. Chung Hua Shen Ching Shen Ko Tsa Chih 1986; 19(5):275–278.

25. Zhao JP. A controlled study of clomipramine and amitriptyline for treating obsessive compulsive disorder. Chung Hua Shen Ching Shen Ko Tsa Chih 1991; 24(2):68–70.

26. Perse TL, Greist JH, Jefferson JW, et al. Fluvoxamine treatment of obsessive compulsive disorder. Am J Psychiatry 1987; 144:1543–1548.

27. Goodman WK, Price LH, Rasmussen SA, et al. Efficacy of fluvoxamine in obsessive compulsive disorder: a double-blind comparison with placebo. Arch Gen Psychiatry 1989; 46:36–44.

28. Jenike MA, Hyman SE, Baer L, et al. A controlled trial of fluvoxamine for obsessive compulsive disorder: implications for a serotonergic theory. Am J Psychiatry 1990; 147:1209–1215.

29. Rasmussen SA, Goodman WK, Greist JH, et al. Fluvoxamine in the treatment of obsessive-compulsive disorder: a multi-center, double-blind placebo-controlled study in outpatients. Am J Psychiatry. In press.

30. Goodman WK, Price LH, Delgado PL, et al. Specificity of serotonin reuptake inhibitors in the treatment of obsessive compulsive disorder. Arch Gen Psychiatry 1990; 47:577–585.

31. Chouinard G, Goodman W, Greist J, et al. Results of a double-blind placebo-controlled trial using a new serotonin reuptake inhibitor, sertraline, in obsessive compulsive disorder. Psychopharmacol Bull 1990; 26:279–284.

32. Jenike MA, Baer L, Summergrad P, et al. Sertraline in obsessive compulsive disorder: a double-blind comparison with placebo. Am J Psychiatry 1990; 147:923–928.

33. Greist J, Chouinard G, DuBoff E, et al. Double-blind comparison of three doses of sertraline and placebo in the treatment of outpatients with obsessive compulsive disorder. Arch Gen Psychiatry 1995; 52(4):289–295.

34. Tollefson GD, Rampey AH, Potvin JH, et al. A multicenter investigation of fixed-dose fluoxetine in the treatment of obsessive compulsive disorder. Arch Gen Psychiatry 1994; 51(7):559–567.

35. Den Boer JA, Westenberg HGM, Kamerbeek WDJ, et al. Effect of serotonin uptake inhibitors in anxiety disorders: a double-blind comparison of clomipramine and fluvoxamine. Int Clin Psychopharmacol 1987; 2(1):21–32.

36. Freeman CPL, Trimble MR, Deakin JFW, et al. Fluvoxamine versus clomipramine in the treatment of obsessive compulsive disorder: a multicenter, randomized, double-blind, parallel group comparison. J Clin Psychiatry 1994; 55(7):301–305.

37. Pigott TA, Pato MT, Bernstein SE, et al. Controlled comparisons of clomipramine and fluoxetine in the treatment of obsessive compulsive disorder. Arch Gen Psychiatry 1990; 47:926–932.
38. Flament MF, Rapoport JL, Berg CJ, et al. A controlled trial of clomipramine in childhood obsessive compulsive disorder. Psychopharm Bull 1985; 21(1):150–151.
39. Flament MF, Rapoport JL, Berg CJ, et al. Clomipramine treatment of childhood obsessive compulsive disorder. Arch Gen Psychiatry 1985; 42:977–983.
40. DeVaugh-Geiss J, Moroz G, Biederman J, et al. Clomipramine hydrochloride in childhood and adolescent obsessive compulsive disorder: a multicenter trial. J Am Acad Child Adolesc Psychiatry 1992; 31(1):45–49.
41. Rapoport J, Elkins R, Mikkelsen E, et al. Clinical controlled trial of chorimipramine in adolescents with obsessive compulsive disorder. Psychopharmacol Bull 1980; 16(3):61–63.
42. Leonard HL, Swedo SE, Rapoport JL, et al. Treatment of childhood obsessive compulsive disorder with clomipramine and desmethylimipramine: a double-blind crossover comparison. Psychopharmacol Bull 1988; 24:93–95.
43. Leonard HL, Swedo SE, Lenane MC, et al. A double-blind desipramine substitution during long-term clomipramine treatment in children and adolescents with obsessive compulsive disorder. Arch Gen Psychiatry 1991; 48:922–927.
44. Riddle MA, Scahill L, King RA, et al. Fluoxetine in the treatment of obsessive compulsive disorder in children and adolescents. J Am Acad Child Adolesc Psychiatry 1992; 31(3):575.
45. Montgomery SA, McIntyre A, Osterheider M, et al. A double-blind placebo-controlled study of fluoxetine in patients with DSM-IIIR obsessive compulsive disorder. Eur Neuropsychopharmacol 1993; 3:143–152.
46. Pato MT, Zohar-Kaduch R, Zohar J, et al. Return of symptoms after discontinuation of clomipramine in patients with obsessive compulsive disorder. Am J Psychiatry 1988; 145:1521–1525.
47. Glassman AH, Preudhomme XA. Review of the cardiovascular effects of heterocyclic antidepressants. J Clin Psychiatry 1993; 54(suppl):16–22.
48. Herman JB, Brotman AW, Pollack MH, et al. Treatment emergent sexual dysfunction with fluoxetine. J Clin Psychiatry 1990; 51:25–27.
49. Pollack MH, Smoller JW. Management of antidepressant-induced side effects. In: Challenges in Clinical Practice New York: Guilford Press, 1996:451–480.
50. Rosenstein DL, Nelson C, Jacobs SC. Seizures associated with antidepressants: a review. J Clin Psychiatry 1993; 54:289.
51. Baldessarini RJ. Drugs and the treatment of psychiatric disorders: depression and mania. In: Hardman JG, Limbird LE, Molinoff PB, Ruddon RW, Gilman AG, eds. Goodman and Gilman's The Pharmacological Basis of Therapeutics. 9th ed. New York: McGraw-Hill, 1996:431–459.
52. Shen WW, Lin KM. Cytochrome P450 monooxygenases and interactions of psychotropic drugs. Int J Psych Med 1991; 21:47–56.

53. von Moltke LL, Greenblatt DJ, Harmatz JS, et al. Cytochromes in psychopharmacology. J Clin Psychopharmacol 1994; 14:1–4.
54. Nemeroff CB, DeVane L, Pollack BG. Newer antidepressants and the cytochrome P450 system. Am J Psychiatry 1996; 153:311–320.
55. Stoudamire A, Fogel BS. Psychopharmacology in the medically ill. In: Principles of Medical Psychiatry. Orlando, FL: Grune & Stratton, 1987:79–112.
56. Fallon BA, Campeas R, Schneier FR, et al. Open trial of intravenous clomipramine in five treatment refractory patients with obsessive compulsive disorder. J Neuropsychiatry Clin Neurosci 1992; 4:70–75.

8

Novel Pharmacological Treatments of OCD

William A. Hewlett
Vanderbilt University School of Medicine
Nashville, Tennessee

INTRODUCTION

For years obsessive compulsive disorder (OCD) was considered to have a poor treatment outcome. Traditional insight-oriented psychotherapies had little effect on the core symptoms of the illness (1). While pharmacological therapies were reported, they did not capture the interest of the psychiatric community. Medications that we now know to be beneficial in the treatment of OCD were first reported to be efficacious in the late 1960s. It wasn't until the early '80s that trials of these medications began in the United States. These studies, reviewed in Chapter 7, demonstrated that clomipramine, which preferentially inhibits the uptake of serotonin, was effective in the treatment of OCD and was superior to antidepressants that inhibited norepinephrine uptake or that inactivated monoamine oxidase. Subsequently, more selective serotonin-reuptake inhibitors (SRIs) became available, and large trials, reviewed in Chapter 7, have demonstrated their efficacy in OCD. Pharmacological treatment of uncomplicated OCD has now become possible for primary physicians with little knowledge of the disorder.

Alternative treatments of OCD have been limited. While insight-oriented therapies have had little success in reducing the primary symptoms of OCD, behavioral treatment involving exposure and response prevention has been found to be highly effective (Chapter 10). Unfortunately, such treatment requires a therapist who has had significant training and experience with this modality. Such therapists can be found in cities associated with academic centers; however, in many areas of the country, patients are left solely with pharmacotherapeutic options— specifically, with the preferential serotonin reuptake inhibitors (PSRIs*).

Although the PSRIs represent a significant improvement over other pharmacotherapeutic options, they have limitations that dismay both patients and physicians. Some patients cannot tolerate the side effects; moreover, these medications do not completely alleviate the symptoms of OCD. It is a rare patient who will tell his physician that he is no longer troubled by obsessive-compulsive symptoms. Most patients treated with PSRIs will experience, at best, a 50–60% reduction in symptoms. Other patients will not respond to treatment at all, or have such severe OCD that even a 50% reduction in symptoms leaves them unable to function effectively. For these patients, and for those who cannot tolerate treatment with PSRIs, the physician must have a new strategy. The most common and appropriate approach is the addition of an augmenting agent, reviewed in Chapter 9. An augmentation strategy cannot be employed in patients who do not tolerate the PSRIs. In addition, there are patients who simply do not respond to current combination therapies. For these patients, one must consider the use of novel (non-PSRI) medications to treat OCD symptoms. It is these strategies that are reviewed in this chapter.

It is important to note at the outset that treatment studies must be evaluated in the context of the time at which they were undertaken. OCD has gone from being virtually untreatable to a point at which a clinically significant partial response can be expected. This means that the standards of successful treatment have changed over the last 20 years. Medications used in previous decades that might have produced a minimal improvement by current standards would, at that time, have been reported as having a significant effect on OCD. Prior to the use of PSRIs, medications that might have affected a secondary component of OCD, such as anxiety or depression, would have been reported as being efficacious for the syndrome, although they had limited efficacy in reducing the core symptoms of OCD. Similarly, the definition of OCD has changed over the years. A clear delineation of obsessive-compulsive personality disorder (OCPD) and OCD has now been developed. In the earlier literature, phobias, excessive anxiety, and OCPD, as well as true OCD, were all considered together and treated as phobic neuroses.

PSRIs refers to clomipramine plus the more selective serotonin reuptake inhibitors (SSRIs).

Finally, it must be noted that the pool of patients available for treatment studies has changed over time. When the benefits of PSRIs in the treatment of OCD were first publicized, thousands of never-medicated patients with clear-cut OCD symptoms emerged to take part in the clinical trials. Once they were successfully treated, many patients never again participated in these trials. Subsequently PSRIs became available to general practitioners for the treatment of uncomplicated OCD. Secondary- and tertiary-care providers were called on more frequently to treat a mixed group of OCD patients who were more refractory to treatment. As a result, treatment-refractory patients are now more highly represented in the pool on which academic centers rely to study this illness, and results from recent trials may therefore not be comparable to those of earlier studies. The changes in diagnostic criteria, in definitions of successful treatment, and in the character of the research pool make it imperative that one be cognizant of the period during which pharmacological treatments were undertaken when interpreting findings of efficacy for those treatments.

Our group has surveyed reports documenting treatment outcomes for individual patients. In the following sections, we summarize case studies for treatments that do not employ PSRIs and review treatment trials of these agents. We do not include experimental challenge paradigms that attempt to produce acute changes in OCD, but focus on treatment instituted for the purpose of long-term changes. We have also tabulated treatment successes and failures for non-PSRI pharmacological treatments from 98 reports that document treatment outcomes for individual patients (see Table 1). Finally, in an attempt to estimate the frequency of response in clinical practice, we polled 12 OCD treatment centers and report their success rate with different non-PSRI pharmacological treatments. The results of this survey are summarized in Table 2.

SEROTONERGIC TREATMENTS

Intravenous Clomipramine

It is ironic that intravenous (i.v.) clomipramine is considered a novel treatment for OCD when much of the early work with clomipramine in obsessional illness was done with this parenteral preparation. The use of i.v. clomipramine was initially reported in 1966 by Lopez-Ibor at the Fourth World Congress of Psychiatry in Madrid and published one year later (2). This was followed by multiple reports confirming this initial finding (3–15). By 1977, however, oral clomipramine had become the

Table 1 Positive and Negative Medication Case Outcomes from 98 References Documenting Treatment Outcomes of Novel Medications in Individual OCD Patients

Drug	Neg.	Pos.	Drug	Neg.	Pos.
Amitriptyline	21	8	Alprazolam	15	8
Amoxapine	1	0	Bromazepam	19	18
Desipramine	33	3	Chlordiazepoxide	19	10
Doxepin	13	9	Clonazepam	13	18
Imipramine	23	3	Diazepam	20	12
Maprotiline	3	0	Lorazepam	3	0
Mianserin	12	11	Oxazepam	7	13
Nortriptyline	5	4	Other benzodiazepines	100	1
Trazodone	19	17	*Total benzodiazepines*	196	80
Venlafaxine	0	1	Amytal	1	0
Other tricyclics (non-PSRI)	52	13	Buspirone	21	7
Other heterocyclics (non-PSRI)	34	0	Clonidine	23	6
Total heterocyclics (non-PSRI)	216	69	Clonidine/low-dose clomipramine	0	3
			Diphenhydramine	19	7
Clorgyline	2	2	Hydroxyzine	1	0
Phenelzine	8	13	Meprobamate	1	0
Tranylcypromine	11	5	Propranolol	1	0
Other MAOIs	31	7	Unnamed sedative/anxiolytics	18	0
Total MAOIs	52	27	*Total other sedative/anxiolytics*	85	23
Trazodone + MAOI	1	6	Bromocriptine	1	3
Trazodone + tryptophan	9	2	d-Amphetamine	0	4
Unnamed antidepressants	14	0	Ergot mesylates	1	0
Total antidepressants (non-PSRI)	292	104	LSD	0	1
Lithium	15	3	Methylphenidate	4	0
Rubidium	0	1	Sernyl	3	2
Total alkalis	15	4	*Total stimulants/hallucinogens*	9	10

	Neg.	Pos.		Neg.	Pos.
Chlorpromazine	23	8	Cyproterone	1	6
Fluphenazine	1	0	Estrogen	1	1
Haloperidol	8	2	Levothyroxine	2	0
Loxapine	1	1	Oxytocin	10	2
Molindone	2	0	Tryptophan/pyridoxine/± niacin	0	8
Pimozide	1	0	Pyridoxine	0	1
Perphenazine	3	0	ddAVP	3	0
Thioridazine	9	1	Vasopressin	3	0
Thiothixene	2	0	*Total hormones*	20	18
Trifluoperazine	7	1	Carbamazepine	17	3
Other neuroleptics	61	1	Diphenylhydantoin	1	0
Total neuroleptics	118	14	Valproic acid	1	0
IV immunoglobulin	1	0	Dilantin	4	0
Plasmapheresis	0	2	*Total anticonvulsants*	23	3
Prophylactic PCN	0	1			
Total immunosuppressants	1	3			

Totals

No. pts. having neg. trials	512	No. pts. having pos. trials	390
Neg. trials (non-PSRI)	759	Pos. trials (non-PSRI)	259
Total PSRI failures in the patients	174	Total PSRI successes in these patients	115
Total neg. trials	933	*Total pos. trials*	374

Table 2 OCD Center Poll: Treatment Response Frequencies

Treatment drug	No. of centers	No. of patients	% favorable
Analysis for all responses			
Tryptophan[a]	4	117	60
i.v. clomipramine	2	17	47
Antistreptococcal rx	3	29	38
Clonazepam[a]	10	123	30
Diphenhydramine[a]	2	29	24
Valproate[a]	3	26	23
Buspirone[a]	8	121	19
MAOIs[a]	6	79	19
d-Amphetamine	3	26	19
Clonidine	5	49	18
Carbamazepine	2	12	17
Neuroleptics[a]	6	69	11
Venlafaxine[a]	7	56	11
Trazodone[a]	7	115	9
Alprazolam	5	85	8
Lithium	6	46	0
Methylphenidate	3	17	0
Bupropion	3	15	0
Benzodiazepines	1	10	0
Oxytocin	2	8	0
Bromocriptine	2	2	0
Ondansetron	1	1	0
Other (fenfluramine)[b]	1	20	45
Totals	*12*	*1072*	*22*
Reanalysis without extraordinary responses			
Clonazepam	9	95	23
MAOIs	5	59	10
Venlafaxine	6	46	7
Buspirone	7	81	6
Trazodone	6	95	5
Neuroleptics	5	49	4
Tryptophan	3	17	0
Valproate	2	6	0
Diphenhydramine	1	3	0
Reanalyzed totals	*12*	*768*	*11*

12 centers estimated the no. of patients treated with the listed medications and, for each drug, the percentage of trials with favorable outcomes, defined as response equal to or better than the typical favorable response to climipramine. Dosage information was not given.

[a] Response rate extraordinarily affected by results from one center.

[b] Additional novel treatment medication reported by one center.

standard treatment in Europe for obsessional illness (16), with i.v. administration reserved for partial responders.

Intravenous clomipramine was rediscovered in the Western Hemisphere in 1984, with a report by Warneke (17) of five responsive OCD cases (200–300 mg*). Warneke has subsequently reported four additional cases (9,18), while others have reported another nine North American cases (19–21). Warneke (22) also reported, in passing, 40 additional successful cases without further description. In all, there are well over 100 cases of successful treatment with this preparation. Our poll of OCD sites found eight of 17 patients at two sites achieving a clinically significant response with this preparation.

The relative efficacy of i.v. clomipramine and oral PSRIs has never been systematically addressed. Rack and Chir (16) reported that 37 of 39 patients who improved on oral clomipramine improved further on i.v. preparation. In his opinion, only three patients improved "adequately" on oral clomipramine alone. It is unclear whether the patients cited received adequate trials of the oral preparation since improvement on the oral preparation continues for at least 12 weeks. Warneke (22) reported 60 cases of severe OCD not responsive to "oral medications." Two-thirds of these achieved a significant reduction in their Yale-Brown Obsessive Compulsive Scale (Y-BOCS) scores when treated with i.v. clomipramine. He cited similar response rates from unpublished trials in New York and Denmark. Again, there are no data regarding the dose and duration of treatment, nor is it even stated unequivocally that these patients had failed a PSRI.

Tryptophan

Tryptophan is the precursor amino acid from which serotonin is derived. Its presence is rate-limiting in central serotonin synthesis. Tryptophan was first reported as a pharmacological therapy in seven patients in 1977 (23). Patients were given tryptophan (3–9 g, mean 6.3 g), pyridoxine phosphate (400 mg), and nicotinic acid (2000 mg), all in divided doses. Patients showed "considerable improvement" at 1 month, 6 months. and 1 year. No information was given concerning the measurement of improvement. Two cases were complicated by histories of aggressive behavior that worsened on tryptophan.

Tryptophan is not currently available in the United States because of reports of eosinophilic myalgia, later found to be associated with contaminants in the amino acid preparation. In our review, only these

---

*All doses are reported as total daily doses.

seven successful cases have been reported, with no treatment failures reported. Our poll of OCD sites found that 60% of patients (70 of 117) had a good response with this medication; however, a single site having substantial success with this medication accounted for 85% of the patient trials. At the other three sites (17 patients), there were no responders to tryptophan. It is unclear whether the success of the center using tryptophan may be in some way related to the addition of pyridoxine to the treatment regimen. In this regard, Koizumi (24) reported an ADD patient having OCD-like symptoms precipitated by methylphenidate whose symptoms abated with L-tryptophan and pyridoxine. In fact, Frye and Arnold (25) reported a similar case of amphetamine-induced OCD-like symptoms that were successfully treated with pyridoxine alone. Although tryptophan has also been used with mixed success as an adjunct in PSRI therapy, the efficacy of this treatment in the group of PSRI non-responders has not been addressed. While one group appears to have had significant success with tryptophan, it has not been studied in a double-blind protocol, and questions remain regarding its use in modern-day settings.

Trazodone

Trazodone is a weak inhibitor of serotonin uptake and an antagonist at 5-HT2 and α-adrenergic sites. A metabolite of this medication, m-CPP, acts at multiple serotonin-receptor subtypes as well as at receptors for other neurotransmitters. The successful use of trazodone in OCD was first reported by Prasad in 1984 (26) in a patient with contamination concerns and concurrent depression. Trazodone treatment (100 mg) improved OCD symptoms by 70% over 4 weeks, as measured by the total symptom score on the Leyton Obsessional Inventory. These improvements were maintained for 5 months on the medication. Baxter (27) reported two patients with clear OCD symptoms and comorbid depression responding to trazodone. One patient failed several non-PSRI pharmacological treatments, as well as low-dose trazodone (300 mg). Treatment with trazodone at a higher dose (400 mg) produced a "marked improvement" in mood and OCD symptoms. Tranylcypromine (30 mg) added after 6 weeks further improved his mood. A second patient having similar treatment failures was able to terminate his compulsive rituals after trazodone treatment (300 mg). This patient relapsed on discontinuing the medication and regained his level of functioning on restarting the medication.

Lydiard (28) described a patient with clear OCD symptoms who had failed trials of two non-PSRI antidepressants and a benzodiazepine.

He was hospitalized with depression and treated for 2 weeks with trazo-done (350 mg), with improvement in mood and slight improvement in OCD symptoms. Upon stopping treatment, his obsessions returned. They diminished again with treatment at 200 mg, reappeared at 50 mg, and subsided with subsequent treatment at 150 mg. Kim (29) reported a patient with clear OCD and secondary depression who responded to tra-zodone (150 mg). This patient also relapsed upon discontinuing the medication and improved with retreatment. Ramchandani (30) reported a case of an individual with fears of constipation who could induce bowel movements by going into a supermarket. Although this case was termed a "bowel obsession" that responded to trazodone, it was clearly not a case of OCD since the behavior produced the desired autonomic result, and was not egodystonic.

An open-label trial (31) was conducted in eight patients with no more than "mild" depression. Six of these showed improvement that was sustained for 10 weeks of follow-up, using the Leyton obsessional total symptom score as a measure. No doses were given in this report. Baxter et al. (32) described the treatment of 10 OCD patients (six with Major Depression, four without) treated with trazodone, or trazodone plus an MAOI (mean trazodone dose 445 mg). Eight responded to treat-ment. There was a significant difference between the doses of trazodone for responders (481 mg) and those for nonresponders (300 mg), sug-gesting that higher doses might have been more effective. All six pa-tients with Major Depression responded to treatment, two taking trazo-done alone and four taking trazodone plus an MAOI. Only two of the four patients without Major Depression responded to treatment. No pa-tient without depression responded to trazodone alone. In another open-label study, Hermesh et al. (33) treated nine patients having clom-ipramine-resistant OCD with trazodone (500 mg). He used nonstandard behavioral indices to measure efficacy. Although the presence of Major Depression was not documented, higher levels of depression were asso-ciated with a poorer treatment response in this study. Withdrawal of trazodone in responders resulted in relapse, and reinstitution resulted in a resolution of symptoms. Mattes (34) reported the use of trazodone (mean 425 mg) in 11 patients augmented by tryptophan (5 g). Only four patients were able to complete a 4-week trial, and only two of these improved. Both patients remained well after stopping both medi-cations. One further report (35) involved OCD with concurrent trichotil-lomania. Both problems responded to trazodone (200 mg).

The only double-blind, placebo-controlled trial of trazodone was conducted by Pigott et al. (36) in nondepressed patients using low-dose (mean 235 mg) trazodone. There was no effect of trazodone on OCD symptoms in this study. It was not reported whether any patients were responders in the trazodone treatment group. Interestingly, there was no effect of trazodone on depression scores in this study.

A total of 17 successes and 19 treatment failures were found in our literature review. In our survey, however, only 11 of 115 cases (10%) were reported as having good or excellent responses. While case studies might indicate that there are patients with trazodone-sensitive OCD symptoms, a controlled double-blind trial of low-dose trazodone found no evidence of efficacy in nondepressed subjects. It appears that high doses of trazodone and the presence of depression may be important factors in treatment with this medication. High-dose trazodone might be an option for PSRI nonresponders, since one-third of clomipramine-resistant patients appeared to respond to such treatment in one study.

Buspirone

Buspirone is a partial agonist at 5-HT1A receptors. It has been used in the treatment of generalized anxiety disorder. Open trials of buspirone were initiated by Jenike and Baer (37) in an 8-week study of 14 patients using doses of up to 60 mg daily. None of these patients improved. A subsequent case report (38) described the efficacy of buspirone (30 mg) in a case of new-onset OCD. Improvement continued over 4 weeks until "all his symptoms were gone." Improvement was maintained over 6 months, at which time buspirone was discontinued without recurrence of symptoms. Realmuto et al. (39) reported no benefit of buspirone treatment in an autistic child with obsessive ideation. It is unclear whether this patient had true OCD. Farid and Bulto (40) report a single case unresponsive to multiple therapies, including ECT, leukotomy, and three PSRIs, who responded to buspirone (30 mg) over a period of 2 months and at 6-month follow-up (15 mg). Improvement was measured by a nonstandard adaptation of the Leyton Obsessional Inventory in which the symptoms were classified according to the degree of associated resistance and interference. The need to resist was considered disadvantageous in this analysis. Before treatment 47% of symptoms interfered with functioning (with or without resistance), while at 6 months 26% of symptoms were so categorized. No global measure of OCD was reported.

Murphy et al. (41) described a parallel treatment study of clomipramine versus buspirone (10 patients in each group). There was no difference between the treatments, each of which was reported to be effective. Pato et al. (42), reporting on the expanded analysis of this study, found benefits of both clomipramine and buspirone treatment.

The criterion for clinically significant improvement in this study (20% reduction of Y-BOCS score) was low by today's standards. Using this criterion, six subjects improved on clomipramine and five improved with buspirone treatment. The average Y-BOCS decline for buspirone over the 6-week period was 27% and that for clomipramine was 28%. The latter figure contrasts with more extensive studies finding aggregate improvement of up to 50% with clomipramine treatment over 12 weeks. It is unclear whether improvement on buspirone would continue to that degree in a longer study, making interpretation of these results problematic.

In total, we found seven reported cases of successful treatment with buspirone and 21 reported failures (not including the negative result in the autistic child). Our survey found 23 of 121 (19%) cases having a good or excellent response to buspirone. While the double-blind comparison trial raises the possibility that buspirone may be helpful in OCD, it does not appear to have the efficacy of a PSRI. It is unclear how effective the medication might be in PSRI non- or partial responders. The addition of buspirone to an PSRI seems to have limited benefit (see review in Chapter 9). A larger and longer study in PSRI treatment failures is required to determine whether buspirone has any benefit in this population.

Mianserin

Mianserin is an antidepressant that has been available for use outside the United States. Mianserin has multiple effects at serotonergic and nonserotonergic receptors. It has highest affinities as an antagonist at 5-HT2 and histamine-1 receptors. Vaisanen et al. (43) reported the use of mianserin (60 mg) in a four week trial in nine patients with obsessional illness. One patient was rated as very much improved and two were moderately improved. A fourth patient was unchanged during the trial, but "improved considerably" after 2 months' treatment. A follow-up study from this group (44) compared mianserin (60 mg, 13 patients) with clomipramine (150 mg, 15 patients) in a 4-week, double-blind, placebo-controlled trial. Only patients with "compulsive neurosis" and "polymorphic neurosis with compulsive neurotic symptoms predominating" were included in the study. Patients with clear depressive symptoms were excluded. Six of 10 subjects completing mianserin treatment were rated as having a good response (symptomless or near symptomless). One patient became psychotic. In contrast, four of nine patients completing clomipramine treatment improved.

No statistical conclusions were drawn as the authors discovered that their primary evaluation tool (Lynfield Obsessional/Compulsive Questionnaire) was insensitive as a measure of change. This report also provided a 3-year follow-up on two of the cases previously reported. Neither case involved OCD as a single diagnosis. One patient having "obsessive blinking of the eyes," severe aggressiveness, and social phobias, as well as severe OCD, had a complete remission of symptoms after 2.5 months of treatment (60 mg), and was subsequently maintained symptom-free on 30 mg mianserin. The second patient with severe OCD symptoms also suffered from psychosomatic illness (migraine headaches and diarrhea). Her psychosomatic symptoms disappeared with 5 weeks of treatment (60 mg), while her obsessive-compulsive thoughts disappeared after 4 months of treatment (20 mg). Stressful situations and an attempt to discontinue the medication caused recurrence of symptoms, which were alleviated by temporary increases in dosages.

In all, 11 successful trials of this medication and 12 failed trials have been reported. Our OCD center poll did not include this medication since it has not been available at these centers. Both trials of this medication were conducted prior to studies based on current criteria and ratings. As such, although these data are difficult to interpret, it does appear that this medication merits further study.

Other Serotonergic Agents

5-HT3 receptor antagonists have been found in animal models to increase an animal's ability to tolerate situations involving risk. These studies suggest that 5-HT acting at these receptors may increase an animal's perception of risk, and as such may have significant relevance in the etiology of OCD. Himmelhoch (45) has described a patient meeting DSM diagnostic criteria for OCD and Panic Disorder whose OCD symptoms were markedly reduced with ondansetron (4 mg), a 5-HT3 antagonist currently marketed as an antiemetic agent. He also described a second patient with compulsive rituals and ruminations whose symptoms were reduced on this medication. No other reports are available for this medication, which is in Phase III trials for use in other anxiety disorders. One OCD center reported a single treatment failure with this medication. Although clinical experience with ondansetron in the treatment of OCD is very limited, future trials of this medication seem warranted.

Fenfluramine is a substituted amphetamine that selectively releases serotonin from neuronal vesicles and competes with serotonin for reuptake into the neuron. Prolonged administration depletes the synapse of serotonin. One center in our poll estimated that nine of 20 patients taking fenfluramine as a monotherapy achieved a good or excellent reduction of their OCD symptoms. No other details are available regarding the use of this medication. Although it is unclear by what means this medication might act to reduce OCD symptoms, further investigation seems warranted.

Agonists at the 5-HT2 class of receptors, including LSD (46–48), psilocin (48), and mescaline (48), have also been reported to reduce the symptoms of OCD. We have seen a similar case of improvement in a 19-year-old patient with moderate to severe OCD, several tic-like compulsions, and polysubstance abuse. This patient abused cocaine, amphetamines, barbiturates, and marijuana, in addition to LSD. He reported that the only time he was free of both obsessions and compulsions in the last several years was when he had taken LSD. He said that for several hours after ingestion he was completely free of obsessive thoughts. No other substance produced this effect for him. 5-HT2 agonists are hallucinogenic and not available for use in treatment; however, these reports may suggest a role for 5-HT2 receptors in future serotonergic treatments of OCD.

OTHER MEDICATIONS AFFECTING MONOAMINES

Early Tricyclic Antidepressants

The use of tricyclic antidepressants other than clomipramine would be considered novel at this point, given the wealth of information relating to the efficacy of the PSRIs. While they have been used for three decades with only marginal success, there have been scattered case reports of dramatic improvements associated with these medications (49–52). Although not all tricyclics have been studied individually, there is little evidence that tricyclics other than clomipramine have significant benefits in treating the core symptoms of OCD. Because most studies comparing tricyclics and PSRIs have not employed a crossover design, it is not clear whether those patients responding to tricyclics might also have responded to PSRIs. In all, we found 151 reported cases of tricyclic failures and only 27 reported successes, the majority of which were reported before the universal availability of PSRIs. OCD sites were not polled on their use of tricyclics. In the absence of studies demonstrating a clear subset of PSRI nonresponders who respond to tricyclics, the use of these medications as monotherapy for uncomplicated OCD cannot be recommended at this time.

Venlafaxine

Venlafaxine is a novel tricyclic antidepressant that inhibits the reuptake of norepinephrine, serotonin, and dopamine. Zajecka et al. (53) have recently reported efficacy of venlafaxine (375 mg) in reducing OCD in a single patient with depression. This patient had been refractory to treatment with amitriptyline, fluoxetine, and clomipramine. After 4 weeks of treatment, her OCD symptoms improved significantly, but not her depressive symptoms. OCD improvement was maintained for another 8 weeks, at which time she discontinued the medication because of lack of efficacy for her depression. Her OCD symptoms then returned. In our poll of centers, six of 56 cases (11%) were reported as having good or excellent results. While the single reported case was refractory to two PSRIs, it remains to be seen whether this will be an effective medication for PSRI nonresponders.

C. MAOIs

Monoamine oxidase inhibitors (MAOIs) block the breakdown of norepinephrine, dopamine, and serotonin. The antidepressant action of MAOIs is thought to lie in their ability to increase the concentration of these monoamines in the synapse, although the relative contribution of the different monoamines is not clear. Joel (54) reported efficacy of iproniazid in a 20-month study of patients with multiple psychiatric disorders. Six of these were said to have had severe OCD symptoms for 5 to 25 years. In a review of the cases, at least four of these would qualify for a modern diagnosis of OCD. Patients took iproniazid for 5 to 25 months, with initial doses ranging from 30 to 150 mg and maintenance doses ranging from 8 to 75 mg daily. An unspecified number of patients were also given pyridoxine 25–50 mg daily, and some patients were also initially given barbiturates or amphetamines. All patients with OCD showed marked improvement in this trial. Ten years later, Annesley (55) reported a case of OCD refractory to bilateral rostral leukotomy who obtained substantial improvement when treated with phenelzine (60 mg) and chlordiazepoxide (50 mg). Jain et al. (56) reported a similar case that was refractory to frontal leukotomy but responsive to phenelzine (45 mg). Ananth (57) reported the use of phenelzine in combination with trimipramine as having good results, without further details.

Jenike (58) reported two cases responsive to tranylcypromine (20 mg) as well as a third case not responsive to tranylcypromine. Jenike noted that cases that were responsive appeared to be associated with phobias, although the phobic symptoms described might now be considered simple obsessive fears. Jenike et al. (59) subsequently reported four additional cases responsive to phenelzine or tranylcypromine, all of whom had panic attacks and severe anxiety. Two of these relapsed off MAOIs and responded again when the medication was reintroduced. None of the four nonresponders had panic or severe anxiety. Isberg (60) reported a case responsive to phenelzine but not to imipramine. He maintained that the obsessions may have been triggered by the panic symptoms; however, the "panic-like episodes" occurred exclusively in association with contamination fears, and as such may not have been true panic attacks. Rihmer et al. (61) described a claustrophobic patient with obsessive fears that resulted in a secondary agoraphobia. This patient responded to treatment with nialamide (150 mg).

Swinson (62) reported a patient with depression and a ruminative state treated with tranylcypromine (30 mg). The depression responded to the MAOI, but the ruminative thoughts required thought-stopping. It is unclear whether the ruminative thoughts represented true OCD. Although thoughts about masturbation had triggered washing rituals in the past, the target symptoms of tranylcypromine treatment were disabling masochistic fantasies, not true obsessions associated with OCD. Mahgoub (63) reported a case of OCD with concurrent suicidal depression, both unrelieved by ECT, clomipramine, chlorpromazine, and the combination of the latter two medications (225 and 200 mg, respectively). This patient had a significant response to phenelzine (90 mg) initially taken with chlordiazepoxide (30 mg). After 13 weeks his obsessive-compulsive symptoms were mild and infrequent. Discontinuing this medication triggered a recurrence of OCD symptoms within 2 weeks.

Two studies have found minimal efficacy of MAOIs in treating obsessive and compulsive symptoms in anxiety disorders other than OCD. Tyrer et al. (64) measured obsessions in a group of simple phobics and agoraphobics treated with phenelzine. He found no benefit. Using the SCL-90 subscale for obsessions and compulsions, Sheehan et al. (65) found that phenelzine reduced these symptoms by a small but statistically significant degree at 6 weeks, but not at 12 weeks, in a series of 57 patients having panic disorder with agoraphobia. Neither of these studies involved patients selected for a diagnosis of OCD.

There have been two double-blind studies of MAOIs in OCD. Neither of these was placebo-controlled. Insel et al. (66) described a trial of clorgyline and clomipramine in a 6-week crossover study. He reported having had initial success with clorgyline prior to this trial, without further details. Clomipramine was found to be superior to clorgyline (30 mg), which did not have a significant effect on aggregate OCD symptoms. Insel notes that individual patients did improve on clorgyline, and that one of the 10 patients who completed trials of both medications improved more on the clorgyline than on clomipramine. The degree of improvement was not given for this case. He subsequently described a comparison of clorgyline and tranylcypromine efficacy in three patients who had responded to some degree during the trial. One patient experi-

enced more side effects on tranylcypromine and was retreated with clorgyline with "continued improvement." The other two showed improvement similar to that on clorgyline. One of these latter patients
discontinued the medication within 6 months because of "attenuation
of therapeutic effects." One additional patient who did not take part in
the medication trials was treated with tranylcypromine (15 mg) for a
period of 2 years with a "marked reduction" in symptoms.

A 12-week double-blind trial (67) compared the efficacy of phenelzine and clomipramine in 30 panic-free patients, consisting of both ritualistic and "ruminating" subjects. Ruminations are currently excluded
from the definition of OCD, and it is unclear whether all patients met
DSM diagnostic criteria for the illness. Fourteen subjects completed trials
of clomipramine (225 mg) and 12 completed trials of phenelzine (75
mg). Seven patients in each group "notably improved." The criteria for
this designation were not specified. One patient in the phenelzine group
was symptom-free at the end of 12 weeks. There were no statistically
significant differences between the two medication conditions, although
baseline-to-endpoint differences for the clomipramine group showed
greater statistical significance in every measure for which changes were
present. The failure to find differences in efficacy could have arisen by
two means. First, three OCD scales were employed as measures of
change that were simple inventories of symptoms—such scales are insensitive to changes in intensity of OCD symptoms. Second, Bonferroni
statistical corrections applied to the large number of comparisons made
reduced the ability to find significant differences that might have been
present. As a result, the findings of this study are difficult to evaluate.

In summary, MAOIs have been studied in the treatment of OCD
for over three decades, and case reports suggest that a subset of individuals with OCD have symptoms that are sensitive to these medications.
Two double-blind studies have reached contradictory conclusions regarding the efficacy of these medications in comparison to the PSRI
clomipramine, although neither study employed both modern measurements and adequate duration of treatment. To date there are 52 reported failures and 27 treatment successes in our literature review. Fif-
teen of 79 patients (19%) achieved a good or excellent response with
these medications. There is little information regarding the relative responses of MAOIs and PSRIs in the same patients, except for Insel's
study, in which only one patient in 10 had a better response to the
MAOI over 6-week trials. The response rate of MAOIs in PSRI nonresponders is not known. Clearly a large placebo-controlled study of these
medications, in patients with documented PSRI response histories, is
warranted.

Neuroleptics

Neuroleptics are dopaminergic antagonists used in the treatment of psychosis, tics, and aggressive behavior. While the lines between psychosis, complex tics, maladaptive urges, and OCD are not always clear, the use of neuroleptics as monotherapy for OCD has been limited, and generally discouraged, because of the risk of tardive dyskinesia. Neuroleptics have been used as adjunctive therapy for selected subsets of OCD patients, as described in Chapter 9, and in conditions in which obsessions have grown to psychotic proportions (68,69).

There are a small number of case reports involving the use of neuroleptics in OCD. The first such report appeared in 1953 (70). Although it is impossible to diagnose the patients in the report according to today's criteria, four patients with clear-cut obsessive fears had a good response to the medication. Of the eight additional patients described as having combinations of obsessions, scruples, doubts, and meticulousness, four patients were described as having a good response. Combining these groups, eight of 12 patients had good outcomes with this medication. The mean maximal dose of chlorpromazine in these patients was 112 mg. Maintenance doses averaged 69 mg, quite low by today's standards.

Garmany et al., in 1954 (71), reported unsuccessful chlorpromazine treatment in three patients with "chronic obsessional state" and three patients having either depression or anxiety with "obsessional features." He employed a maximum dose of 225 mg daily, followed by maintenance doses of 50–100 mg per day. In none of these patients was there an improvement in obsessional thinking. While these patients are classified as obsessional, they are described as having phobias, panic attacks, depression, an inability to read, and a fear of body odor. In short, other than one patient described as having "macabre ruminations," none of their symptoms would be classified as OCD by today's definitions.

Altschuler (72) reported that one of three OCD patients responded to treatment with trifluoperazine (60–120 mg). He also noted that four of seven schizophrenics with compulsive rituals responded to treatment. Responders were maintained on 60–90 mg per day. All relapsed with placebo substitution and responded again with reinstitution of the medication. Insel and Murphy (68) cite an early text on psychopharmacology (73) as reporting efficacy of perphenazine (6 mg) in OCD. O'Regan (74) reported three cases of OCD responsive long-term to haloperidol. One of these patients had had multiple non-PSRI treatments as well as ECT. Improvement on haloperidol (15 mg) was maintained for this patient over a 6-month period. Hussain and Ahad (75) reported a patient with

severe OCD referred for psychosurgery who responded to chlorprothix-
ene (300–400 mg).

Rivers-Bulkely and Hollender (76) reported successful inpatient
treatment of a college student with fears of being poisoned by his roommates that led to decontamination rituals. It is unclear whether this patient was psychotic. He was treated as an outpatient with perphenazine,
with some relief, but stopped the medication because of side effects. He
was then treated with loxapine (100 mg). After 3 weeks, he reported
that he was free of obsessions and compulsions. Knesevich (77) reported
a case responsive to fluphenazine combined with an inpatient behavioral program that included threat of transfer to a locked ward. When
medication was discontinued, the patient returned to her premorbid
state. This patient subsequently improved with a 3-week course of loxapine treatment (dose unknown). Her symptoms returned when loxapine
was withdrawn. More recently, Ross and Pigott (78) described a 14-
year-old boy whose OCD responded to thioridazine (125 mg) over 14
days. The medication was discontinued after 2 weeks, however, because
of side effects and decreasing efficacy.

The only OCD-related placebo-controlled trial of neuroleptics involved 4- to 6-week trials of chlorpromazine (150–200 mg) in a complex
single-blind crossover study (79). This study examined the presence, severity, and persistence of multiple symptoms, including obsessive or
compulsive symptoms, in a broad group of patients with psychoneurosis
and personality disorders monitored as a group. The authors did not
attempt to classify patients by diagnosis. They noted that six of the 59
study patients exhibited "classical obsessive-compulsive neurosis."
Twenty-seven patients experienced a greater decrease in at least some
symptoms when taking chlorpromazine than when on placebo. Compulsive rituals, present in 19 patients, did not respond to this medication, in aggregate. Aggressive urges toward self or others, also present in
19 patients, showed a significant response to chlorpromazine as compared to placebo, while intellectual ruminations showed "some response." All patients had a return of some symptoms 3 to 5 days after
stopping chlorpromazine; however, the symptoms that returned (e.g.,
insomnia, restlessness) were not specified. No information was presented regarding the responses of patients with classic obsessive-compulsive neurosis. Placebo trials following chlorpromazine treatment were as
short as 1 week long, and placebo ratings were conducted immediately
after drug discontinuation without allowing for washout. Only placebo-
drug differences were reported. Although no differences between medication and placebo conditions were found, it is unclear whether sufficient time elapsed for symptoms of interest to reappear during placebo
trials.

In total, there are only 14 successful cases of neuroleptic treatment in our literature survey and 118 cases of probable failure. Our poll of OCD centers found only eight of 69 patients (12%) treated with neuroleptics having a significant response. It should be noted that many Tourette's patients with concomitant OCD who are treated with neuroleptics for their tics require a PSRI to achieve a reduction of their OCD symptoms, suggesting that neuroleptics alone are not sufficient to treat OCD in this population (80). As with most novel monotherapies, however, the use of neuroleptics has not been studied in any detail. The percentage of PSRI nonresponders who might have a reduction of symptoms on this medication as a monotherapy is also not known. In light of the potential tardive effects of these medications, it is unlikely that neuroleptics will play a major role as monotherapies in the treatment of OCD, regardless of any potential efficacy in a subpopulation of OCD patients.

Stimulants

Paradoxically, while most attention has focused on the blockade of dopaminergic receptors in OCD, there are reports that facilitators of dopamine release and dopamine receptor agonists may also have efficacy in OCD. Insel et al. (81) reported that two patients treated with amphetamines (10–20 mg) achieved a "persistent benefit" for a period of several weeks. He reported an additional two patients treated with "low-dose" amphetamines for several months who reported a decrease in obsessional symptoms. More recently, Ceccherini-Nelli and Guazzelli (82) described three cases of OCD with concurrent depression responding to the dopaminergic agonist bromocriptine (15–30 mg). These reports must be reconciled with reports that chronic administration of methylphenidate and amphetamine may induce ritualized behaviors and other OCD-like symptoms (24,25).

In total, there are only these seven cases of reported improvement and one reported failure on chronic dopaminergic agonists. In our survey, five of 28 subjects (19%) achieved a good response with chronic amphetamine. Neither of two patients treated with bromocriptine had any improvement. One other medication, bupropion, an antidepressant with an unknown mechanism of action, has the capacity to inhibit dopaminergic reuptake. Our review did not find reports of efficacy or failure for this medication; however, our poll found no positive responses with this medication, and 15 failed treatments.

Clearly dopaminergic mechanisms of symptom alleviation in OCD are not well explained, with both agonists and antagonists having reported benefits in OCD. The fact that agonists may precipitate OCD-like symptoms in patients with ADHD further complicates the issue, although it is conceivable that the OCD-like behaviors induced by chronic amphetamine may represent stereotopies, perseverative behaviors, complex tics, or overfocusing of attention rather than compulsions that are performed to alleviate fear or internal distress. Insel and colleagues (66) argue that a dearth of dopamine may adversely affect OCD, and notes that clomipramine is a potent inhibitor of dopamine uptake. He additionally notes that encephalitis lethargica, which results in deterioration of nigrostriatal dopamine pathways, was associated with OCD. To reconcile the apparent efficacy of neuroleptic augmentation of PSRI treatment, it has been suggested that low-dose neuroleptics may block presynaptic dopamine D-2 receptors, increasing dopamine release (82). This would be consistent with the efficacy of very low-dose chlorpromazine reported by Sigwald and Bouttier (70). If this is true, one should avoid the use of high-dose, high-potency neuroleptics in OCD.

Clonidine

This medication, initially used as a antihypertensive, acts as an agonist at presynaptic α_2-receptors to decrease the release of norepinephrine. It was first reported by Cohen et al. (83) to be helpful in Tourette's syndrome, and subsequently reported to be helpful in treating obsessional symptoms associated with Tourette's syndrome (84). Knesevich (77) later reported a single case of OCD responding to clonidine (0.3 mg). This report indicated that the patient's condition deteriorated after increasing the dose to 0.4 mg/day. Lipsedge and Prothero (85) reported improvement using clonidine (0.25–0.75 mg) in three patients in association with low-dose clomipramine (20–75 mg). In this report, the authors allude to a double-blind study in progress, not found in our literature search.

The only double-blind controlled trial of clonidine (0.4–1.0 mg; mean ~0.65 mg) found this medication to be without efficacy in treating OCD symptoms in 26 adult subjects (86). Although a number of patients experienced a significant worsening of symptoms, clonidine produced a significant improvement (25% decrease in Y-BOCS) in five patients (19%) during this trial. Four of these patients also responded to clomipramine as well as diphenhydramine and, as such, do not represent the typical spectrum of PSRI nonresponders for whom novel treatments might be indicated.

There are a total of nine case reports of OCD patients without Tourette's syndrome responding to clonidine alone or in combination with very-low-dose clomipramine. There are 23 reported failures. Nine of 49 patients (20%) had a good response in our survey. One should note that there might be a biphasic response to this medication, with a better response at lower doses. This might account for the improvement in OCD reported in children with Tourette's syndrome treated with lower doses of the medication. Alternatively, it is possible that the "compulsions" reported in the Tourette's literature are actually complex tics that are responding to this treatment. Finally, it is possible that children with tics and OCD respond differently than adults so affected, since in the above-mentioned study adults with tics showed a significant worsening of their OCD on clonidine (86). All this taken together, there is little evidence that clonidine as a monotherapy, particularly in doses greater than 0.4 mg, has any value in the treatment of adult OCD.

Diphenhydramine

Diphenhydramine is an antagonist at histamine-1 receptors. In addition, it is a muscarinic cholinergic antagonist. Hewlett et al. (86) included diphenhydramine (100–250 mg; mean ~225 mg) in a 6-week, double-blind, multimedication controlled trial in 26 OCD patients. Diphenhydramine was inferior to clomipramine, although there was a significant decline in symptoms from baseline. Seven patients (27%) taking diphenhydramine had a significant reduction (25%) in OCD symptoms. One additional patient, dropped from the study after a psychotic episode, experienced a complete cessation of his obsessions during the diphenhydramine trial.

Diphenhydramine was not included as a medication in the poll OCD site. The mechanism by which it might exert its minor effect is not clear. Diphenhydramine is a weak inhibitor of serotonin reuptake, and five of the six responders or near-responders who also took clomipramine in a separate trial also had significant responses to that PSRI. As such, it is unlikely that this is an effective medication in PSRI nonresponders. At this time there is little to recommend this agent as an antiobsessive treatment.

BENZODIAZEPINES

Early Studies

The use of benzodiazepines in OCD has been extensively reviewed elsewhere (69). Early case studies focused on high doses of benzodiazepines in treating OCD symptoms (75,87–93). Bromazepam (also known as Medazepam, Lexotan, Lexotanil, and Ro 5-3350), a medication not available in the United States, was the focus of significant early interest

(94–105). No modern studies of this medication have been undertaken. Two early studies compared the efficacy of clomipramine and diazepam. One involved a head-to-head comparison (106) and the other examined the effect of diazepam as an adjunct to clomipramine therapy (107). Although both studies were flawed by today's criteria, clomipramine was found to be superior to diazepam as a monotherapy, and treatment with diazepam in addition to clomipramine was worse than clomipramine treatment alone.

Alprazolam

More recent reports have focused on two benzodiazepines: alprazolam and clonazepam. Tesar and Jenike (108) reported a single patient with obsessional fears responding to alprazolam (12 mg). This patient had a single panic attack, unrelated to his obsessions, which had prompted the original treatment. At 2 months follow-up, this patient had occasional obsessions that were no longer bothersome. Tollefson (109) subsequently reported on four cases responding to alprazolam (1.25–6 mg). From the descriptions given, only one of these four cases appears to have had classic OCD. Ketter et al. (110) reported on an unusual case of a 56-year-old individual with fecal and urinary incontinence, and obsessions and compulsions centered on cleanliness. The patient was described as having secondary anxiety and depression and no history of panic. Obsessions and compulsions responded to alprazolam at 3 mg/ day. Cognitive status was not reported in this case; however, the individual was discharged to a skilled nursing facility where he was maintained on alprazolam, and intermittent haloperidol for agitation, suggestive of a dementing illness. Stein et al. (111) conducted an open 12-week trial of alprazolam in 14 subjects. Doses were raised as clinically indicated, to up to 10 mg per day. Average dose was not reported. Two of 14 patients responded to this medication, similar to the placebo rate found in an earlier study from this group.

Clonazepam

Clonazepam is a benzodiazepine unique in its effects on the serotonergic system (112). Bodkin and White (113) reported the use of clonazepam (3 mg) in a single patient with panic disorder. This patient had previously been treated with lorazepam, which reduced his panic symptoms but not his OCD. Improvement on clonazepam was maintained for as long as 6 months. Hewlett et al. (112) reported patients having obsessions and compulsions that responded to doses of 4–5 mg/day. One of these trials, although successful in reducing OCD symptoms, was termi-

Novel Pharmacological Treatments

nated due to side effects associated with high-dose benzodiazepines. The second case was complicated by depression and a secondary eating disorder. The third case involved a patient whose obsessions became delusions under stress, necessitating brief additions of neuroleptics. Improvement on clonazepam lasted up to 1 year in follow-up. Bacher (114) reported a patient with "recurrent obsessional thinking" who responded to clonazepam (1.5 mg). No further details were given concerning symptomatology, other diagnoses, or duration-improved status; however, it was reported that he had not responded to other benzodiazepines. Finally, Ross and Pigott (78) reported the case of a 14-year-old boy whose obsessions were not responsive to clomipramine or fluoxetine but responded to clonazepam (2 mg).

The only double-blind controlled trial of clonazepam as a monotherapy compared the efficacy of clonazepam, clonidine, clomipramine, and diphenhydramine in 28 patients in crossover design using 6-week trials (86). This study employed high doses of clonazepam (4–10 mg; mean 6.85 mg). Clonazepam was found to be as effective as clomipramine and significantly more effective than clonidine and diphenhydramine. Of those who completed the trial of clonazepam, 60% experienced a clinically significant (25%) reduction in their YB-OCS score. In addition, four of 10 patients failing to improve on clomipramine experienced a clinically significant reduction of symptoms on clonazepam. This study had the limitation of being only 6 weeks in duration. Since clomipramine treatment is known to continue over an additional 6 weeks, and since clonazepam efficacy appeared to level out after 4 weeks, it is unclear whether the two medications would have been equally effective at a 12-week time point. It should also be noted that side effects, including depression and disinhibition, resulted in a 20% dropout rate as opposed to a 4% dropout rate for clomipramine.

Overall, there are 80 successful reports of benzodiazepine treatment and 196 failures. These data are somewhat skewed by the high percentage of reports occurring in the early literature. Looking at alprazolam and clonazepam separately, there have been eight successes and 15 failures reported for alprazolam treatment. Our OCD poll found that only seven of 85 (8%) cases treated with alprazolam resulted in a positive outcome. For clonazepam, there have been 18 successful cases reported and 13 failures. In our poll of OCD sites, 37 of 123 cases (30%) at 10 sites reported successful treatment with clonazepam as a monotherapy. It should be noted that 15 of these successful cases were reported at one site. The success rate for the other nine sites was 23%. None of the 10 cases treated with other benzodiazepines showed significant improvement in our poll.

Bromazepam and clonazepam are clearly the benzodiazepines most frequently reported as being efficacious. Unfortunately, bromazepam is not available in this country, and most of the data for this medication were derived from studies using outdated criteria for diagnosis and efficacy. A good study of this medication using modern criteria would be helpful in establishing its efficacy. Clonazepam is the most successful benzodiazepine treatment reported. Its success rate in the literature and across centers, however, is less than that reported for PSRIs. Although an extended, placebo-controlled trial of this medication has not been completed, there is evidence that it may be useful in PSRI failures, and in patients with seizure disorders (112).

ALKALI METALS

Lithium

Lithium, commonly employed in the treatment of bipolar illness, is known to augment serotonergic neurotransmission. Baastrup (115) originally noted that patients with manic-depressive illness and personalities characterized by "psychic rigidity" and "overconcern for orderliness" became "less tense with regard to their duties" when taking lithium. He further noted that patients without bipolar illness having obsessive-compulsive symptoms experienced an improvement in those symptoms. It is unclear whether these patients had OCD or OCPD. Forssman and Walender (116) reported the effective use of lithium at unknown doses in 18 patients, six of whom experienced symptoms suggestive of obsessive-compulsive illness. Only one of these, however, was free of other psychiatric symptoms. The others experienced either paranoia or auditory hallucinations. There are few other modern reports of lithium treatment in OCD. Jefferson et al. (117) cite the work of Kukopulos and colleagues (118) as reporting that OCD patients had a poor response to lithium in an open trial. No other details were given. Van Putten and Sanders (119) treated a group of patients with "intractable illness" in a double-blind, placebo-controlled trial. The only patient having OCD, a severe obsessional with a facial tic, exhibited a "dramatic response" to the lithium treatment. Stern and Jenike (120) reported the use of lithium in a single patient whose symptoms continually returned following withdrawal from the medication. Finally, Coleman and Cesnik (121) reported the successful use of lithium in two patients with obsessional gender dysphoria. It is unclear whether these individuals actually had OCD.

Only two controlled trials of lithium as a monotherapy have been conducted. Both suffer from poor design by modern standards. Both were double-blind placebo-controlled crossover trials that employed small numbers of patients. Geisler and Schou (122) studied 12 patients with mixed diagnoses. Six of these experienced "severe anachastic symptoms," five were described as having a "neurotic state," and one patient experienced "periodic psychosis-like symptoms." The subjects were treated for 6 to 12 weeks with alternating 2-week intervals of either lithium or placebo. Lithium levels were maintained between 0.6 and 1.4 mEq. Patients rated their own symptoms at the end of each 2-week interval. Only one patient experienced a clear improvement over a period of 2 months of alternating treatment. Hesso and Thorell (123) reported a placebo-controlled crossover study of lithium in eight patients having compulsive neurosis. The patients were randomly assigned to sequential 3–5-week trials of lithium (0.5–1.2 mEq) or placebo. Six patients improved during the initial trial. Three of these relapsed during the crossover trial. No information was provided as to whether lithium was given in the first or second trial for these patients. The paper states that only four of the eight improved more on lithium than on placebo, and concluded on that basis that there was no benefit to lithium treatment. The degree of improvement on lithium was not reported, nor were any statistical comparisons of OCD symptoms during the two treatment conditions. The study attributes improvement in the first trial to nonspecific expectations. The report did state that one patient having compulsive thoughts was "completely improved" at the conclusion of the crossover trial.

In our literature survey there are three cases of successful treatment attributable to lithium as a monotherapy and 14 reported failures. No properly controlled trials of lithium in OCD have been conducted. National OCD sites reported 46 patients treated at six sites. None of the patients achieved a significant improvement with this medication as a monotherapy. Given these data, it is unlikely that, overall, lithium has any primary role as a monotherapy in OCD.

Rubidium

The other alkali metal that has been employed in the treatment of mental illness is rubidium. Rubidium chloride has been used as an antidepressant in open trials (124,125). There is a single case report of effective treatment of obsessive neurosis with rubidium (125). None of the OCD sites has used this medication and it is not generally available in the United States.

ANTICONVULSANTS

Anticonvulsants are a heterogeneous group of medications of different classes used to treat different forms of epileptic illness. They have in common the ability to moderate synchronized firing of neuronal populations in different brain regions. Most results with nonbenzodiazepine anticonvulsants have been disappointing. Pacella et al. (126) treated four OCD patients having abnormal electroencephalograms (EEGs) with dilantin (4.5 grains) for 3 weeks without improvement. Uhlenhuth et al. (127) found no effect of an 8-week trial of either diphenylhydantoin (300 mg) or phenobarbital (90 mg) on compulsive symptoms in a heterogeneous group of 80 patients with psychoneurotic illness. Joffe and Swinson (128) reported that one of nine patients in an open-label trial of carbamazepine achieved a significant reduction in obsessive-compulsive symptoms. No EEGs were performed on this group of subjects.

Khanna (129) screened 50 OCD patients for EEG abnormalities. He treated seven patients having abnormal EEGs with carbamazepine (600–1000 mg). No patient without an epileptic history responded to carbamazepine. Two of the three cases with coexistent clinical epilepsy did respond to treatment. The author surmised that OCD symptoms were probably a manifestation of the epileptic process. Jenike and Brotman (130) reported a retrospective chart review of 12 patients with severe OCD who had EEGs. Five of these showed abnormalities over the temporal lobes and were treated with carbamazepine. None of these patients achieved a significant response on carbamazepine. One patient also failed a trial of chlorazepate and another failed a second trial of diphenylhydantoin. In a retrospective review of 36 patients treated with sodium valproate, McElroy et al. (131) reported that a single patient with OCD and no EEG abnormalities had no benefit from 12 weeks of valproate treatment (1300 mg) in conjunction with a neuroleptic. Patients with seizure disorders or paroxysmal EEG abnormalities were excluded from this review.

In total, there are three case reports of significant response to nonbenzodiazepine-related anticonvulsants, all with carbamazepine, and 23 treatment failures. Two of these had clinical epilepsy. It should be noted that two other patients with OCD and clinical epilepsy have responded to clonazepam treatment (112). Clearly, selection bias may affect anticonvulsant treatment outcome. Only one study selected patients purely on the basis OCD criteria. Three of the reports selected patients on the basis of abnormal EEGs; a fourth selected patients on the basis of valproate treatment, in patients without paroxysmal EEGs. Only one of 21 patients without known epilepsy responded to non-benzodiazepine-related anticonvulsants, and none of 12 patients with abnormal EEGs without clinical epilepsy responded to these medications. On the basis of this analysis, the utility of anticonvulsants in OCD appears questionable, outside of the subpopulation having clinical epilepsy. Actual clinical experience with anticonvulsants may be more positive. Two of 12 patients (17%) at two sites had successful trials of carbamazepine, and six of 26 patients (23%) at three sites had positive outcomes with sodium valproate. It is not clear, however, whether any of these cases had EEG abnormalities or clinical epilepsy.

GONADAL STEROIDS

The use of gonadal steroids in the treatment of OCD is derived from serendipitous findings of improvement in OCD symptoms in patients treated for other medical disorders. Most of these reports have involved cyclical treatment of symptoms in females. Surprisingly, there are two case reports of estrogen derivatives in OCD. Von Wieczorek (132) reported that the ovulation inhibitor mestranol (0.1 mg), given with the progesterone derivative chloro-dehydro-acetoxy-progesterone (3 mg), reduced premenstrually associated symptoms in a female with anachastic syndrome. In contrast, Tollefson (109) reported a woman with aggressive obsessions and paranoid ideation who did not respond to estrogen treatment.

Two papers report results of antiandrogen treatments. Casas et al. (133) describe a male with OCD and a sexual-identification disorder. This patient achieved "spectacular" improvement in symptoms when treated with antiandrogens. His OCD symptoms gradually returned over 4–5 months after the medication was discontinued. This same report describes a female with moderate OCD who improved significantly over 2–3 months when treated with antiandrogens for hirsutism. No information was given regarding symptoms, medication, or medication dose for either case. The author conducted a 5-month trial of cyproterone in six female patients: four with severe OCD, one with a "schizophrenia-like illness" associated with obsessive symptoms, and one with a phobic disorder associated with a "complex ritual-like behavior." A 10-day course of cyproterone was given during the follicular phase of the menstrual cycle, beginning at 25 mg and increasing by 25 mg each month to 100 mg daily. In addition, a 21-day course of cyproterone (2 mg) and ethinyl estradiol (0.05 mg) was taken as an anovulatory precaution. The 10-day cyproterone dose was reduced to 75 mg in the fourth month when depressive symptoms appeared. Over the first 3 months, the four patients with OCD reported a decrease in symptoms during the follicular phase of treatment and gradual reappearance of symptoms during the 18-day period off cyproterone. The method for determining OCD severity was not specified, and no attempt was made to assess cyclic changes in symptoms that might have been present off medication. Obsessive symptoms during the 10-day treatment period began to reappear over the next 2 months; however, OCD-related distress and the urge to carry out ritual behaviors reportedly remained greatly reduced. The two other patients in the trial did not respond in this open trial.

Feldman et al. (134) subsequently reported a single patient with well-described OCD symptoms who did not respond to cyproterone in a single-blind trial. The patient was treated continuously with cyproterone for 3 months (50 mg for 1 month, then 75 mg), then switched to placebo for 2 months. Cyproterone and ethinyl estradiol were given as anovulatory agents as in the previous study. Unfortunately, to assess changes in OCD this study used scales (Maudsly) that are insensitive to changes in the severity of OCD symptoms. The investigators found no differences between the treatment and placebo conditions. More recently, Perciaccante and Perciaccante (135) reported efficacy of levonorgestrel (0.15 mg) in treating OCD in one patient; however, this paper clearly describes symptoms of trichotillomania as the target symptoms, and does not describe a patient with OCD.

In total, there have been six reported cases of improvement associated with antiandrogen treatment, four of which were menstrually related, and one menstrually related improvement with an anovulatory medication. Only one antiandrogen failure has been reported, and one failure of estrogen treatment alone. None of the OCD centers has reported using this modality in treating OCD. As such, this treatment has not been well studied. In practice, the feminizing effects of these treatments in males limit their use in this population. In females, it is unclear whether treatment efficacy, if present at all, is limited to specific phases of the menstrual cycle. Although it has been poorly studied, this treatment is unlikely to become a mainstream therapy for OCD.

PEPTIDE HORMONES

Oxytocin is a hormone released by the posterior pituitary that regulates uterine and lactiferous duct contraction. It has been implicated in certain ritualized behaviors and in the extinction of active avoidance behavior in animals (136). Ansseau et al. (137) reported a single patient with well-described OCD symptoms showing improvement in symptoms after treatment with intranasal oxytocin (approximately 8–17 IU) over a 4-week period as compared to a 4-week trial of intranasal placebo treatment. Unfortunately, this treatment was associated with hyponatremia, hypo-osmolarity, and psychotic symptoms. There were also profound disturbances in memory.

Den Boer and Westenberg (138) reported a second case of a patient treated intranasally with oxytocin whose OCD symptoms improved, without any details. This paper then describes a 6-week double-blind placebo-controlled trial of intranasal oxytocin treatment (18 IU) in 12 DSM-III-diagnosed OCD patients who used low doses of benzodiazepines, and had had a course of behavior therapy at least 6 months prior to the study. Depressed patients and any patient previously treated with an antidepressant were excluded from this study. This study found no difference in the number of rituals performed during oxytocin treatment. There were no measures of obsessive thoughts. The paper does not report whether individual patients benefited from the procedure. As an extension, two patients were treated open-label (approximately 53 IU). One patient had a 38% decrease in the number of rituals, while the other had a 22% decrease over 6 weeks, surprisingly reported as a "slight change" and "virtually no change," respectively.

Two additional studies attempted to employ acute administration of peptide hormones to produce a longer-term change in behavior. Salzberg and Swedo (139) investigated changes associated with two doses of either intranasal oxytocin (8 IU) or vasopressin (80 IU) 90 minutes apart. In an acute trial in three OCD patients, no significant changes were noted as compared to placebo inhalation for either treatment regimen; however, because one patient did not carry out one of his normal compulsions after the oxytocin treatment, he continued this treatment in his home environment for an unspecified period of time. This latter treatment was without benefit. The second study (140) involved DDAVP, a synthetic analog of the antidiuretic hormone vasopressin, reported to enhance learning in humans (141,142). Intranasal DDAVP (60 μg) was administered in a placebo-controlled, double-blind crossover study in three patients with a DSM-III diagnosis of OCD to determine whether such pretreatment improved the efficacy of exposure therapy carried out over the subsequent week. No overall change was found in anxiety associated with exposure or in avoidance of feared situations, and no individual OCD patient showed any improvement on these measures. No measure of obsessions or compulsions or their severity was obtained for analysis in this study.

In all, there have been three reported cases of improvement with chronic intranasal oxytocin and 12 failures. There have been no reports of improvement with vasopressin; however, this medication has not been administered chronically. None of eight patients at two OCD sites improved with oxytocin treatment. Although experience is limited with this modality, it does not appear to be a promising treatment.

IMMUNOSUPPRESSANTS AND ANTISTREPTOCOCCALS

Perhaps the most intriguing of reports of non-PSRI treatments are those related to pediatric infection–triggered autoimmune responses resulting in acute onset of OCD symptoms. Swedo and Leonard (143) reported that individuals with Sydenham's chorea, a transient choreiform movement disorder related to an inappropriate immune response triggered by group A β-hemolytic streptococci, developed OCD during the period that their chorea was present. This group also found that the level of autoimmune antibodies in the sera of children with a severe episodic form of OCD correlated with OCD episodes (144). Theorizing that episodic forms of OCD and Tourette's syndrome might be related to CNS autoimmune reactions, this group undertook trials of immunosuppressant treatments in these disorders. Allen et al. (145) describe a 14-year-old boy with a history of OCD who exhibited a significant exacerbation of OCD symptoms after a streptococcal infection, accompanied by motoric hyperactivity and mild choreiform movements. He was treated with plasmapheresis six times over 2 weeks, with a marked decline in OCD symptoms. An MRI scan showed a 25% decrease in the size of the head of his caudate nucleus as compared to a scan taken before treatment. A second case of sudden-onset OCD following a non-streptococcal-related flulike illness also responded to treatment with plasma exchange. A third case occurred in a 13-year-old male with OCD, Tourette's syndrome, and hyperactivity. He was treated with i.v. immunoglobulin (1 mg/kg/day for 2 days), with a subsequent improvement in his tics. His OCD symptoms were unchanged. A subsequent viral infection associated temporally with an allergic reaction to influenza immunization resulted in an exacerbation in symptoms that did not respond to immunosuppressant therapy. This paper also noted the benefit of chronic prophylactic penicillin in one patient subject to episodes of OCD. There is no evidence that autoimmune exacerbations of OCD can occur in adults; however, individuals with a history of Sydenham's chorea have an increased risk of developing OCD (146).

These three patients (two successful, one unsuccessful with respect to OCD symptoms) are the only cases yet reported. In our survey of OCD sites, 11 of 29 patients (38%) at three sites had a positive response to this treatment. It should be noted that 24 of these subjects, including nine of the 11 successes, came from one site. Two of the remaining five patients at the other sites responded. This treatment modality clearly requires more study. An investigation of the possible benefits of prophylactic penicillin is reportedly in progress (145). This work is important not only for its value in determining the potential therapeutic benefits of immunosuppressant therapies, but also because it may shed light on an etiological process for symptom development and could potentially lead to prophylactic treatments to reduce the incidence of new-onset OCD.

CONCLUSIONS

OCD has devastating effects on the lives of those afflicted. OCD symptoms can be reduced in many individuals by a combination of pharmacological and behavioral therapies. The primary pharmacological treatment for this disorder involves the use of medications that inhibit the reuptake of serotonin. If these medications are inadequate, one should add adjunctive medications that might enhance or complement the effects of the PSRIs. For those patients who cannot tolerate the PSRIs or do not respond adequately to these treatments, one must consider the use of novel pharmacological therapies. The utility of available novel treatments is summarized below and in Table 3.

Serotonergic Treatments

Of all the novel treatments, only i.v. clomipramine has stood the test of time, having been used to treat OCD over a span of two and a half decades. It has reported efficacy in individuals who have failed previous PSRIs. Tryptophan (used in conjunction with pyridoxine and niacin), mianserin, fenfluramine, ondansetron, and 5-HT2 receptor agonists may have benefits in OCD; however; there has been little research on these agents, and they are not generally available for use. Trazodone and buspirone appear to have marginal benefit as monotherapies except in isolated cases.

Other Monaminergic Treatments

MAOIs have had mixed success in the treatment of OCD with and without panic and phobic symptoms. Little information is available as to the benefits of this medication in PSRI nonresponders. There is little indication that clonidine, diphenhydramine, neuroleptics, or classical tricyclics have any benefit in OCD as monotherapies except in isolated cases. There is too little information about the use of stimulants and venlafaxine to say whether these are effective agents in any subpopulation of OCD patients.

Table 3 Novel Medication Summary

Treatment	Population
Treatments that may be useful	
IV clomipramine	Failed SSRIs with augmentation
Clonazepam	Failed SSRIs with augmentation; OCD in setting of clinical epilepsy; OCD with Panic
MAOIs	Failed SSRIs with augmentation; OCD with Panic
Carbamazepine	OCD in setting of clinical epilepsy
Valproic acid	OCD in setting of clinical epilepsy
Treatments that require further research	
Tryptophan/pyridoxine/niacin	
Mianserin	
Ondansetron	
Fenfluramine	
LSD	
d-Amphetamine	
Bromocriptine	
Bromazepam	
Trazodone (high-dose)	Patients with OCD and major depression
Immunosuppessants	Children with chronic postinfectious exacerbation of OCD
Prophylactic PCN	Children with chronic postinfectious exacerbation of OCD
Treatments that are rarely useful	
Antiandrogens, bupropion, buspirone, clonidine, diphenhydramine, lithium, methylphenidate, neuroleptics, non-PSRI heterocyclic antidepressants, oxytocin, other benzodiazepines, trazodone (low-dose), vasopressin analogs, venlafaxine	

Benzodiazepines

Clonazepam is the only benzodiazepine that has had consistent reports of efficacy in the modern literature. There is some evidence to suggest that this medication may have efficacy in PSRI nonresponders; however, side effects may limit its usage. Bromazepam received significant early attention, but there are no modern data for his medication, which is not available in the United States. There is little evidence that any other benzodiazepine has any benefit in treating the core symptoms of OCD.

D. Immunosuppressants

Although early work with these treatments appears to be promising, the efficacy of these treatment must still be demonstrated. Efficacy at this time appears to be limited to a subgroup of children having an episodic form of OCD related to an autoimmune response.

Other Psychopharmacological Treatments

None of the other novel treatments—alkali metals, gonadal steroids, anticonvulsants, or peptide hormones—has shown much promise in the treatment of uncomplicated OCD. Anticonvulsants may be useful in treating OCD symptoms in the setting of clinical epilepsy, however.

The recent discovery of multiple serotonergic receptors should spawn a host of new medications that may be useful in the treatment of OCD. In addition, as the circuitry of OCD becomes more clear, medications affecting other neurotransmitters and neuromodulators may become important in treatment. Future studies of novel OCD pharmacological treatments should consider the existence of subgroups of OCD patients. The most important of these subgroups would be the PSRI nonresponders. It will be important to document the effects of treatments in both PSRI responders and nonresponders. Medications that benefit only PSRI responders are of little use for physicians trying to treat refractory cases. It will also be important to document the success rate of individuals taking part in trials, even if the trial medications as a whole are ineffective in treating OCD. The possibility exists that selected subgroups of patients may respond to certain medications that are ineffective for the general OCD patient population. Hopefully, as a greater understanding develops of processes underlying the etiology and phenomenology of OCD, physicians will be able to treat refractory cases with greater efficacy, and potentially employ treatments having prophylactic or curative effects.

ACKNOWLEDGMENTS

We thank R. Dominguez (University of Miami), W. Goodman (University of Florida), J. Greist (Dean Foundation, Wisconsin), L. Koran (Stanford University), E. Hollander (Mount Sinai Medical Center, New York), S-W Kim (University of Minnesota), C. McDougal (Yale University), T. Pigott (University of Texas—Galveston), S. Rasmussen (Brown University), S. Swedo and H. Leonard (NIMH Child Branch), and J. Yaryura-Tobias (Institute for Biobehavioral Therapy and Research, New York) for providing information on their experience with novel pharmacological treatments at their centers.

REFERENCES

1. Jenike MA. Obsessive-compulsive disorder: efficacy of specific treatments as assessed by controlled trials. Psychopharmacol Bull 1993; 29:487–499.
2. Cordoba EF, Lopez-Ibor J. La monoclorimipramina en enfermos psiquiatricos resistentes a otros tratamientos. Actas Luso-espanolas de neurologia y psiquiatria 1967; 26:119–147.
3. Amat Aguirre E. Our experience in the treatment of depressive states with 3-chloro-5-(3-dimethylaminopropyl)-10,11-dihydro-5H-dibenzodiazpine hydrochloride, preparation F 34586—Anafranil, Geigy: comparative study of the results obtained with venous perfusion and single daily oral dose. Revista Folia Neuropsiquiatrica del Sur de Espana 1968; 3:1.
4. Guyotat J, et al. A clinical trial with a new anti-depressant (G34586). Congres de Psychiatrie et de Neurologie (1967). Dijon, France: Masson, 1968.
5. Jimenez F. Experiencia clinica con clorimipramina, Anafranil (Geigy), en enfermos psiquiatricos (depresivos, obsesivos y esquizofrenicos.). Folia Neuropsiquiatrica 1968; 3:189–211.
6. van Renynghe de Voxrie GV. Anafranil (G34586) in obsessive neurosis. Acta Neurol Belg 1968; 68:787–792.
7. Dickhaut HH, Galiatsatos P. Neuartige Wege in der Pharmakotherapie von Verstimmungszustanden mit Anafranil. Der Nervenarzi 1968; 39:552–536.
8. Lopez-Ibor J. Intravenous perfusions of monochlorimipramine: technique and results. Sixth International Congress of the C.I.W.P. Amsterdam: Medica Foundation, 1969.
9. Warneke L. Intravenous chlorimipramine therapy in obsessive-compulsive disorder. Can J Psychiatry 1989; 34:853–859.
10. Marshall WK. Treatment of obsessional illnesses and phobic anxiety states with clomipramine [letter]. Br J Psychiatry 1971; 119:467–471.
11. Collins GH. The use of parenteral and oral chlorimipramine (Anafranil) in the treatment of depressive states. Br J Psychiatry 1973; 122:189–190.
12. Allen JJ, Rack PH. Changes in obsessive/compulsive patients as measured by the Leyton Inventory before and after treatment with clomipramine. Scot Med J 1975; 20:41–44.
13. Marshall WK, Micev V. Clomipramine (Anafranil) in the treatment of obsessional illnesses and phobic anxiety states. J Int Med Res 1973; 1:403–412.
14. Rack PH. Clomipramine (Anafranil) in the treatment of obsessional states with special reference to the Leyton Obsessional Inventory. J Int Med Res 1973; 1:397–402.
15. Collins G. Intravenous chlorimipramine in the treatment of severe depression. Br J Psychiatry 1970; 117:211–212.

16. Rack PH, Chir B. Clinical experience in the treatment of obsessional states (2). J Int Med Res 1977; 5:81–90.
17. Warneke LB. The use of intravenous chlorimipramine in the treatment of obsessive compulsive disorder. Can J Psychiatry 1984; 29:138–141.
18. Warneke LB. Intravenous chlorimipramine in the treatment of obsessional disorder in adolescence: case report. J Clin Psychiatry 1985; 46:100–103.
19. Thakur AK, et al. Intravenous clomipramine and obsessive-compulsive disorder. Can J Psychiatry 1991; 36:521–524.
20. Fallon B, et al. Open trial of intravenous clomipramine in five treatment-refractory patients with obsessive-compulsive disorder. J Neuropsychiatry 1992; 4:70–75.
21. Koran LM, et al. Intravenous clomipramine for obsessive-compulsive disorder [letter]. J Clin Psychopharmacol 1994; 14:216–218.
22. Warneke LB. Intravenous clomipramine for OCD [letter; comment]. Can J Psychiatry 1992; 37:522–523.
23. Yaryura-Tobias JA, Bhagavan HN. L-tryptophan in obsessive-compulsive disorder. Am J Psychiatry 1977; 134:1298–1299.
24. Koizumi HM. Obsessive-compulsive symptoms following stimulants [letter]. Biol Psychiatry 1985; 20:1332–1333.
25. Frye PE, Arnold LE. Persistent amphetamine-induced compulsive rituals: response to pyridoxine (B6). Biol Psychiatry 1981; 16:583–587.
26. Prasad AJ. Obsessive-compulsive disorder and trazodone [letter]. Am J Psychiatry 1984; 141:612–613.
27. Baxter L. Two cases of obsessive-compulsive disorder with depression responsive to trazodone. J Nerv Ment Dis 1985; 173:432–433.
28. Lydiard RB. Obsessive-compulsive disorder successfully treated with trazodone. Psychosomatics 1986; 27:858–859.
29. Kim SW. Trazodone in the treatment of obsessive-compulsive disorder: a case report [letter]. J Clin Psychopharmacol 1987; 7:278–279.
30. Ramchandani D. Trazodone for bowel obsession [letter]. Am J Psychiatry 1990; 147:124.
31. Prasad A. Efficacy of trazodone as an anti-obsessional agent. Neuropsychobiology 1986; 15:19–21.
32. Baxter LRJ, et al. Trazodone treatment response in obsessive-compulsive disorder—correlated with shifts in glucose metabolism in the caudate nuclei. Psychopathology 1987; 1:114–122.
33. Hermesh H, et al. Trazodone treatment in clomipramine-resistant obsessive-compulsive disorder. Clin Neuropharmacol 1990; 13:322–328.
34. Mattes JA. A pilot study of combined trazodone and tryptophan in obsessive-compulsive disorder. Int Clin Psychopharmacol 1986; 1:170–173.
35. Sunkureddi K, Markovitz P. Trazodone treatment of obsessive-compulsive disorder and trichotillomania [letter]. Am J Psychiatry 1993; 150:523–524.
36. Pigott TA, et al. A double-blind, placebo controlled study of trazodone in patients with obsessive-compulsive disorder. J Clin Psychopharmacol 1992; 12:156–162.

37. Jenike MA, Baer L. An open trial of buspirone in obsessive-compulsive disorder. Am J Psychiatry 1988; 145:1285–1286.
38. Watts VS, Neill JR. Buspirone in obsessive-compulsive disorder [letter]. Am J Psychiatry 1988; 145:1606.
39. Realmuto GM, et al. Clinical effect of buspirone in autistic children. J Clin Psychopharmacol 1989; 9:122–125.
40. Farid B, Bulto M. Buspirone in obsessional compulsive disorder: a prospective case study. Pharmacopsychiatry 1994; 27:207–209.
41. Murphy DL, et al. Obsessive-compulsive disorder: treatment with serotonin-selective uptake inhibitors, azapirones, and other agents. J Clin Psychopharmacol 1990; 10:91s–100s.
42. Pato MT, et al. Controlled comparison of buspirone and clomipramine in obsessive-compulsive disorder. Am J Psychiatry 1991; 148:127–129.
43. Vaisanen E, et al. Mianserin hydrochloride (org gb 94) in the treatment of obsessional states. J Int Med Res 1977; 5:289–291.
44. Jaskari MO. Observations on mianserin in the treatment of obsessive neuroses. Curr Med Res Opin 1980; 6:128–131.
45. Himmelhoch J. Personal communication, 1995.
46. Solursh LP. The use of LSD-25 in psychotherapy—an evaluation. Int J Neuropsychiatry 1965; Nov–Dec:651–656.
47. Brandrup E, Vanggaard T. LSD treatment in a severe case of compulsive neurosis. Acta Psychiat Scand 1975; 55:127–141.
48. Leonard HL, Rapoport JL. Relief of obsessive-compulsive symptoms by LSD and psilocin [letter]. Am J Psychiatry 1987; 144:1239–1240.
49. Bauer G, Nowak H. Doxepine ein neues antidepressivum wirkeingsvergleich mit amitriptyline. Arzrreunittelforschung 1969; 19:1642–1646.
50. Freed A, et al. The treatment of obsessional neurosis. Br J Psychiatry 1972; 120:590–591.
51. Snyder S. Amitriptyline therapy of obsessive-compulsive neurosis. J Clin Psychiatry 1980; 41:286–289.
52. Bartucci RJ, et al. Trimipramine in the treatment of obsessive-compulsive disorder [letter]. Am J Psychiatry 1987; 144:964–965.
53. Zajecka JM, et al. Coexisting major depression and obsessive-compulsive disorder treated with venlafaxine [letter]. J Clin Psychopharmacol 1990; 10:152–153.
54. Joel S. Twenty month study of iproniazid therapy. Dis Nerv Sys 1959; 20:521–524.
55. Annesley PT. Nardil response in a chronic obsessive compulsive. Br J Psychiatry 1969; 115:748.
56. Jain V, et al. Phenelzine in obsessional neurosis. Br J Psychiatry 1970; 117:237–238.
57. Ananth J. Treatment of obsessive compulsive neurosis: pharmacological approach. Psychosomatics 1976; 17:180–184.
58. Jenike MA. Rapid response of severe obsessive-compulsive disorder to tranylcypromine. Am J Psychiatry 1981; 138:1249–1250.

59. Jenike MA, et al. Monoamine oxidase inhibitors in obsessive-compulsive disorder. J Clin Psychiatry 1983; 44:131–132.

60. Isberg RS. A comparison of phenelzine and imipramine in an obsessive-compulsive patient. Am J Psychiatry 1981; 138:1250–1251.

61. Rihmer Z, et al. Response of phobic disorders with obsessive symptoms to MAO inhibitors [letter]. Am J Psychiatry 1982; 139:1374.

62. Swinson RP. Response to tranylcypromine and thought stopping in obsessional disorder. Br J Psychiatry 1984; 144:425–427.

63. Mahgoub OM. A remarkable response of chronic severe obsessive-compulsive neurosis to phenelzine. Acta Psychiatr Scand 1987; 75:222–223.

64. Tyrer P, et al. A study of the clinical effects of phenelzine and placebo in the treatment of phobic anxiety. Psychopharmacologia (Berlin) 1973; 32:237–254.

65. Sheehan DV, et al. Treatment of endogenous anxiety with phobic, hysterical and hypochondriacal symptoms. Arch Gen Psychiatry 1980; 37:51–59.

66. Insel TR, et al. Obsessive-compulsive disorder: a double-blind trial of clomipramine and clorgyline. Arch Gen Psychiatry 1983; 40:605–612.

67. Vallejo J, et al. Clomipramine versus phenelzine in obsessive-compulsive disorder: a controlled clinical trial. Br J Psychiatry 1992; 161:665–670.

68. Insel TR, Murphy DL. The psychopharmacological treatment of obsessive-compulsive disorder: a review. J Clin Psychopharmacol 1981; 1:304–311.

69. Hewlett WA. Use of benzodiazepines in obsessive compulsive disorder and Tourette's syndrome. Psychiatric Ann 1993; 23:309–316.

70. Sigwald J, Bouttier D. Le chlorhydrate de chloro-3 (dimethylamino-3'-propyl)-10-phenothiazine en pratique neuro-psychiatrique courante. Ann de Medecine 1953; 54:150–182.

71. Garmany G, et al. The use and action of chlorpromazine in psychoneuroses. Br Med J 1954; 8:439–441.

72. Altschuler M. Massive doses of trifluoperazine in the treatment of compulsive rituals. Am J Psychiatry 1962; 119:367–368.

73. Dally P. Chemotherapy of Psychiatric Disorders. London: Logos Press, 1967.

74. O'Regan JB. Treatment of obsessive-compulsive neurosis with haloperidol. CMA J 1970; 103:167–168.

75. Hussain M, Ahad A. Treatment of obsessive-compulsive neurosis. CMA J 1970; 103:648–650.

76. Rivers-Bulkeley N, Hollender MH. Successful treatment of obsessive-compulsive disorder with loxapine. Am J Psychiatry 1982; 139:1345–1346.

77. Knesevich JW. Successful treatment of obsessive-compulsive disorder with clonidine hydrochloride. Am J Psychiatry 1982; 139:364–365.

78. Ross D, Pigott L. Clonazepam for OCD [letter]. J Am Acad Child Adolesc Psychiatry 1993; 32:470–471.

79. Trethowan WH, Scott PAL. Chlorpromazine in obsessive-compulsive and allied disorders. Lancet 1955; i:781–785.

80. Delgado PL, et al. Fluvoxamine/pimozide treatment of concurrent Tourette's and obsessive-compulsive disorder. Br J Psychiatry 1990; 157:762–765.

81. Insel TR, et al. D-amphetamine in obsessive-compulsive disorder. Psychopharmacology (Berlin) 1983; 80:231–235.

82. Ceccherini-Nelli A, Guazzelli M. Treatment of refractory OCD with the dopamine agonist bromocriptine [letter]. J Clin Psychiatry 1994; 55:415–416.

83. Cohen DJ, et al. Clonidine in Tourette's syndrome. Lancet 1979; ii:551–553.

84. Cohen DJ, et al. Clonidine ameliorates Gilles de la Tourette syndrome. Arch Gen Psychiatry 1980; 37:1350–1356.

85. Lipsedge MS, Prothero W. Clonidine and clomipramine in obsessive-compulsive disorder [letter]. Am J Psychiatry 1987; 144:965–966.

86. Hewlett WA, et al. Clomipramine, clonazepam, and clonidine treatment of obsessive-compulsive disorder. J Clin Psychopharmacol 1992; 12:420–430.

87. Breitner C. Drug therapy in obsessional states and other psychiatric problems. Dis Nerv Sys 1960; 21:31–35.

88. Denham J. Psychotherapy of obsessional neurosis assisted by lithium. Topic Probl Psychother 1963; 4:195–198.

89. Bethune HC, et al. A new compound in the treatment of severe anxiety states: report on the use of diazepam. NZ Med J 1964; 63:153–156.

90. Rao AV. A controlled trial with "valium" in obsessive compulsive state. J Ind Med Assoc 1964; 42:564–567.

91. Orvin GH. Treatment of the phobic obsessive-compulsive patient with oxazepam, an improved benzodiazepine compound. Psychosomatics 1967; 8:278–280.

92. De Buck R. Clinical experience with lorazepam in the treatment of neurotic patients. Curr Med Res Opin 1973; 1:291–295.

93. Haward LRC. Multivariate symptom analysis related to response to lorazepam treatment. Curr Med Res Opin 1979; 6:20–23.

94. Lopez-Nogueira J. Terapeutica de la neurosis obsessiva con el Ro 5-3350. 5th World Congress of Psychiatry. Mexico, 1971.

95. Okuma T, et al. Effect of 7-bromo-5-(2-pyridyl)-3H-1,4-benzodiazepine-2(1H)-one, bromazepam (Ro 5-3350), a new minor tranquilizer, on psychoneurosis with special reference to the obsessive-compulsive symptoms. Folia Psychiatrica et Neurologica 1971; 25:181–193.

96. Kerry R, et al. A double blind cross over comparison of Ro 5-3350, bromazepam, diazepam (Valium) and chlordiazepoxide (Librium) in the treatment of neurotic anxiety. Psychosomatics 1972; 13:122.

97. Salmoni G, et al. Clinical and therapeutic considerations on the use of a benzodiazepine derivative, bromazepam (Ro 5-3350), in the treatment of obsessive-phobic disorders. Acta Neurol (Napoli) 1973; 28:588–609.

98. Grattarola FR, Morgando E. Clinical trial of a new derivative of the series of benzodiazepines: bromazepam (Ro 5-3350) in the treatment of phobic-obsessive symptoms. Minerva Med 1973; 64:2107–2111.

99. Deberdt R. Le traitement des nevroses obsessionnelles et phobiques par le Ro 5-3350. Therapie 1974.

100. De Giacomo P, Pierri G. Clinical evaluation of bromazepam with special reference to obsessive syndromes and phobias. Acta Neurol (Napoli) 1974; 29:307–313.

101. Burrell RH, et al. Use of bromazepam in obsessional, phobic and related states. Curr Med Res Opin 1974; 2:430–436.

102. Sonne LM, Holm P. A comparison between bromazepam (Ro 5-3350, Lexotan) and diazepam (Valium) in anxiety neurosis: a controlled, double-blind clinical trial. Int Pharmacopsychiatry 1975; 10:125–128.

103. Draper R. Clinical experience with Ro 5-3350 (bromazepam). J Int Med Res 1975; 3:214–222.

104. Cassano GB, et al. Bromazepam versus diazepam in psychoneurotic inpatients. Pharmakopsychiat 1975; 1:1–7.

105. Lin HN, Chen CC. A double-blind test on the effect of bromazepam in obsessive-compulsive neurosis. Taiwan I Hsueh Hui Tsa Chih 1979; 78:267–275.

106. Waxman D. A clinical trial of clomipramine and diazepam in the treatment of phobic and obsessional illness. J Int Med Res 1977; 5:99–110.

107. Cassano GB, et al. A multicenter controlled trial in phobic-obsessive psychoneurosis: the effect of chlorimipramine and its combinations with haloperidol and diazepam. Prog Neuro-Psychopharmacol 1981; 5:129–138.

108. Tesar GE, Jenike MA. Alprazolam as treatment for a case of obsessive-compulsive disorder. Am J Psychiatry 1984; 141:689–690.

109. Tollefson G. Alprazolam in the treatment of obsessive symptoms. J Clin Psychopharmacol 1985; 5:39–42.

110. Ketter T, et al. Alprazolam in the treatment of compulsive symptoms [letter]. J Clin Psychopharmacol 1986; 6:59–60.

111. Stein DJ, et al. Comparison of clomipramine, alprazolam and placebo in the treatment of obsessive-compulsive disorder. Hum Psychopharm 1992; 7:389–395.

112. Hewlett WA, et al. Clonazepam treatment of obsessions and compulsions. J Clin Psychiatry 1990; 51:158–161.

113. Bodkin JA, White K. Clonazepam in the treatment of obsessive compulsive disorder associated with panic disorder in one patient. J Clin Psychiatry 1989; 50:265–266.

114. Bacher NM. Clonazepam treatment of obsessive compulsive disorder [letter]. J Clin Psychiatry 1990; 51:168–169.

115. Baastrup P. Lithium in psychiatry. Acta Psychiat Scand 1969; 207(suppl):12.

116. Forssman H, Walender J. Lithium treatment on atypical indication. Acta Psychiatr Scand 1969; 207:34–40.

117. Jefferson JW, et al. Lithium for obsessive-compulsive disorder? [letter]. Psychosomatics 1984; 25:493.

118. Kukopulos A, et al. Prophylactic lithium in chronic phobic and obsessive syndromes. Eleventh CINP Conference. Vienna, 1978.

119. Van Putten T, Sanders D. Lithium in treatment failures. J Nerv Mental Dis 1975; 161:255–264.
120. Stern TA, Jenike MA. Treatment of obsessive-compulsive disorder with lithium carbonate. Psychosomatics 1983; 24:671–673.
121. Coleman E, Cesnik J. Skoptic syndrome: the treatment of an obsessional gender dysphoria with lithium carbonate and psychotherapy. Am J Psychother 1990; 44:204–217.
122. Geisler A, Schou M. Lithium and obsessive-compulsive neurosis: a double-blind therapeutic trial. Nordisk Psykiatrisk Tidsskrift 1970; 23:493–495.
123. Hesso R, Thorell L. Lithium and obsessive-compulsive neurosis. A double-blind cross-over clinical-therapeutic pilot-trial. Nordisk Psykiatrisk Tidsskrift, 1970; 23:496–499.
124. Platman SR. Lithium and rubidium: a role in the affective disorders. Dis Nerv System Sept 1971; 604–606.
125. Perez AR, Pillado LV. Estudio sobre el traiamiento con cloruro de rubidio en dos enfermas con depresion encronizada y una neurosis obsesiva. Actas Luso-Espanol de Neurol, Psiqui y cien afines 1981; IX:507–510.
126. Pacella B, et al. Clinical and EEG studies in obsessive-compulsive states. Am J Psychiatry 1944; 100:830–838.
127. Uhlenhuth E, et al. Diphenylhydantoin and phenobarbital in the relief of psychoneurotic symptoms. Psychopharmacologia (Berlin) 1972; 27:67–84.
128. Joffe RTK, Swinson RP. Methylphenidate in primary obsessive-compulsive disorder. J Clin Psychopharmacol 1987; 7:420–422.
129. Khanna S. Carbamazepine in obsessive-compulsive disorder. Clin Neuropharmacol 1988; 11:478–481.
130. Jenike MA, Brotman AW. The EEG in obsessive-compulsive disorder. J Clin Psychiatry 1984; 45:122–124.
131. McElroy SL, et al. Sodium valproate: its use in primary psychiatric disorders. J Clin Psychopharmacol 1987; 7:16–24.
132. von Wieczorek V. Anwendung von ovulationshemmern bei epileptikerinnen und psyhiatrischen kranken. Munchener Medizinische Wochenschrift 1969; 254–257.
133. Casas M, et al. Antiandrogenic treatment of obsessive-compulsive neurosis. Acta Psychiatr Scand 1986; 73:221–222.
134. Feldman JD, et al. Improvement in female patients with severe obsessions and/or compulsions treated with cyproterone acetate [letter]. Acta Psychiatr Scand 1988; 78:254.
135. Perciaccante M, Perciaccante RG. Progestin treatment for obsessive-compulsive disorder [letter]. Psychosomatics 1993; 34:284–285.
136. Kovacs G, Telegdy G. Role of oxytocin in memory and amnesia. Pharm Ther 1987; 18:375–395.
137. Ansseau M, et al. Intranasal oxytocin in obsessive-compulsive disorder. Psychoneuroendocrinology 1987; 12:231–236.
138. Den Boer JA, Westenberg HG. Oxytocin in obsessive compulsive disorder. Peptides 1992; 13:1083–1085.

139. Salzberg AD, Swedo SE. Oxytocin and vasopressin in obsessive-compulsive disorder [letter]. Am J Psychiatry 1992; 149:713–714.

140. Greenberg D, Belmaker RH. DDAVP as a possible method to enhance positive benefit of behavior therapy. Br J Psychiatry 1985; 147:713–715.

141. Weingartner H, et al. Effects of vasopressin on human memory function. Science 1981; 211:601–603.

142. Beckwith B, et al. DDAVP facilitates concept learning in human males. Peptides 1982; 3:627–630.

143. Swedo SE, Leonard HL. Childhood movement disorders and obsessive compulsive disorder. J Clin Psychiatry 1994; 55:32–37.

144. Swedo S, et al. Meeting of the American Psychiatric Association. San Francisco, 1993.

145. Allen AJ, et al. Case study: a new infection-triggered, autoimmune subtype of pediatric OCD and Tourette's syndrome. J Am Acad Child Adolesc Psychiatry 1995; 34:307–311.

146. Swedo SE, et al. High prevalence of obsessive-compulsive symptoms in patients with Sydenham's chorea. Am J Psychiatry 1989; 146:246–249.

9

Combination Pharmacological Treatment Strategies

Christopher J. McDougle
Yale University School of Medicine
New Haven, Connecticut

Wayne K. Goodman
University of Florida College of Medicine
Gainesville, Florida

INTRODUCTION

Despite significant advances in pharmacological treatment with potent serotonin [5-hydroxytryptamine (5-HT)] reuptake inhibitors (SRIs), as many as 40 to 60% of obsessive-compulsive disorder (OCD) patients are clinically unchanged after an adequate trial with these agents (1). Moreover, for most patients who "respond" to SRIs, the improvement is incomplete. In many large-scale clinical trials, for example, a 25 to 35% decrease in severity of OC symptoms as measured by the Yale-Brown Obsessive Compulsive Scale (Y-BOCS) (2,3) corresponds to a categorical treatment response. While this modest degree of reduction in symptom severity may enhance a patient's functional capacity, few patients become asymptomatic.

The lack of significant improvement in OC symptoms in the large group of SRI-refractory OCD patients suggests that the disorder may be neurobiologically heterogeneous and that many patients may require pharmacological treatments other than SRI monotherapy for maximal symptom control. It is conceivable that SRI-refractory patients may have alterations in 5-HT neurotransmission that are different from those in patients who are responsive to SRIs. Alternatively, these patients may have OCD as a result of abnormalities in neurochemical systems different from or in addition to those involving 5-HT, e.g., dopamine (DA) (4,5).

The OCD patient who has had only a partial response (less than 35% reduction in total Y-BOCS score) or is unimproved following 8- to 12-week trials of two different SRIs at adequate dosages should be considered for combination pharmacological treatment. To date, researchers have been pursuing two primary approaches to the psychopharmacology of the SRI-refractory OCD patient. The first involves adding to ongoing treatment with an SRI drugs that may further enhance 5-HT function. This strategy has proven particularly effective in refractory major depression, in which lithium augmentation of ongoing antidepressant treatment has been shown to be a useful pharmacological intervention (6). The second approach has been to add a DA receptor antagonist, such as pimozide (7) or haloperidol (8), to ongoing SRI therapy. The neuroleptic addition strategy is based largely on phenomenological (9,10) and genetic (11,12) evidence linking some forms of OCD with chronic tic disorders, such as Tourette's syndrome. Although associated with the potential development of significant side effects, including tardive dyskinesia, low-dose DA receptor antagonists are currently the most effective drug treatment for tics (13).

SRIs PLUS DRUGS AFFECTING SEROTONIN FUNCTION

A number of agents affecting 5-HT function, including tryptophan (14,15), fenfluramine (16), lithium (15,17–23), and buspirone (24–26), have been investigated for their potential to decrease OC symptoms when added to ongoing treatment with SRIs. The addition of the benzodiazepine clonazepam and combinations of two SRIs are also reviewed in this section.

Tryptophan

Rasmussen reported in a case study that the addition of tryptophan, the amino acid precursor of 5-HT, to ongoing clomipramine treatment led to a significant improvement in OC symptoms (15). However, others have found no improvement with this approach (14), and no controlled studies evaluating the efficacy of adding tryptophan to ongoing SRI therapy have been published in patients with OCD. Adverse neurological reactions resembling the 5-HT syndrome observed in laboratory animals have been reported when tryptophan is used in combination with fluoxetine (27). In addition, oral tryptophan is currently unavailable in the United States because of evidence linking some preparations with the eosinophilia myalgia syndrome (28,29).

Fenfluramine

Fenfluramine is marketed in the United States for the treatment of obesity under the trade name Pondimin. Hollander et al. (16) observed that the addition of open-label *d,l*-fenfluramine, an indirect 5-HT agonist, to ongoing SRI treatment led to improvement in OC symptoms in six of seven patients. Subsequently, two clomipramine-treated patients were reported to improve following addition of *d*-fenfluramine (30), which is believed to have more specific effects on 5-HT transport and release than the racemic mixture, but which is unavailable in the United States.

Some studies in laboratory animals have suggested that fenfluramine may be neurotoxic (31). Although there is no direct evidence that fenfluramine is toxic to 5-HT neurons in humans, this may reflect the difficulty in determining subtle neurological changes upon routine clinical examination. The preadministration of an SRI appears to prevent fenfluramine-induced 5-HT neurotoxicity by blocking entry of fenfluramine into 5-HT nerve terminals (32). Thus, the combined administration of an SRI and fenfluramine may be safer than fenfluramine alone with regard to 5-HT neurotoxicity. However, no controlled studies have been published that indicate that fenfluramine addition is efficacious in SRI-refractory OCD.

Lithium

Lithium has been hypothesized to potentiate antidepressant-induced increases in 5-HT neurotransmission by enhancing presynaptic 5-HT release in some areas of the brain (33). Based on the "serotonin hypothesis of OCD" (34) and the efficacy of lithium augmentation in refractory major depression (6), adding lithium to ongoing antidepressants has been investigated as a potential treatment approach in OCD.

In individual cases, lithium has been reported to augment the antiobsessional effect of chronic treatment with imipramine (23), clomipramine (15,18,19), desipramine (17), and doxepin (19) in patients with OCD. Also, the addition of open-label lithium to ongoing fluoxetine treatment reportedly led to an improvement in OC symptoms in three of four patients with OCD (22).

In contrast, no significant improvement in OC symptoms has been shown in controlled studies of lithium addition in OCD. Following 4 weeks of double-blind lithium augmentation of ongoing clomipramine treatment in 16 OCD patients who had demonstrated a partial response to clomipramine, Pigott et al. (21) observed no further reduction in OC symptoms. In a study by the Yale group (20), 2- and 4-week double-blind, placebo-controlled trials of lithium augmentation of ongoing fluvoxamine treatment were conducted in 20 and 10 patients with primary OCD, respectively, who had not responded to fluvoxamine monotherapy. Two weeks of double-blind lithium augmentation produced a small but statistically significant reduction in OC symptoms, although most patients did not have a clinically meaningful response. Furthermore, during the subsequent 4-week, double-blind, placebo-controlled trial, there was no significant statistical or clinical improvement in OC symptoms. Only 18% and 0% of the patients met criteria for a response to lithium augmentation during the 2- and 4-week treatment trials, respectively.

Based on these controlled studies, the addition of lithium in SRI-refractory OCD does not appear to approach the rate or quality of response typically observed with this strategy in antidepressant-resistant depression (6). This finding parallels the marked difference in behavioral response to acute tryptophan depletion between patients with major depression (35) and OCD (36) who are stabilized on SRIs, and suggests that the role of 5-HT in the mechanism of drug response in these disorders is different. Clinical experience suggests that lithium augmentation of ongoing SRI therapy may remain a viable treatment option for those patients who have primary major depression with secondary OC symptoms.

Buspirone

Buspirone is a 5-HT1A receptor partial agonist that, following chronic treatment, has been shown in preclinical studies to enhance 5-HT neurotransmission (37). Two open-label studies have investigated the use of buspirone as an adjunct to ongoing SRI treatment in patients with OCD. Markovitz et al. (38) and Jenike et al. (39) reported that the addition of buspirone to ongoing fluoxetine treatment led to greater improvement in OC symptoms than did treatment with fluoxetine alone. Also, an open-label case study described positive results with this approach in an 11-year-old girl with OCD and comorbid major depression (40).

Results from controlled studies of buspirone addition in OCD patients refractory to SRI monotherapy, however, have not corroborated these initial reports. Pigott et al. (25) found that the addition of buspirone, up to 60 mg/day for 10 weeks, to 14 patients who had partially improved following at least 3 months of clomipramine did not produce significant further improvement in ratings of OCD compared with the baseline period. Similarly, in a double-blind, placebo-controlled investigation of 6 weeks of buspirone addition to ongoing fluvoxamine treatment, McDougle et al. (24) found buspirone (up to 60 mg/day) no better than placebo in reducing OC, depressive, or anxiety symptoms in OCD patients. On the basis of conservative treatment response criteria, two of 19 (11%) patients who received 6 weeks of buspirone addition to ongoing fluvoxamine demonstrated a response (one marked, one partial), whereas two of the 14 (14%) patients treated with placebo showed a response (one marked, one partial). Negative results have also been reported from a controlled study evaluating the efficacy of buspirone addition in fluoxetine-refractory OCD patients (26).

In addition to the general lack of efficacy for this approach as determined in controlled studies, case reports have described a paradoxical worsening of OC symptoms (41) and the induction of a seizure (42), respectively, in OCD patients following the addition of buspirone to fluoxetine. Based on our clinical experience, the addition of buspirone to ongoing SRI treatment can at times result in an improvement in depressive symptoms in OCD patients with comorbid major depression.

In consideration of the "serotonin hypothesis of OCD" (34), a better response to lithium and buspirone addition to ongoing SRI treatment might have been predicted in these controlled treatment studies. Lithium, for example, is hypothesized to potentiate tricyclic antidepressants (TCAs) by enhancing the function of presynaptic 5-HT neurons, which interact with postsynaptic 5-HT receptors sensitized by long-term TCA treatment (33). Although selective SRIs do not cause postsynaptic sensitization to 5-HT, Chaput and colleagues (43) have suggested that chronic administration of these agents enhances net 5-HT neurotransmission by desensitizing inhibitory presynaptic 5-HT autoreceptors. Combining this presumed action of SRIs with lithium's facilitatory effect on presynaptic 5-HT neurons, the net effect would still be to enhance 5-HT neurotransmission (44).

The chronic administration of buspirone has also been shown in preclinical studies to enhance 5-HT neurotransmission (37). 5-HT1A binding sites have been identified both on the cell body of 5-HT neurons in the raphe nuclei and on postsynaptic neurons in the limbic system (45). Two days of treatment with the 5-HT1A agonist gepirone, which is similar to buspirone, markedly decreases the firing rate of dorsal raphe 5-HT neurons. After 7 days of treatment, there is partial recovery of baseline firing rates, and after 14 days of treatment, recovery is complete. This progressive adaptation of the firing rate of 5-HT neurons has been shown to be due to somatodendritic 5-HT autoreceptor desensitization. Postsynaptic 5-HT1A receptors are less responsive to microiontophoretically applied 5-HT during short-term treatment with gepirone. However, with long-term treatment this normalizes, resulting in a net increase in 5-HT neurotransmission during 5-HT1A agonist administration.

The facilitation of 5-HT function by a drug, however, may not be a sufficient condition for efficacy in the treatment of OCD. As Blier and de Montigny (46) observed, the lack of response to lithium augmentation in OCD patients may be related to the differential regional effects of lithium on 5-HT release in the central nervous system. For example, preclinical studies indicate that lithium administration can enhance 5-HT release in the spinal cord (47), the hypothalamus (48), and the hippocampus (49), whereas negative results have been consistently shown for the capacity of lithium to enhance 5-HT release in the cerebral cortex (50) and in the striatum (51), areas of the brain hypothesized to be involved in the pathophysiology of OCD (52–54). Similarly, with respect to the lack of efficacy of buspirone addition in SRI-refractory OCD patients, quantitative autoradiographic techniques have been used to demonstrate high densities of 5-HT1A receptors in hippocampal areas, lateral septum, entorhinal cortex, and central amygdala (55). In contrast, only very low densities of 5-HT1A receptors have been identified in areas such as the caudate-putamen, globus pallidus, and substantia nigra (55), which are believed to mediate some forms of OC phenomena (52–54). Thus, although buspirone administration may be affecting 5-HT function, this activity may not be occurring in areas of the brain relevant to the treatment of OCD.

Clonazepam

Evidence from studies in laboratory animals and humans suggests that the benzodiazepine clonazepam may have effects on 5-HT function unlike those of other drugs in its class (56). To date, little has been published regarding the addition of clonazepam to SRIs in the treatment of refractory OCD. Only one of seven patients with OCD had more than a 20% reduction on the Y-BOCS when open-label clonazepam (1–1.5 mg/day) was added to ongoing fluoxetine treatment (57). Cohen and Rosenbaum (58) described a 30-year-old man with OCD who experienced a significant reduction in OC symptoms following the addition of clonazepam 2 mg/day to ongoing imipramine 300 mg/day. Leonard et al. (59) reported that a 16-year-old male had a 75% reduction in OC symptoms after clonazepam 4–6 mg/day was added to ongoing fluoxetine 60 mg/

day. In a 4-week double-blind, placebo-controlled, crossover trial of clonazepam addition (3–4 mg/day) to ongoing fluoxetine or clomipramine, Pigott et al. (60) found significant improvement on one of three measures of OCD, not including the Y-BOCS. The patients did show a significant reduction in ratings of anxiety. In general, benzodiazepines may help secondary anxiety but are usually not effective for reducing the core symptoms of OCD.

Combining SRIs

No controlled studies of the simultaneous administration of two potent SRIs have been published in the treatment of OCD. A small open-label case series has described encouraging results with the coadministration of fluoxetine and clomipramine in adolescents with OCD (61). Because of the risks of selective SRI-induced elevations of plasma levels of TCAs (62), including clomipramine, caution should be used when giving these drugs concurrently. Due to clomipramine's potential to lower the seizure threshold and to impede cardiac conduction, it is important to obtain clomipramine blood levels before and after the addition of a selective SRI. Without controlled data that demonstrate efficacy for this combination treatment approach, this strategy cannot be routinely recommended.

In light of the heterogeneous clinical presentation (63), the inconsistent treatment outcome with SRI monotherapy (64), and the variation in behavioral and neurochemical responses to neuropharmacological probes of 5-HT function (65–68), it would be simplistic to assume that abnormalities in the 5-HT system alone could fully explain the complex neurobiological processes mediating OC symptoms. Several lines of evidence suggest, for example, that the brain DA system may contribute significantly to the pathophysiology and treatment of OC phenomena (4).

SRIs PLUS DRUGS AFFECTING DOPAMINE FUNCTION

Several lines of evidence from preclinical and clinical investigations implicate DA in the mediation of some forms of OCD (4). Considerable preclinical data suggest the existence of significant anatomical and functional interactions between 5-HT and DA systems in the brain, particularly in the basal ganglia (69,70). For some, but not all, brain regions, 5-HT neurons are believed to maintain a tonic inhibitory influence on DA function (71,72).

The Relationship Between Some Forms of OCD and Tourette's Syndrome

Tourette's syndrome (TS) is a chronic neuropsychiatric disorder of childhood onset characterized by multiple motor and phonic tics that wax and wane in severity (73). In addition to tics, many patients with TS have comorbid OCD. However, although the tics of TS are often reduced with DA receptor antagonists (13), comorbid OC symptoms are typically resistant to treatment with neuroleptic alone (5). Similarly, the frequency and intensity of OC symptoms in patients with a principal diagnosis of OCD are rarely decreased with neuroleptic monotherapy (4,5).

That OCD and TS are related conditions is not a new observation. Indeed, Frankel et al. (74) reported OC symptoms in 52%, Pitman et al. (75) in 63%, Nee et al. (76) in 68%, and Stefl (77) in 74% of TS patients studied. Family genetic studies provide evidence that TS and some forms of OCD are related (11,12).

While the etiology of TS remains unknown, neurobiological (78), pharmacological (13), neuroanatomic (79), brain imaging (80), and genetic (81) data implicate the DA system, in part, in the pathobiology of TS. The DA receptor antagonists haloperidol and pimozide partially reduce TS symptoms (13), whereas stimulants, which increase DA release, can acutely exacerbate symptoms in some patients with TS (82–84). It may be that some forms of OCD, particularly those comorbid with chronic tic disorders, are associated with dysregulated DA function.

To our knowledge, there have been no published controlled trials of DA receptor antagonist monotherapy in the treatment of OCD as it is currently defined in DSM-IV. Most experienced clinicians agree that, in general, DA receptor antagonists alone are not effective in the treatment of the core symptoms of OCD.

DA Receptor Antagonists

In light of the phenomenological (9,10), neurobiological (85), and genetic (11,12) overlap between some forms of OCD and chronic tic disorders, and the extensive preclinical literature documenting functionally coupled interactions between the 5-HT and DA systems in the brain (71,72), some investigators have been pursuing SRI/DA receptor antagonist combination treatment strategies in subgroups of OCD patients with SRI-refractory symptoms. Riddle et al. (86) reported on the anti-OC benefits of adding fluoxetine to neuroleptic in two cases of concomitant TS and OCD. Subsequently, the case of a 25-year-old man with comorbid TS who presented for treatment of OCD was described (87).

Fluvoxamine treatment worsened tics, led to coprolalia, and did not help the OC symptoms. The addition of the DA receptor antagonist pimozide, however, dramatically reduced both OC and tic symptoms. Double-blind sequential discontinuation of fluvoxamine and pimozide confirmed that pimozide alone reduced only tics, and that the combination of fluvoxamine and pimozide was required for the improvement in OC symptoms.

Pimozide

In an open case series by our group at Yale (7), neuroleptic, primarily pimozide, was added to ongoing treatment in 17 nonpsychotic OCD patients unresponsive to fluvoxamine with or without lithium. These cases were reviewed by a rater blind to treatment outcome to determine whether comorbid chronic tic disorders or schizotypal personality disorder (SPD) were associated with a positive response to pimozide addition. According to stringent criteria, nine of 17 (53%) patients were judged responders to this combination treatment strategy. A concurrent diagnosis of chronic tics or SPD was associated with a positive response to addition of pimozide. Seven of eight (88%) patients with these comorbid diagnoses were responders, whereas only two of nine (22%) patients without these comorbid diagnoses were responders.

Haloperidol

In a double-blind, placebo-controlled study in OCD patients with and without comorbid chronic tic disorders, the DA receptor antagonist haloperidol (mean dose = 6.2 ± 3.0 mg/day) was significantly more effective than placebo when added to ongoing fluvoxamine treatment in OCD patients unimproved with fluvoxamine monotherapy (8). The superiority of haloperidol over placebo in reducing the severity of OC symptoms was shown with the Y-BOCS. There was significant improvement in OC symptoms beginning at week 3 in the fluvoxamine-haloperidol-treated group. In contrast, there was no significant change in OC symptom severity at any time during the 4 weeks of placebo addition to ongoing fluvoxamine treatment. Based on conservative treatment response criteria, 11 of 17 (65%) patients randomly assigned to receive haloperidol were rated as responders after 4 weeks of treatment, compared with none of 17 patients who received placebo. Furthermore, as hypothesized, those OCD patients with a concurrent chronic tic disorder, such as TS, demonstrated a preferential response to the fluvoxamine-haloperidol combination treatment strategy. In fact, eight of eight patients with comorbid chronic tic disorders responded to double-blind haloperidol addition to ongoing fluvoxamine treatment. These results suggest that OCD patients with a comorbid chronic tic disorder may represent a valid and reliable subtype of OCD that requires conjoint SRI-DA receptor antagonist therapy for effective symptom reduction. Moreover, these drug response data indicate that both the brain 5-HT and DA systems may contribute to the treatment response and, perhaps, the pathophysiology of this "tic-related" subtype of OCD. While the relationship between OCD with comorbid chronic tic disorders and response to neuroleptic addition was substantiated in this study, it was not possible to make definitive conclusions about the usefulness of this treatment strategy in OCD patients with comorbid SPD because our sample included only two such patients.

In a related study, McDougle et al. (88) found that SRI monotherapy in OCD patients with comorbid chronic tics was less effective than in those without. In a retrospective case-controlled analysis, 33 fluvoxamine-treated OCD patients with a concurrent chronic tic disorder were compared with 33 age- and sex-matched OCD patients without chronic tics who had received fluvoxamine treatment in the same setting during the same period of time and in a similar manner. Although both groups of patients demonstrated statistically significant reductions in OC, depressive, and anxiety symptoms with fluvoxamine treatment, the frequency and magnitude of response of OC symptoms were significantly different between the two groups. A clinically meaningful improvement in OC symptoms occurred in only 21% of OCD patients with comorbid chronic tics compared with a 52% response rate in OCD patients without chronic tics. OCD patients with a concurrent chronic tic disorder showed only a 17% reduction in Y-BOCS scores compared with a 32% decrease in severity of OC symptoms in those OCD patients without chronic tics. This differential treatment response to SRI monotherapy between tic-related and non-tic-related OCD suggests that the pathophysiology of these two types of OCD may be dissimilar. Combined with evidence demonstrating significant differences in the phenomenology (9,10), neurobiology (89), and family genetics (11,12) of these disorders, these treatment response data indicate that tic-related forms of OCD may represent a clinically and biologically meaningful subtype of OCD. Because of the significant differences in response to pharmacological interventions between these two types of OCD, it is critical for clinicians to obtain a detailed personal lifetime and family history of tics in all OCD patients whom they are evaluating. As is true for many patients with psychotic depression (90), for example, those with tic-related OCD may have a different response to standard treatment approaches and may require combination pharmacological management for maximal symptom reduction.

Although neuroleptic addition was found to be effective in reducing OC symptoms in a significant number of patients, it should not be used indiscriminately in the treatment of OCD because these patients often require prolonged pharmacotherapy for continued symptom reduction. Because of the substantial risks of tardive dyskinesia, adequate trials of at least two SRIs, including clomipramine, should be completed before neuroleptic addition is considered. Furthermore, a time-limited trial of neuroleptic addition should be attempted, with reassessment of the risk/benefit ratio of ongoing neuroleptic treatment at regular intervals.

Based on our clinical experience since completion of the double-blind, placebo-controlled study of haloperidol addition described above, we now typically begin haloperidol 0.5 mg/day, with subsequent increases every 4–7 days to a maximum of 2–4 mg/day, as clinically indicated. We have found that when this combination treatment strategy is effective, the response will usually occur with lower doses of the DA receptor antagonist than previously described. The recent development of alternative drug treatments that modulate DA transmission without such high risks of toxic extrapyramidal side effects (e.g., clozapine and risperidone) may prove useful in some patients with OCD (see below).

Clozapine Monotherapy

Clozapine is an atypical neuroleptic that is effective for treatment-refractory schizophrenia (91). The drug's ability to block 5-HT2A, 5-HT2C, 5-HT3, and DA (D4 > D3 > D2 = D1) receptors has been proposed as its mechanism of action. Based on the efficacy of combined SRI-DA receptor antagonist treatment in some forms of SRI-refractory OCD (8) and clozapine's neurochemical profile, our group recently completed a 10-week systematic investigation of clozapine monotherapy in adults with treatment-refractory OCD (92). Ten of 12 patients who entered the study completed the 10-week trial of clozapine. Two patients discontinued the trial prematurely due to sedation (100 mg/day for 3 weeks) and hypotension (125 mg/day for 2 weeks), respectively. The mean dose of clozapine in the 10 completers was 462.5 ± 93.7 mg/day. Clozapine was not associated with statistically significant improvement in scores on the Y-BOCS, the Y-BOCS obsession subscale, the Y-BOCS compulsion subscale, the Hamilton Depression Rating Scale, or the Clinical Global Impression global improvement item. None of the 10 patients met criteria for treatment response. Two patients who had comorbid chronic motor tic disorder showed no significant reduction in tics. The results of this systematic investigation suggest that clozapine monotherapy is not an effective intervention for most adult patients with treatment-refractory OCD. The role of clozapine addition in SRI-refractory OCD remains undetermined.

Risperidone

Risperidone is a highly potent and selective 5-HT2 receptor antagonist that also acts as an antagonist at the alpha-1, histamine-1, D2, and alpha-2 receptor sites (93). It has no peripheral or central anticholinergic activity, nor does it have significant interactions with opioid, benzodiazepine, substance P, or neurotensin receptors (94). Its side-effect profile appears to offer advantages over that of D2 receptor antagonists currently used to treat SRI-refractory OCD, such as haloperidol and pimozide. Our group recently described our initial experience in adding risperidone to ongoing fluvoxamine treatment in three patients with SRI-refractory OCD (95). The following case exemplifies our preliminary observations.

Ms. A, a 52-year-old married woman, first developed OC symptoms at the age of 20 years. Her primary symptoms consisted of contamination and sexual obsessions and repeating and washing compulsions. At the age of 23 she developed a secondary major depressive episode. Her OC symptoms persisted without significant improvement until her presentation to our clinic 32 years after the onset of her OCD. Ms. A had received numerous somatic treatments prior to entering our program. At the age of 25 she had a course of ECT without improvement. She received subsequent treatment with tranylcypromine 60 mg/day, phenelzine 60 mg/day plus lithium carbonate 900 mg/day, phenelzine plus lithium and fluphenazine 10 mg/day, clomipramine 250 mg/day with clonazepam 1 mg/day, clomipramine plus lithium, clomipramine plus haloperidol 1 mg/day, clozapine 600 mg/day, fluvoxamine 300 mg/day, and fluvoxamine plus desipramine 150 mg/day plus 6 months of in-home exposure and response prevention behavior therapy, with no improvement in her OC symptoms.

Risperidone 1 mg/day was added to fluvoxamine 250 mg/day, and within 2 weeks Ms. A reported a marked reduction in her level of anxiety, improved mood, and increased ability to resist performing compulsions. She showered unassisted for the first time in 3 years, ate dinner with her husband in a restaurant for the first time in 8 years, had sex with her husband for the first time in 6 years, began assisting her housekeeper in cleaning her home, and started to look for volunteer work. Four weeks following risperidone addition, Ms. A had a reduction in her Y-BOCS score from 31 to 11. She has retained this treatment response, with mild sedation being the only side effect. Interestingly, Ms. A had a family history of chronic tics. The two other OCD patients in this preliminary report who had a similar treatment response had comorbid schizotypal personality disorder and body dysmorphic disorder, respectively.

The addition of risperidone to ongoing SRI may also be an effective treatment for some children with SRI-refractory OCD. In a recently completed open-label trial, we found that risperidone in doses of 1.5–2.5 mg/day was effective in reducing children's Y-BOCS scores by 16%, 100%, and 30% when added to ongoing paroxetine 60 mg/day, sertraline 100 mg/day, and paroxetine 30 mg/day, respectively, in children with chronic tic disorders with comorbid OCD (96). We are currently conducting double-blind, placebo-controlled studies of risperidone addition in children and adults with SRI-refractory OCD.

Bromocriptine

A recent open-label case series described a significant reduction in OC and depressive symptoms during chronic treatment with the DA receptor agonist bromocriptine (12.5–30 mg/day), in three of four adults with OCD and comorbid major depression (97). These results are consistent with an earlier report by Insel et al. (98) that described improvement in OC symptoms in OCD patients given an acute dose of dextroamphetamine and contrast with reports describing induction or exacerbation of OC symptoms in some subjects following dextroamphetamine (99), bupropion (100), and cocaine use (101,102). Like bromocriptine, dextroamphetamine, bupropion, and cocaine enhance central DA function although other neurochemical systems are also affected. Controlled studies of bromocriptine in OCD patients with and without comorbid conditions, including major depression and chronic tics, are needed before the efficacy of this approach can be determined.

SUMMARY AND FUTURE DIRECTIONS

To date, two primary lines of approach have been taken in the development of pharmacological treatments for the SRI-refractory OCD patient. Controlled studies of the first approach—adding drugs that further enhance 5-HT function, such as lithium and buspirone—have not yielded consistently encouraging results. However, preliminary reports suggest that additional agents that affect 5-HT function may be worthy of further study. For example, Chouinard et al. (103) described a man with SRI-refractory OCD who had a robust and sustained response following the addition of the steroid suppressant aminoglutethimide 250 four times per day to ongoing fluoxetine 40 mg/day. Steroid antagonists, such as aminoglutethimide, ketoconazole, and metyrapone, work to enhance 5-HT function and have been reported to be effective in some cases of treatment-refractory depression (104).

Pindolol, a beta-blocker with potent 5-HT1A receptor antagonism properties, has been reported to induce a dramatic and rapid improvement in depressive symptoms when added to ongoing drug treatment in some patients with major depression who are unimproved on SRIs or monoamine oxidase inhibitors (105). The drug is believed to increase 5-HT function by blocking the inhibitory feedback to somatodendritic 5-HT1A autoreceptors induced by SRI-generated increases in extracellular 5-HT (106). Controlled studies of pindolol coadministered with an SRI should be conducted in patients with OCD to evaluate the potential efficacy of the treatment and to determine if a more rapid onset of action can be achieved.

The second major line of investigation has involved the addition of DA receptor antagonists, such as haloperidol and pimozide, to the treatment regimen of SRI-refractory OCD patients. This combination treatment strategy has been shown to be effective for reducing OC symptoms, primarily in SRI-refractory patients who have comorbid personal or family histories of chronic tics. Preliminary reports describing the effectiveness of risperidone addition to SRIs are encouraging—this drug has been associated with fewer acute and chronic extrapyramidal side effects than the typical neuroleptics. Controlled studies of risperidone addition are needed in children and adults with SRI-refractory OCD. Finally, the addition of other drugs with demonstrated efficacy for reducing tics, such as the alpha$_2$ adrenoreceptor agonists clonidine (107) and, possibly, guanfacine (108), may be worthy of study as adjuncts to SRIs in the treatment of tic-related forms of OCD.

ACKNOWLEDGMENTS

This work was supported in part by grants MH25642, MH30929, MH45802, and MH49351 from the National Institute of Mental Health, the State of Connecticut Department of Mental Health and Addiction Services, and a 1994–96 National Alliance for Research on Schizophrenia and Depression Young Investigators Award (C.J.M.). The authors wish to thank Elizabeth Kyle for her assistance in the preparation of the manuscript.

REFERENCES

1. McDougle CJ, et al. The psychopharmacology of obsessive compulsive disorder: implications for treatment and pathogenesis. In: Dunner DL, ed. Psychopharmacology II. Psychiatric Clinics of North America. Vol 16(4). Philadelphia: WB Saunders, 1993:749–766.
2. Goodman WK, et al. The Yale-Brown Obsessive Compulsive Scale (Y-BOCS). Part I. Development, use, and reliability. Arch Gen Psychiatry 1989; 46:1006–1011.
3. Goodman WK, et al: The Yale-Brown Obsessive Compulsive Scale (Y-BOCS). Part II. Validity. Arch Gen Psychiatry 1989; 46:1012–1016.
4. Goodman WK, et al: Beyond the serotonin hypothesis: a role for dopamine in some forms of obsessive compulsive disorder? J Clin Psychiatry 1990; 51:36–43.
5. McDougle CJ, et al. Dopamine antagonists in tic-related and psychotic spectrum OCD. J Clin Psychiatry 1994; 55(3 suppl):24–31.
6. Price LH. Lithium augmentation of tricyclic antidepressants. In: Extein I, ed. Treatment of Tricyclic Resistant Depression. Washington, DC: American Psychiatric Press, 1989:49–79.
7. McDougle CJ, et al. Neuroleptic addition in fluvoxamine-refractory obsessive-compulsive disorder. Am J Psychiatry 1990; 147:652–654.
8. McDougle CJ, et al. Haloperidol addition in fluvoxamine-refractory obsessive compulsive disorder: a double-blind, placebo-controlled study in patients with and without tics. Arch Gen Psychiatry 1994; 51:302–308.
9. Holzer JC, et al. Obsessive compulsive disorder with and without a chronic tic disorder: a comparison of symptoms in 70 patients. Br J Psychiatry 1994; 164:469–473.
10. Leckman JF, et al. Tic-related vs. non-tic-related obsessive compulsive disorder. Anxiety 1995; 1:208–215.
11. Pauls DL, Leckman JF. The inheritance of Gilles de la Tourette's syndrome and associated behaviors: evidence for autosomal dominant transmission. N Engl J Med 1986; 315:993–997.
12. Pauls DL, et al. Gilles de la Tourette's syndrome and obsessive-compulsive disorder. Arch Gen Psychiatry 1986; 43:1180–1182.
13. Shapiro E, et al. Controlled study of haloperidol, pimozide, and placebo for the treatment of Gilles de la Tourette's syndrome. Arch Gen Psychiatry 1989; 46:722–730.
14. Mattes J. A pilot study of combined trazodone and tryptophan in obsessive-compulsive disorder. Int Clin Psychopharmacol 1986; 1:170–173.
15. Rasmussen SA. Lithium and tryptophan augmentation in clomipramine resistant obsessive-compulsive disorder. Am J Psychiatry 1987; 141:1283–1285.

16. Hollander E, et al. Fenfluramine augmentation of serotonin reuptake blockade antiobsessional treatment. J Clin Psychiatry 1990; 51:119–123.
17. Eisenberg J, Asnis G. Lithium as an adjunct treatment in obsessive-compulsive disorder. Am J Psychiatry 1985; 142:663.
18. Feder R. Lithium augmentation of clomipramine. J Clin Psychiatry 1988; 49:458.
19. Golden RN, et al. Combined lithium-tricyclic treatment of obsessive-compulsive disorder. Biol Psychiatry 1988; 23:181–185.
20. McDougle CJ, et al. A controlled trial of lithium augmentation in fluvoxamine-refractory obsessive compulsive disorder: lack of efficacy. J Clin Psychopharmacol 1991; 11:175–184.
21. Pigott TA, et al. A controlled comparison of adjuvant lithium carbonate or thyroid hormone in clomipramine-treated patients with obsessive-compulsive disorder. J Clin Psychopharmacol 1991; 11:242–248.
22. Ruegg RG, et al. Lithium plus fluoxetine treatment of obsessive compulsive disorder. New Research Abstr 92. 143rd Annual Meeting of the American Psychiatric Association, New York, 1990.
23. Stern TA, Jenike MA. Treatment of obsessive-compulsive disorder with lithium carbonate. Psychosomatics 1983; 24:671–673.
24. McDougle CJ, et al. Limited therapeutic effect of addition of buspirone in fluvoxamine-refractory obsessive compulsive disorder. Am J Psychiatry 1993; 150:647–649.
25. Pigott TA, et al. A double-blind study of adjuvant buspirone hydrochloride in clomipramine-treated patients with obsessive-compulsive disorder. J Clin Psychopharmacol 1992; 12:11–18.
26. Grady TA, et al. Double-blind study of adjuvant buspirone for fluoxetine-treated patients with obsessive-compulsive disorder. Am J Psychiatry 1993; 150:819–821.
27. Steiner W, Fontaine R. Toxic reaction following the combined administration of fluoxetine and L-tryptophan: five case reports. Biol Psychiatry 1986; 21:1067–1071.
28. Hertzman PA, et al. Association of the eosinophilia-myalgia syndrome with the ingestion of tryptophan. N Engl J Med 1990; 322:869–73.
29. Slutsker L, et al. Eosinophilia-myalgia syndrome associated with exposure to tryptophan from a single manufacturer. JAMA 1990; 264:213–217.
30. Judd FK, et al. Fenfluramine augmentation of clomipramine treatment of obsessive compulsive disorder. Aust NZ J Psychiatry 1991; 25:412–414.
31. Schuster CR, et al. Fenfluramine: Neurotoxicity. Psychopharmacol Bull 1986; 22:148–151.
32. Clineschmidt BV, et al. Fenfluramine and brain serotonin. Ann NY Acad Sci 1978; 305:222–241.
33. de Montigny C. Enhancement of the 5-HT neurotransmission by antidepressant treatments. J Physiol 1981; 77:455–461.
34. Insel TR, et al. Obsessive-compulsive disorder and serotonin: is there a connection? Biol Psychiatry 1985; 20:1174–1188.

35. Delgado PL, et al. Serotonin function and the mechanism of antidepressant action: reversal of antidepressant induced remission by rapid depletion of plasma tryptophan. Arch Gen Psychiatry 1990; 47:411–418.

36. Barr LC, et al. Tryptophan depletion in patients with obsessive-compulsive disorder who respond to serotonin reuptake inhibitors. Arch Gen Psychiatry 1994; 51:3009–317.

37. Blier P, et al. A role for the serotonin system in the mechanism of action of antidepressant treatments: preclinical evidence. J Clin Psychiatry 1990; 51(4 suppl):14–20.

38. Markovitz PJ, et al. Buspirone augmentation of fluoxetine in obsessive-compulsive disorder. Am J Psychiatry 1990; 147:798–800.

39. Jenike MA, et al. Buspirone augmentation of fluoxetine in patients with obsessive compulsive disorder. J Clin Psychiatry 1991; 52:13–14.

40. Alessi N, Bos T. Buspirone augmentation of fluoxetine in a depressed child with obsessive-compulsive disorder. Am J Psychiatry 1991; 148(11):1605–1606.

41. Tanquary J, Masand P. Paradoxical reaction to buspirone augmentation of fluoxetine [letter]. J Clin Psychopharmacol 1990; 10:377.

42. Grady TA, et al. Seizure associated with fluoxetine and adjuvant buspirone therapy [letter]. J Clin Psychopharmacol 1992; 12:70–71.

43. Chaput Y, et al. Effects of a selective 5-HT reuptake blocker, citalopram, on the sensitivity of 5-HT autoreceptors: electrophysiological studies in the rat. Naunyn Schmiedebergs Arch Pharmacol 1986; 333:342–345.

44. de Montigny C, et al. Lithium carbonate addition in tricyclic antidepressant-resistant unipolar depression: correlations with the neurobiologic actions of tricyclic antidepressant drugs and lithium ion on the serotonin system. Arch Gen Psychiatry 1983; 40:1327–1334.

45. Vergé D, et al. Presynaptic 5-HT autoreceptors on serotonergic cell bodies and/or dendrites but not terminals are of the 5-HT1A subtype. Eur J Pharmacol 1985; 113:463–464.

46. Blier P, de Montigny C. Lack of efficacy of lithium augmentation in obsessive-compulsive disorder: the perspective of different regional effects of lithium on serotonin release in the central nervous system [letter]. J Clin Psychopharmacol 1992; 12:65–66.

47. Sangdee C, Franz DN. Lithium enhancement of 5-HT transmission induced by 5-HT precursors. Biol Psychiatry 1980; 15:59–75.

48. Baptista TJ, et al. Chronic lithium administration enhances serotonin release in the lateral hypothalamus but not in the hippocampus in rats: a microdialysis study. J Neural Transm 1990; 82:31–41.

49. Treiser SL, et al. Lithium increases serotonin release and decreases serotonin receptors in the hippocampus. Science 1981; 213:1529–1531.

50. Friedman E, Hoau-Yan W. Effect of chronic lithium treatment of 5-hydroxytryptamine autoreceptors and release of 5[3H]hydroxytryptamine from rat brain cortical, hippocampal, and hypothalamic slices. J Neurochem 1988; 50:195–201.

220   McDougle and Goodman

51. Katz RJ, et al. Evoked release of norepinephrine and serotonin from brain slices: inhibition by lithium. Science 1968; 162:466–467.
52. Modell JG, et al. Neurophysiologic dysfunction in basal ganglia/limbic striatal and thalamocortical circuits as a pathogenetic mechanism of obsessive-compulsive disorder. J Neuropsychiatry 1989; 1:27–36.
53. Rapoport JL, Wise SP. Obsessive-compulsive disorder: evidence for basal ganglia dysfunction. Psychopharmacol Bull 1988; 24:380–384.
54. Stahl SM. Basal ganglia neuropharmacology and obsessive-compulsive disorder: the obsessive-compulsive disorder hypothesis of basal ganglia dysfunction. Psychopharmacol Bull 1988; 24:370–374.
55. Radja F, et al. Autoradiography of serotonin receptor subtypes in the central nervous system. Neurochem Int 1991; 18:1–15.
56. Wagner HR, et al. Clonazepam-induced up-regulation of serotonin-1 and serotonin-2 binding sites in rat frontal cortex. Adv Neurol 1986; 43:645–651.
57. Jenike MA. Drug treatment of obsessive-compulsive disorder. In: Jenike MJ, Baer L, Minichiello WE, eds. Obsessive Compulsive Disorders: Theory and Management. 2nd ed. Littleton, MA: PSG Publishing, 1990:249–282.
58. Cohen LS, Rosenbaum JF. Clonazepam: new uses and potential problems. J Clin Psychiatry 1987; 48(suppl 10):50–55.
59. Leonard HL, et al. Clonazepam as an augmenting agent in the treatment of childhood-onset obsessive-compulsive disorder. J Am Acad Child Adolesc Psychiatry 1994; 33(6):792–794.
60. Pigott TA, et al. A controlled trial of clonazepam augmentation in OCD patients treated with clomipramine or fluoxetine. New Research Abstr 144. 145th Annual Meeting of the American Psychiatric Association, Washington, DC, May 4, 1992.
61. Simeon JG, et al. Treatment of adolescent obsessive-compulsive disorder with a clomipramine-fluoxetine combination. Psychopharmacol Bull 1990; 26:285–292.
62. Preskorn SH. Pharmacokinetics of antidepressants: why and how they are relevant to treatment. J Clin Psychiatry 1993; 54(suppl 9):14–34.
63. Goodman WK, et al. Types of symptoms and response to clomipramine in obsessive compulsive disorder. New Research Program and Abstract. 143rd Annual Meeting of the American Psychiatry Association, New York, 1990.
64. Goodman WK, et al. Biological approaches to treatment-resistant obsessive compulsive disorder. J Clin Psychiatry 1993; 54(6 suppl):16–26.
65. Charney DS, et al. Serotonin function in obsessive compulsive disorder: a comparison of the effects of tryptophan and m-chlorophenylpiperazine in patients and healthy subjects. Arch Gen Psychiatry 1988; 45:177–185.
66. Hollander E, et al. Effects of chronic fluoxetine treatment on behavioral and neuroendocrine responses to meta-chloro-phenylpiperazine in obsessive-compulsive disorder. Psychiatry Res 1991; 36:1–17.
67. Zohar J, et al. Serotonergic responsivity in obsessive-compulsive disorder. Arch Gen Psychiatry 1987; 44:946–951.

68. Goodman WK, et al. M-chlorophenylpiperazine in patients with obsessive compulsive disorder: absence of symptom exacerbation. Biol Psychiatry 1995; 38:138–149.

69. Crespi F, et al. Simultaneous in vivo voltametric measurement of striatal extracellular DOPAC and 5-HIAA levels: effect of electrical stimulation of dopamine and 5-HT neuronal pathways. Neurosci Lett 1988; 90:285–291.

70. Parent A. Mammalian pallidum: a source of redundancy. In: Parent A, ed. Comparative Neurobiology of the Basal Ganglia. New York: John Wiley, 1986.

71. Baldessarini RJ, Marsh E. Fluoxetine and side effects [letter]. Arch Gen Psychiatry 1990; 47:191–192.

72. Korsgaard S, et al. Behavioral aspects of serotonin-dopamine interaction in the monkey. Eur J Pharmacol 1985; 118:245–252.

73. American Psychiatric Association Committee on Nomenclature and Statistics. Diagnostic and Statistical Manual of Mental Disorders. 4th ed. Washington, DC: American Psychiatric Association, 1994.

74. Frankel M, et al. Obsessions and compulsions in Gilles de la Tourette's syndrome. Neurology 1986; 36:378–382.

75. Pitman RK, et al. Clinical comparison of Tourette's disorder and obsessive-compulsive disorder. Am J Psychiatry 1987; 144:1166–1171.

76. Nee LE, et al. Gilles de la Tourette syndrome: clinical and family study of 50 cases. Ann Neurol 1980; 7:41–49.

77. Stefl ME. Mental health needs associated with Tourette syndrome. Am J Public Health 1984; 74:1310–1313.

78. Cohen DJ, et al. Chronic, multiple tics of Gilles de la Tourette's disease: CSF acid monoamine metabolites after probenecid administration. Arch Gen Psychiatry 1978; 35:245–250.

79. Singer HS, et al. Abnormal dopamine uptake sites in postmortem striatum from patients with Tourette's syndrome. Ann Neurol 1991; 30:558–562.

80. Malison RT, et al. [^{123}I]β-CIT SPECT imaging demonstrates increased striatal dopamine transporter binding in Tourette's syndrome. Am J Psychiatry 1995; 152:1359–1361.

81. Grice DE, et al. haplotype relative risk association study of Tourette's syndrome. 33rd Annual Meeting of the American College of Neuropsychopharmacology, December 12–16, 1994.

82. Factor SA, et al. Cocaine and Tourette's syndrome. Ann Neurol 1988; 23:423–424.

83. Golden GS. Gilles de la Tourette syndrome following methylphenidate administration. Develop Med Child Neurol 1974; 16:76–78.

84. Mesulam MM. Cocaine and Tourette's syndrome. N Engl J Med 1986; 315:398.

85. Leckman JF, et al. CSF biogenic amines in obsessive compulsive disorder, Tourette's syndrome, and healthy controls. Neuropsychopharmacology 1995; 12:73–86.

86. Riddle MA, et al. Fluoxetine treatment of obsessions and compulsions in

patients with Tourette's syndrome. Am J Psychiatry 1988; 145:1173–1174.

87. Delgado PL, et al. Fluvoxamine/pimozide treatment of concurrent Tourette's and obsessive-compulsive disorder. Br J Psychiatry 1990; 157:762–765.

88. McDougle CJ, et al. The efficacy of fluvoxamine in obsessive-compulsive disorder: effects of comorbid chronic tic disorder. J Clin Psychopharmacol 1993; 13:354–358.

89. Leckman JF, et al. Elevated levels of CSF oxytocin in obsessive compulsive disorder patients without a personal or family history of tics. Arch Gen Psychiatry 1994; 51:782–792.

90. Nelson JC, Bowers MB. Delusional unipolar depression. Arch Gen Psychiatry 1978; 35:1321–1328.

91. Kane J, et al. Clozapine for the treatment-resistant schizophrenic. Arch Gen Psychiatry 1988; 45:789–796.

92. McDougle CJ, et al. Lack of efficacy of clozapine monotherapy in refractory obsessive compulsive disorder. Am J Psychiatry 1995; 152:1812–1814.

93. Leysen JE, et al. Biochemical profile of risperidone, a new antipsychotic. J Pharmacol Exp Ther 1988; 247:661–670.

94. Moller HJ, et al. Efficacy and tolerability of a new antipsychotic compound (risperidone): results of a pilot study. Pharmacopsychiatry 1991; 24:185–189.

95. McDougle CJ, et al. Risperidone addition in fluvoxamine-refractory obsessive compulsive disorder: three cases. J Clin Psychiatry 1995; 56:526–528.

96. Lombroso PJ, et al. Risperidone treatment of children and adolescents with chronic tic disorders: a preliminary report. J Am Acad Child Adolesc Psychiatry 1995; 34(9):1147–1152.

97. Ceccherini-Nelli A, Guazzelli M. Treatment of refractory OCD with the dopamine agonist bromocriptine. J Clin Psychiatry 1994; 55(9):415–416.

98. Insel TR, et al. D-amphetamine in obsessive-compulsive disorder. Psychopharmacology 1983; 80:231–235.

99. Frye PE, Arnold LE. Persistent amphetamine-induced compulsive rituals: response to pyridoxine (B6). Biol Psychiatry 1981; 16:583–587.

100. Jacobsen LK, et al. Bupropion and compulsive behavior [letter]. J Am Acad Child Adolesc Psychiatry 1994; 33:143–144.

101. McDougle CJ, et al. Pathophysiology of obsessive-compulsive disorder [letter]. Am J Psychiatry 1989; 146:1350–1351.

102. Satel SL, McDougle CJ. Obsessions and compulsions associated with cocaine abuse [letter]. Am J Psychiatry 1991; 148:947.

103. Chouinard G, et al. Potentiation of fluoxetine by steroid suppression in obsessive compulsive disorder resistant to SSRIs: a case report. 33rd Annual Meeting of the American College of Neuropsychopharmacology, Dec 12–16, 1994.

104. Anand A, et al. Antiglucocorticoid treatment of refractory depression with ketoconazole: a controlled case study. Biol Psychiatry 1995; 37:338–340.
105. Artigas F, et al. Pindolol induces a rapid improvement of depressed patients treated with serotonin reuptake inhibitors. Arch Gen Psychiatry 1994; 51:248–251.
106. Wong DT, et al. Augmentation of fluoxetine induced elevation of extracellular 5-HT levels by pindolol, an antagonist at 5-HT1A receptor. 33rd Annual Meeting of the American College of Neuropsychopharmacology, Dec 12–16, 1994.
107. Leckman JF, et al. Clonidine treatment of Gilles de la Tourette's syndrome. Arch Gen Psychiatry 1991; 48:324–328.
108. Chappell PB, et al. Guanfacine treatment of comorbid attention deficit hyperactivity disorder in Tourette's syndrome: preliminary clinical experience. J Am Acad Child Adolesc Psychiatry 1995; 34(9):1140–1146.

10

Behavioral Treatment of OCD

Joao Silvestre
New York State Psychiatric Institute
New York, New York

Bonnie R. Aronowitz
The Mount Sinai Medical Center
New York, New York

INTRODUCTION

Research over the past two decades has confirmed that obsessive-compulsive disorder (OCD), once considered treatment-refractory, is now amenable to treatment. Corroborated by controlled double-blind clinical trials, the pharmacological treatments for OCD thought to be most efficacious are medications with potent serotonergic properties, such as clomipramine, fluoxetine, fluvoxamine, sertraline and paroxetine (1–5; Goodman et al., in review). In addition to these pharmacological studies of OCD, there has been a vast increase and development of behavioral interventions in OCD treatment and assessment of their efficacy (6). Behavioral treatments, either alone or in combination with these medications, may have dramatic effects on the alleviation of even moderate to severe OCD symptomatology. Behavior therapy (BT) is composed mainly of the two procedures of exposure and response prevention. Exposure consists of either self- or therapist-guided confrontation with patients' feared objects or circumstances. Once confronted with feared stimuli, patients are asked to refrain from the performance of rituals, which is known as response prevention.

In this chapter, we briefly summarize the current status and application to OCD of established behavioral approaches and alternative treatment methodologies such as cognitive approaches. Special issues in OCD behavioral treatment such as religiosity, home visits, familial involvement, and relapse prevention are addressed. Application of behavioral techniques employed in research trials to clinical practice is highlighted. Finally, we present three case presentations in a private-practice context.

THEORETICAL MODEL OF BEHAVIOR THERAPY

Learning theory underlying the acquisition and modern treatment of OCD is understood as the result of the interplay of classic and operant conditioning theories. The two-stage theory of Mowrer (7) describes mechanisms by which fear is learned. In the first stage, previously neutral stimuli become temporally associated with fearful stimuli (unconditioned stimuli) such that the former acquire anxiety-provoking properties, resulting in a conditioned fear response. When this occurs at the second stage, due to the aversive characteristics of the stimuli, avoidance or escape responses are developed, later reinforced by the removal of anxiety, or negative reinforcement. Finally, higher-order conditioning occurs when other neutral stimuli such as words, numbers, images, thoughts, or situations are associated with the conditioned stimuli. The first stage of fear acquisition is less defensible since patients typically cannot recall specific aversive events connecting to the onset of their symptomatology (8). The second stage is more clearly explicative of how OCD symptoms are maintained because it is readily observable in patients' behavior and forms the basis of BT.

One main shift in conceptualization of OCD maintenance may be viewed in the changes in the OCD diagnosis in DSM-IV. Unlike DSM-III-R, in which the OCD definition postulated a mutually exclusive relationship between obsessions and compulsions, DSM-IV defines compulsions, in addition to being behavioral events, as mental acts, previously classified as obsessions. This new definition is consonant with the findings of Foa and Tillmanns (9), who postulated a functional relationship between obsessions and compulsions. According to Foa's model, obsessions or ruminations are defined as thoughts, images, urges, or impulses that generate anxiety. In contrast, compulsions are viewed as newly learned anxiety-reducing strategies caused by obsessions and may be either overt actions or covert cognitive (neutralizing) events. Thus, OCD is composed by a set of either overt or covert anxiety-provoking events (obsessions). To reduce anxiety caused by obsessions, certain overt or covert behaviors, or compulsions, are performed. This new DSM-IV conceptualization is consistent with the behavioral model of OCD and the techniques of exposure and response prevention (ERP) developed from this model.

BEHAVIOR THERAPY: DESCRIPTION

In Vivo vs. Imaginal Exposure

Exposure is a behavioral technique used to confront patients with feared stimuli, objects, or situations with the goal of ultimate reduction of unpleasant reactions, anxiety, and affect. In "in vivo" exposure, the actual anxiety-producing stimuli are presented to patients until anxiety is reduced to a tolerable level. In imaginal exposure, anxiety-provoking stimuli are presented in imagination only, until feared stimuli lose their fear-provoking properties. In vivo exposure has been found to be more effective than imaginal exposure by some investigators (10).

Steketee et al. (11) matched the content of the exposure situation to patients' fears. They hypothesized that OCD patients with extreme avoidance or fear of catastrophic consequences who were unable to tolerate in vivo exposure, or for whom in vivo exposure is not feasible for practical reasons, might benefit from imaginal exposure and more readily agree to undertake BT (12). They suggested that imaginal exposure does not affect treatment gains initially but aids in the maintenance of treatment gains and may therefore be used to supplement in vivo exposure. In addition, imaginal exposure facilitates the processing of fear cues and thus facilitates the habituation to the feared stimuli.

Response Prevention

Response prevention, based on an extinction model, is used as an adjuvant strategy to exposure in behavior therapy. Following exposure, patients are prevented from engaging in rituals that initially caused increases in obsessions and anxiety, thereby allowing them to remain in their feared situations. Typically, response prevention leads to a gradual reduction in anxiety and obsessions. Prolonged exposure to the feared situation and response prevention of avoidance or rituals lead to habituation.

Efficacy of Behavioral Treatment of OCD

Studies indicate that BT is an effective treatment modality for approximately 70–80% of OCD patients (6,13–16). Behavioral approaches are particularly appealing because they have the highest risk–benefit profile of all OCD treatments (17). Moreover, research indicates that BT results in better maintenance of therapeutic benefits in comparison to pharmacotherapy.

Meyer (18), in the earliest study of BT, provided OCD patients with continuous 24-hour daily ERP and found improvement in symptomatology. Marks (19) compared four BT studies (20–23) of three techniques: 1) rapid exposure (exposure to the highest-anxiety-provoking stimuli at the outset of treatment) with response prevention, 2) slow exposure with response prevention, and 3) relaxation. In vivo exposure was significantly more effective than the 3-week relaxation condition, which yielded almost no benefit; 70% of OCD patients were reported as very much improved and treatment gains were maintained at 6-month and 2-year follow-ups. In contrast, Pato et al. (24) reported a recurrence of obsessions in 89% of patients following clomipramine discontinuation and substitution with placebo.

Stanley and Turner (25) found that BT incorporating ERP produces higher response rates in comparison with pharmacotherapy, particularly when relapse and dropout rates are considered. Foa et al. (6) summarized results from 18 studies involving 273 subjects treated in different countries by different therapists with ERP. Fifty-one percent had reductions of at least 70% in obsessions and rituals and were rated much improved. An additional 39% had reductions between 31% and 69% in obsessions and rituals while 10% had no more than 30% reduction in obsessions and rituals and were considered unimproved. In follow-ups ranging from months to years, three-fourths of subjects were found to remain at least moderately improved. Methodological limitations of these studies include variable outcome measures, use of booster BT and medication by some subjects during follow-up periods, retrospective reports, exclusion of the 25% of subjects who refused BT, and uncontrolled investigation. Finally, these results should be interpreted in light of the fact that research programs typically select highly motivated patients able to tolerate exposure to their most feared situations and that 20 to 30% of patients refuse or drop out of treatment (26). This may serve as a selection bias in favor of less ill patients, and may not be readily generalizable to the larger population of OCD patients.

Behavioral treatment is most effective in OCD patients with contamination fears leading to cleaning or hand-washing compulsions (27). In contrast, patients with checking compulsions may not have as positive a response to BT or may respond more slowly than do those with cleaning rituals (28).

In general, BT is far less effective with patients with severe obsessions in the absence of compulsions. Intuitively it would appear that if behaviors are less overt, they will remain less amenable to intervention and the clinician will be more dependent on patient account as to the frequency and intensity, and thus clinical change, in obsessions. In the past, covert ritualizers (sometimes called pure obsessionals) presented a great deal of difficulty in BT treatment. However, it has been found that response prevention could be applied with success to even covert ritualizers (29).

The most difficult clinical presentation for behavioral treatment are those patients with neither overt nor covert rituals. In these patients, pharmacotherapy is a good first-line treatment. In primarily obsessional pharmacotherapy nonresponders, however, other types of behavioral and cognitive treatment techniques may be of benefit, e.g., thought-stopping, imaginal flooding, cognitive restructuring, and treatment packages including a combination of these.

Common misconceptions about BT are that it causes symptom substitution and that it is dangerous to interrupt avoidance behavior. The interruption of avoidance by response prevention produces transient increases in anxiety but does not result in loss of control or psychotic behavior.

While BT is remarkably effective over the short term and provides long-term gains for most patients, approximately one-fourth of patients refuse BT and a small minority of BT treatment compliers fail to improve.

FACTORS ASSOCIATED WITH TREATMENT-REFRACTORINESS AND FAILURE

A relative shortcoming of the implementation of BT is that some patients with severe OCD symptoms and/or additional interpersonal difficulties cannot tolerate the distress elicited by ERP. These patients may either be unable to make a commitment to such a program or drop out of treatment. Indeed, Fals-Stewart and Lucente (30) found that high ratings on "schizophrenia," "depression," and "social introversion" on the Minnesota Multiphasic Personality Inventory (MMPI) contributed significantly to prediction of treatment compliance with BT.

Other factors associated with treatment noncompliance may be either the complete failure of patients to comply with treatment instructions (19) or the development of unreported covert novel rituals. In addition, the continuation of older rituals may result in the neutralization or reduced efficacy of exposure therapy (27). Moreover, patients may unwittingly and automatically perform competing rituals that interfere with habituation. For example, patients with successful prevention of a hand-washing response may engage in the automatic repetitive rubbing of hands on clothing to ward off contamination anxiety. Patients may also avoid the discomfort of exposure by engaging in dissociation from the experience of anxiety-provoking stimuli.

There is some controversy over whether OCD patients whose obsessions are ego-syntonic have a poorer treatment outcome than those patients with ego-dystonic obsessions. Some authors and clinicians maintain that a patient subgroup likely to be treatment-resistant is OCD patients with overvalued ideation (OVI) or a strong belief in both the veracity of obsessional content and its ability to ward off feared consequences (31). Many clinicians and researchers claim that unless the irrational beliefs of OCD patients with ego-syntonic obsessions are dispelled, the efficacy of BT is likely to be compromised (32). In contrast, others claim that there is no significant association between OVI and the efficacy of BT (33), and that the relationship between degree of insight and treatment outcome requires clarification (34).

An additional subgroup of treatment-recalcitrant patients who respond more slowly to BT than do both checkers and cleaners includes patients with primary obsessional slowness (35). Behavioral treatment of obsessional slowness consists of shaping procedures in which the patient is given a specified time limit to initiate or complete problematic tasks. Improvement of obsessional slowness with BT is generally time-consuming and progress is slow.

Various comorbid disorders have been implicated as complicating the course of BT with OCD. Examples of such axis I disorders or conditions are the depressive disorders, in which patients, possibly because of low energy or motivation or impaired attention and concentration, fail to habituate during exposure (31). Depression should initially be treated by either pharmacotherapy or cognitive behavioral treatment (CBT), particularly if it is severe or debilitating, prior to the implementation of BT. Finally, to boost motivation and provide support, a companion may be enlisted to engage in BT with OCD patients if depression is manageable.

OCD patients dually diagnosed with certain axis II disorders such as schizotypal personality disorder have an extremely high rate of treatment failure with both pharmacological and nonpharmacological treatments (36,37). A case study of a patient with schizotypal personality disorder reported that "restricted environmental stimulation therapy (REST) used adjunctively to imaginal exposure and response prevention resulted in a substantial reduction of arousal to fear-evoking stimuli in addition to a marked reduction in OCD symptoms" (38). In this treatment, subjects relax in a single-bed, soundproofed chamber with an intercommunications system and a silent positive-pressure ventilation system. Monologs designed to evoke feared stimuli are presented on an endless running tape and other stimulation is minimized. In contrast to these behavioral and cognitive-behavioral techniques, other nonpharmacological treatments such as relaxation, hypnosis, or biofeedback, while not harmful when coupled with BT, have not been found effective when used alone in OCD treatment.

On the Millon Clinical Multiaxial Inventory (MCMI), OCD patients with histrionic/borderline traits demonstrated symptom reduction at posttreatment but failed to maintain treatment gains at follow-up (30). OCD patients with dependent characteristics demonstrated the best outcome.

There are indications that high doses of benzodiazepines or alcohol also interfere with habituation during exposure. State-dependent learning may be one reason that habituation fails to occur because learning that occurs in one mood state, such as an intoxicated or substance-induced state, may be not be readily transferrable to another mood state, e.g., a substance-free state. Therefore, substance-dependent or abusing OCD-patient applicants for BT must first be tapered from substances prior to embarking on exposure therapies. However, the judicious use of benzodiazepines may actually be indicated in particularly recalcitrant OCD cases, such as those with debilitating anxiety, who would otherwise refuse to consider BT.

Inadequate duration of exposure within sessions or patients' failure to gain sufficient practice of exposure between sessions through compliance with homework may result in failure of generalization of fear reduction.

Family members who fail to follow ERP instructions, as in cases of familial overinvolvement, enmeshment, or family members affected with OCD, may complicate or result in modest gains in BT.

Some investigators maintain that it is best to refrain from treating OCD patients who cannot tolerate complete exposure to all obsessions and compulsions in a complete hierarchy. Others argue that such patients may be treated until a tolerable limit on their obsessive and compulsive hierarchy is reached. The types of symptoms and psychiatric comorbidity in patients intolerant of BT require further investigation.

COGNITIVE VS. BEHAVIOR THERAPY

Early studies of cognitive therapy techniques as adjuncts or facilitators of BT have not been encouraging (39,40). Emmelkamp et al. (41) found that confronting irrational beliefs through the application of rational-emotive therapy (RET) was beneficial for OCD patients, suggesting that cognitive interventions were as effective as in vivo self-controlled exposure. Van Oppen et al. (42) evaluated cognitive therapy outcome based on the combination of Beck's and Salkovskis' cognitive treatments in comparison with self-controlled in vivo ERP. Seventy-one patients were randomly assigned to 16 sessions of either treatment, and both therapies led to significant improvements. However, multivariate significant interaction effects on obsessive-compulsive and associated psychopathology measures suggested the superior efficacy of cognitive therapy in comparison to self-controlled in vivo exposure. To date, no additional controlled studies have replicated this finding. James and Blackburn (43) concluded that methodological difficulties in cognitive treatment studies limit optimistic conclusions regarding the relative efficacy of cognitive treatments in comparison to other OCD treatments.

One application of cognitive techniques is the re-education of patients in the more realistic appraisal of situations and encouragement of risk-taking behavior. This may facilitate controlling responses to anxiety in addition to the practice of exposure to feared thoughts and response prevention to compulsive behaviors. Moreover, since compliance with BT is contingent on patients' beliefs regarding treatment, cognitive therapy aimed at the ascertainment of reasons for treatment resistance to BT have also been advocated (44). Once these automatic thoughts or irrational beliefs have been identified, they may be open to challenge by the clinician.

The combination of ERP and cognitive therapy may be effective in some patients in eliminating severe obsessions and compulsions and reducing concomitant anxiety and depression (45,46). This may be particularly applicable to patients presenting with overvalued ideation, e.g., those patients believing in the veracity of obsessions, or to those whose thoughts are ego-syntonic and who are extremely resistant to BT (31). However, according to Foa and Steketee (47), cognitive strategies are so integral to BT that it is difficult to ascertain the relative contribution to treatment outcome of behavioral vs. cognitive interventions.

OTHER BEHAVIORAL INTERVENTIONS

Other techniques have been added to BT, such as thought-stopping and relaxation. Thought-stopping has been useful in BT, but has frequently been misused and may worsen patients' conditions. For example, if thought-stopping is used to interrupt intrusive obsessive cognitions, it may become a ritual form of antiexposure or avoidance. As a ritual, it may provide temporary relief from distress associated with obsessions.

However, rituals do not provide enduring relief and actually lead to more frequent and intense obsessions. Proper application of thought-stopping is the interruption of mental rituals that decrease distress from obsessions. Thought-stopping should be applied to interrupt anxiolytic mental rituals but never for anxiogenic obsessions.

Relaxation has also been added to BT. One rationale for the use of relaxation is as a coping device to encourage patients to enter exposure situations. However, relaxation is time-consuming and may distract patients from essential treatment components and constitute a form of avoidance. Relaxation has been viewed by behavior therapists as being inert or an active placebo in controlled studies of effective elements of ERP in BT.

The extent to which such techniques aid certain OCD patients under certain conditions (e.g., relaxation of OCD patients with comorbid panic disorder) or act as redundant or even distraction measures must be determined. Research is thus needed on these adjunctive techniques to ascertain the necessary and sufficient conditions of successful OCD treatment.

COMBINED BEHAVIORAL TREATMENT AND PHARMACOTHERAPY

Behavioral treatment and pharmacotherapy may yield mutually enhancing and additive effects in OCD and may thus be an efficacious treatment strategy. Their simultaneous administration has been viewed as complementary, and their combination appears to be more effective than either modality used alone (48). Three controlled studies demonstrated that BT in combination with SSRIs was more effective than either treatment alone, with either clomipramine (49,50) or fluvoxamine (51). There is no apparent state-dependent learning when SSRIs are combined with BT. Most other medications, in addition to SSRIs, may be combined with BT. There is little information regarding the combination of MAOIs and BT.

Another use of BT and pharmacotherapy combination is for OCD patients unable to tolerate a BT program. These patients may initiate pharmacological treatment to facilitate their participation in BT. In addition, when OCD patients have a robust response to pharmacotherapy, residual symptoms may benefit from the addition of a BT trial. Finally, there is a high relapse rate in OCD following medication discontinuation. Thus, the addition of BT to the pharmacological regimen may protect patients against symptom recurrence following medication discontinuation (52).

Baxter et al. (53) found that OCD patients treated with BT or fluoxetine demonstrated brain changes on positron emission tomography
(PET) scans. One OCD subject group was treated with fluoxetine; the
second was treated with twice-weekly ERP BT. Subjects were followed
for 10 weeks and pre- and posttreatment PET scans were compared.
Following both treatments, PET scans of six of nine subjects in the BT
condition and seven of nine subjects in the fluoxetine condition exhibited decreased glucose metabolic activity in the right caudate nucleus of
the brain—the area responsible for habit learning and complex movements. Five nonresponders to either treatment and two controls did not
demonstrate such brain changes. This fascinating finding suggests that,
like pharmacotherapy, BT causes metabolic and functional changes in
the brains of OCD subjects. The novel habit learning gathered from BT
may thus alter brain anatomy and hence brain functions. Recent research strongly supports the notion that a specific brain circuit is responsible for OCD (53,54).

OCD ASSESSMENT

Most behavioral treatments (9,12,56,57) are composed of hallmark elements, briefly summarized below. We supplement these descriptions
with observations and rationales derived from our clinical applications
and experience.

Many patients present with an enormous array of unsuccessful
treatments and, despite current motivation, remain hopeless, demoral-
ized, and suspicious regarding the efficacy of new treatments. In the
initial evaluation, these treatment experiences should be probed by the
clinician in detail for several reasons. First, invaluable information is
yielded about potentially inadequate diagnostic assessment or poor understanding of the functional relationship between obsessions and compulsions, leading to inadequate treatment. The identification of an insufficient length of a medication or BT trial or insufficient frequency of
clinician visits in past treatments provides both the OCD patient and the
current clinician with renewed hope regarding the undertaking of a new
treatment. Knowledge of these factors will aid the clinician in understanding the nature of treatments as well as in planning current treatment in light of past therapeutic failures.

Hollander (58) surveyed 701 members of the OC Foundation regarding costs and quality-of-life issues. Of 701 OCD subjects, 60% had
suffered a significant impact on general quality-of-life measures: 60%
had lowered academic achievement, 66% had lowered career aspira-
tions, and 40% were unable to work because of OCD—with an average

loss of 2 years of wages. Finally, 62% of the subjects had difficulty maintaining relationships secondary to OCD. It is thus important to ascertain the relative impact of OCD in comparison to other psychiatric comorbidity on patients' quality of life in the context of the initial assessment.

OCD patients have been found to perform significantly more poorly than normal controls on visuospatial, visuoperceptual, and visual discrimination tasks as well as on set shifting, sequencing, and tracking tasks (59–62). It should be ascertained, in the context of the evaluation, whether OCD patients have additional neuropsychological deficits that may contribute to or exacerbate OCD symptoms; e.g., visuoperceptual impairment may contribute to sensory doubt, which may lead to checking compulsions.

A daily self-monitoring journal of the situations and/or objects that elicit obsessive thoughts or compulsive rituals should be maintained by the OCD patient. The journal both provides a baseline measure and enhances awareness of symptoms for patient and therapist. The journal should include notes on specific triggers for obsessions and/or compulsions—e.g., fear of fire, the death image of a family member—in addition to the ways in which the OC symptoms interfere with daily functioning. An OCD symptom constellation is identified and a detailed functional analysis made for each symptom, e.g., for handwashing: frequency, intensity/severity, duration, and eliciting stimuli (internal cues—thoughts, feelings, physical sensations—or external cues—specific objects or situations), the feared consequences, when OC is prevented, and the situations avoided (see case presentations).

The clinician must carefully ascertain both avoidance patterns and pervasiveness on a continuum to ensure that subtle avoidances are not overlooked. In addition, this detailed inquiry aids in the development of the exposure hierarchy. An example of severe avoidance and pervasiveness is the complete avoidance of opening a door due to contamination obsessions, leading to either dependence on significant others or complete houseboundedness. The next level of avoidance may be the use of a napkin or object to turn the doorknob. A final level may be touching a "less contaminated" part of the doorknob with only the fingertips.

A hierarchy of feared objects and situations is developed in collaboration with the patient and graded in order of difficulty level using the Subjective Units of Discomfort Score (SUDS), with 0 being "no anxiety at all" and 100 being "the most anxiety experienced, close to a panic state." In addition to being a detailed description of a patient's feared items, the hierarchy serves as a general treatment contract between patient and clinician. Patients often require the therapist's assistance in the form of probes in order to deal with difficulty in assigning gradations or specific numbers to their feared situations. The therapist may provide structure in the form of anchors; e.g., a SUDS of 0 would be a state of relaxation or sleep while a SUDS of 50 may be high anxiety while simultaneously being able to work. In contrast, a SUDS of 80 may involve severe distress that significantly interferes with the ability to perform daily activities. The therapist should remain flexible about changing the order of difficulty of items in the hierarchy at any point since patients often over- or underestimate expected discomfort.

Three or four initial sessions are typically devoted to the BT evaluation phase. A sound therapeutic rapport (63) in addition to the detailed explication of the content, frequency, intensity, duration, irrationality, and degree of control and distress over OCD symptoms is essential in this initial evaluation. The use of psychometric assessments and informant information, when available, augment patient data and provide rich information regarding symptoms in a variety of contexts. A structured interview can be employed to assess and monitor severity and change in OCD patients' symptomatology. The Yale-Brown Obsessive Compulsive Scale (Y-BOCS) (64,65) is a widely used assessment instrument that includes a checklist to assess both obsession and compulsion type and severity. A widely used scale to assess improvement in OCD as a result of treatment is the National Institute of Mental Health Obsessive Compulsive Scale (NIMH-OC). The Maudsley Obsessional Compulsive Inventory has 30 true–false questions focused on symptom dimensions (66). It has a total obsessional score and five subscales (checking, slowness, repetition, washing, doubting-conscientiousness, and ruminating). Other widely used OCD scales include the Leyton Obsessional Inventory (LOI) (67) and the Obsessive-Compulsive Disorder Checklist.

BEHAVIORAL TREATMENT IMPLEMENTATION

The necessary ingredients of behavior therapy following assessment, diagnostic determination, and establishment of a hierarchy include:

1. Psychoeducation with patient and/or significant others about OCD, including possible etiologies, mechanisms responsible for maintenance of the disorder, and research findings
2. Rationale for and description of the components of ERP in BT and the setting of realistic treatment expectations; citation of work demonstrating that BT serves as a biological treatment in that its efficacy and demonstrated changes in the brain are comparable to those of pharmacological treatment
3. A behavioral contract between patient and therapist

4. ERP with enlistment of family members, when available or clinically indicated, to serve as BT cotherapists; individualized BT sessions for sufficient habituation to occur
5. Design of daily homework
6. Termination
7. Relapse-prevention strategies
8. Booster sessions

FAMILY INVOLVEMENT

Initial interview and/or enlistment of family members into BT may be beneficial or even essential, depending on the degree of family involvement with the OCD patient. However, patients should not be treated solely at the request of family members. From the vantage point of the clinician, family members often provide information about obsessions and compulsions that patients may minimize or feel uncomfortable discussing initially, or of which they may be unaware because of chronicity or automaticity. Family interviews likewise provide information regarding the impact of OCD symptoms on family members and the role of the family in OCD symptom maintenance. Examples of family involvement in rituals include the removal of work clothing when the patient comes home to avoid contamination; reassurance against dirt, germs, and contaminants; and joint counting, checking, or washing. The situation is further complicated when other family members are also affected with OCD and engage in either joint rituals or vastly discrepant or antagonistic rituals, resulting in significant conflict.

Resentment and emotional conflict are engendered by the constraints placed upon family life by the OCD patient. For these reasons, and out of fear that family members will control the treatment or intrude in the relationship with the therapist, OCD patients may refuse to have family members involved in treatment. When family members are an integral part of BT, the challenge for the clinician is to maintain a strong patient rapport while insisting that family members not provide reassurance or collude with patients' rituals. It is our experience that the establishment of a strong therapeutic alliance ensures that the family will enter BT unremarkably.

Family members are typically knowledgeable about OCD from everyday life with the patient. However, psychoeducation providing corrective information about OCD and explication of BT concepts and rationale is essential to treatment. Instead of the family's enabling the OCD patient by participation in obsessions/compulsions, the role of the family in BT is one of cotherapist and empathic responder to the patient.

However, they should make firm commitments to neither accompany the patient in rituals nor reassure him that obsessions indeed neutralized anxiety or that rituals were performed correctly.

Families may insist that the OCD patient is manipulative with his obsessions and compulsions. This raises a philosophical question regarding the etiology of OCD. If one believes that OCD is a biologically determined illness, then the patient would be viewed as an unfortunate victim of his symptomatology, as with any organic illness. Conversely, if one believes that OCD is a solely psychological disorder under conscious control, then one is more likely to blame the patient for his inability to change. Therefore, in practice, clinicians may confront this issue with families, arguing that OCD is neither a fully biological nor a psychologically determined illness, but that it is more realistically viewed as being mutually interactive. At times patients may use obsessions and compulsions in a manipulative fashion for secondary gain, but at other times symptoms may be more independent of environmental stressors and can be considered more biologically driven.

HOME VISITS

Clinical experience indicates that home visits lead to better generalization of therapeutic gains and outcome (9,31). Not all patients require home visits, but they are appropriate for those with extreme symptom severity or other life circumstances precluding visits to the therapist's office. Moreover, the therapist's office may lack the stimuli necessary to reliably elicit obsessions and compulsions, which may exist solely in the patient's home. Home visits thus enable in vivo observation and identification of patients' OC symptoms, in an excellent environment for the engagement of both the patient and significant others in treatment. In the natural home setting, the therapist may identify OC symptoms that are inherent in the patient's life or have gained sufficient automaticity that patients fail to recognize that they are in fact due to OCD.

In addition, home-based treatment is particularly valuable in the treatment of hoarding. Individuals with saving obsessions will probably require direct supervision by the therapist, or a significant other trained by the therapist, to aid them in the initial disposal of items. The therapist can initially model the disposal of items without undue checking and encourage the patient to continue in structured homework. Frequently the severity of hoarding is such that additional arrangements are required, such as hiring a pickup service for removal of discarded objects.

RELIGIOUS ISSUES IN BT IMPLEMENTATION

Religious beliefs may interfere with patients' willingness to engage in BT. Individuals with intrusive religious images or sexual obsessions often feel them to be sacrilegious and forbidden, and tend to fear and reject such thoughts. Devout patients—particularly those with sexual and religious obsessions, e.g., a devout grade-school teacher obsessed with potentially molesting young children when in close proximity to them—often engage in self-blame and struggle with acceptance of these thoughts as part of their OCD, and thus strongly resist the implementation of exposure. The content of religious and sexual obsessions in devout OCD patients typically involves guilt, immorality, or a state of sin. Otherwise the OCD process is similar to that in other OCD types in that obsessions are triggered by external or internal events and result in anxiety or guilt, and ritualistic or avoidance behavior is an attempt to eliminate such discomfort.

Steketee et al. (68) suggest that type of religion is not predictive of treatment outcome; however, the most religious patients appear to do less well in BT. They also suggest that rigid religious or moral beliefs in OCD may be targeted for exposure with patients' assent. During the BT assessment phase, the therapist often struggles with the wish to both respect the patient's religious beliefs and aid the patient through exposure. Because of the nature of these OC symptoms in religious OCD patients, therapists may hesitate to recognize the legitimacy of targeting these symptoms for BT modification. This treatment impasse may best be resolved by the introduction of clergy or religious leaders as consultants. However, spiritual leaders typically lack the clinical expertise necessary to appropriately address the needs of the religious OCD patients. The ideal form of therapeutic liaison is contact with clergy familiar with mental-health issues—and OCD in particular, if available.

ISSUES SPECIFIC TO BT IN PRIVATE PRACTICE

The application of protocols with demonstrated efficacy in research trials is likewise beneficial in private-practice settings. However, certain adaptations and variations are necessarily required, such as fewer and shorter sessions and greater reliance on homework assignments. Paradoxically, however, patients presenting to clinical practice tend to have more severe OCD than those accepted into controlled BT studies; thus, a particular challenge is presented to the private-practice clinician. One solution is brief but frequent telephone contact with patients between sessions or the incorporation of trained significant others, lay paraprofessionals, or qualified supervised graduate students. This may be more cost-effective and allow for home visits and/or more frequent contact with patients. Various investigations have demonstrated that therapists' intervention can be reduced and patients can partially conduct their own treatments through self-controlled exposure.

Emmelkamp and Kraanen (69) found that self-controlled in vivo exposure proved to be as effective as therapist-controlled in vivo exposure despite the fact that in the latter condition the duration of each treatment session was twice that of the former condition. Emmelkamp and Wessels (70) investigated the efficacy of self-controlled exposure in OCD and agoraphobic patients. Gradual exposure was used because of its ease in self-administration in comparison to flooding.

In a controlled study of severe, unremitting OCD, Marks et al. (50) found that the most significant treament element appeared to be appropriate exposure instructions rather than actual intensive therapist involvement. One group was given clomipramine in addition to antiexposure instructions, or instructions to actually avoid anxiety. Another group received clomipramine plus self-exposure instructions, and a third received placebo plus self-exposure instructions. The clomipramine-plus-self-exposure group was again subdivided so that one-half received therapist-accompanied exposure and the other half continued with self-exposure. Despite the fact that the first half received five times more treatment, they fared no better than the second half, who simply conducted self-exposure. The clomipramine-plus-self-exposure group fared significantly better than the clomipramine-plus-antiexposure group in comparison to exposure with therapist involvement. Kirk (71) treated 36,000 outpatients in a practice setting with ERP and reported that 58% of patients achieved their goals, 17% were found moderately improved, and 25% had poor outcomes. This author reported that in clinical practice he emphasized homework exposures unless a patient required the presence of the clinician.

The effect of individual variables, such as social or family support and symptom type and severity, on intensive inpatient BT vs. private-practice BT has not been investigated. Emmelkamp et al. (72) found that BT directed at the OCD resulted in improvement irrespective of marital quality and partner involvement in therapy. Steketee (55) found that general social support did not predict relapse, but significant others' empathy and postive interactions were associated with positive gains.

TERMINATION AND RELAPSE PREVENTION

The final two BT sessions should focus on relapse prevention and termination; therapist and patient review learned coping skills and anticipate future potentially problematic situations, e.g., changing residences, job relocation or layoff, family death or illness, divorce, or financial problems. Coping skills should be developed in anticipation of these situations and patients should be informed that avoidance signals further exposure to the specific situations and response prevention to the overt or covert rituals. In addition, patients should be reminded that there is no actual cure for OCD, that it is a waxing and waning disorder, with exacerbations at the onset of separation and stress. Instead, the maintenance of therapeutic gains will be contingent on reinforcement through the practice of learned skills combined with high motivation. In addition, family interventions directed at reducing criticism, angry reactions, and misinformation regarding OCD are more likely to aid in the maintenance of gains and the prevention of relapse. In some cases, joining self-help or support groups is recommended in order to consolidate gains.

When OCD is significantly improved, treatment should focus on residual areas of functioning such as social skills. We have observed that chronic OCD sufferers may have developed deficient social skills as well as social anxiety as epiphenomena of their disorder. Social skills training will aid in the cultivation of interpersonal abilities necessary for reintegration into the social environments of work, etc. Social skills will result in improved overall functioning and thus decreased anxiety and probability of relapse.

Sufferers of severe OCD may be accustomed to structuring the majority of their time around their symptom requirements. Moreover, they may exhibit a behavioral style generalizing to a wide range of daily activities, such as workaholism or anhedonia. Thus, it is clinically advisable to develop a counterbalanced life approach including the development of hobbies, vacation planning, interpersonal relationships, and relaxation time. The evaluation of potential obstacles preventing engagement in positive activities may be anticipated with patients.

Finally, patients are encouraged to contact the behavior therapist for booster sessions should relapse occur. Occasional reinforcement of BT principles is often necessary to consolidate gains, particularly in stressful periods.

OCD CASE STUDIES

Case 1

C is a 26-year-old single Hispanic man referred to one of the authors by a leader of an OCD self-help group. The onset of C's symptoms was 2 years prior to his presentation, precipitated by his attendance at a party where he became drunk. He reportedly developed the fear of having contracted AIDS after awakening and failing to recall details of the party, finding an inexplicable bruise on his upper left leg. C worried that his colleagues or a stranger had sexually abused him while he was unconscious, and believed that he had contracted AIDS. For the following 2 years he refrained from sexual intercourse because he feared infecting others, avoided going to the doctor, and kept this secret from his family. Several months prior to seeking BT he tested HIV-negative, but continued to fear contracting AIDS or other viruses and infecting others.

C's symptoms consisted of fears of contracting illnesses, mainly AIDS and TB, and then contaminating others when breathing in the presence of others or touching unknown objects. As a result he was extremely anxious, checked locks repetitively, and suffered from severe insomnia due to his fear that an ill stranger would enter his home and either spread viruses or contaminate or rape him or his sister while they slept. These obsessions intruded despite his repetitive checking of the lock as well as asking his sister to verify that the door was locked. Compulsions included checking objects, praying, and avoiding exposing his mouth in public.

These symptoms significantly interfered with C's occupational and social functioning. He lost his job as a pizza maker because of the "risk" he perceived in working in a public place. He was not seeking employment, and was socially isolated at the time of his presentation. C spent approximately 8 hours a day performing rituals and experiencing germ and contamination obsessions.

After a three-session initial evaluation of his symptoms, family background, and interpersonal relationships, it was ascertained that C was rational, that his symptoms were ego-dystonic, and that his compulsion to perform rituals was due to repetitive doubt and fears. C had had no prior psychiatric treatment with the exception of a single visit to a psychologist in his country. He was both eager and motivated for treatment, yet fearful of revealing his bizarre symptoms, which were maintained as completely secret.

C was treated with BT for 20 90-minute sessions over a 4-month period. He was seen twice weekly for the first eight sessions, once weekly for an additional eight sessions, and every 2 weeks for the remaining four sessions.

At the outset of the sessions, C was instructed to maintain a journal of the time of day at which rituals occurred and their duration, brief descriptions of the thoughts or activities that elicited them, and the anxiety/discomfort level, ranging from 0 (no anxiety at all) to 100 (the worst anxiety ever experienced, as in a panic state). Rituals included hand-washing, washing or cleaning glasses or other objects, checking that the door was closed, and checking under the bed or in the bathroom. With C's active participation, an anxiety hierarchy was developed for his AIDS and illness phobias (Table 1). A list of feared situations, circumstances and objects was ordered by anxiety intensity using the same 1–100 SUDS level scale. The therapists's role was to be empathic to C by probing sensitively and offering feedback and information about OCD, complete with possible etiologies, effective treatments, and other research findings. Finally, constant encouragement about his treatment and psychoeducation was provided. The following explanation was offered:

Table 1   Case 1: Anxiety Hierarchy

Situation	SUDS level
Touching office trashcan	60
Touching street trashcan	65
Eating fruit brought at the local store	70
Selection of damaged-looking packages at the market	73
Drinking directly from soda cans or bottles	75
Walking by high buildings with open windows	75
Touching toilet seat at home	75
Eating in a restaurant	78
Walking in the street with an open mouth passing by an ill-looking person	79
Touching the toilet seat at the therapist's office	80
Touching his own genitals	85
Touching toilet seat in dirty public bathrooms	85
Walking inside a gay bar with his mouth open	90
Opening and closing home doors without double-checking	95
Touching homeless person while giving money	97
Sitting close to and rubbing against an underweight, ill-looking person	99
Visiting infectious-disease department in a large hospital	100

When you come into contact with objects that make you feel contaminated, you feel extremely anxious. Once you feel extremely anxious, you try to avoid or escape as soon as possible from the situation. However, escape from the situation is not good enough if you already feel contaminated, and over time you have developed ways or rituals to reduce your discomfort. With time, rituals that were initially designed to relieve your anxiety become a problem in their own way. For example, you need to wash and clean more and more and it seems that you never feel completely decontaminated, so sometimes even without touching anything you have the urge to wash your hands.

C's treatment began in the office with his touching the edge of the office trashcan. It was of the utmost importance that the therapist model the exposure for the patient. Mr. C initially froze and his hands were sweaty. However, with the therapists's encouragement, C grabbed the trashcan with both hands. He understood that exposure could decrease his high anxiety level by allowing him to habituate or to become less anxious. Thus, he agreed to continue the exposure. C's initial anxiety while touching the trashcan was 60, but after 40 minutes it fell to 45. To approach the multiple items in Table 1, an ERP model was employed, beginning with the lowest item on the hierarchy (touching trash at the office) and progressing to the next item on the list when the initial one did not cause further distress. Prior to exposure in vivo, Mr. C was exposed in imagination to this item. The decision to begin sessions with imaginal exposure was based on our experience and research corroboration that imaginal exposure optimizes the processing of the OCD patient's fears through the focus on feared consequences. The following is an excerpt from the script used on the imaginal exposure tape:

> Imagine as vividly as you can—as if you were living through this situation right now—that you decided that in order to begin confrontation of your symptoms, you will touch different things and stop washing your hands. Today as you look at the green office trashcan you feel scared, your hands are sweaty and trembling, and your heart is racing. You want to leave the room, but instead you near the trash, and touch it with the tips of your fingers; you feel jittery and cannot stop thinking about all the dirt and germs contaminating your hands. Despite this, your hands are now grabbing the sticky walls of the trash can. You cannot believe that by doing this you are allowing all the garbage germs to freely crawl on your skin and penetrate your pores and travel throughout your body through your blood circulation.

The complete script was taped, and C was asked to provide SUDS levels every 5 minutes to the imaginal exposure. The scene was repeatedly read by the therapist for 45 minutes, and C's anxiety declined from 60 at the outset to 40 at the end. The therapist told C that his anxiety was reduced and habituation occurred as he processed his feared consequences. This exercise followed the exposure in vivo, in which C modeled the behavior initially and then, with the therapist's encouragement, grabbed the edges of the trashcan and kept them there for 20 minutes. At that point the exposure was interrupted because C's anxiety level was significantly reduced, from 60 to 20. The remainder of the sessions—the "debriefing"—focused on C's first exposure experience, to reinforce this relatively small success to prepare him for future, more difficult items. C shared his concerns about contaminating his apartment with his dirty hands since he agreed to refrain from hand-washing, and about the homework of contaminating the apartment by touching everything with a napkin that he had brushed firmly against the internal walls of the trashcan. C extended his touching-trash contamination to other designated trashcans of the same difficulty for 2–3 hours per day, with a steady reduction to SUDS levels of 20. When he felt prepared to attempt the next item in the hierarchy, exposure continued with touching trashcans on the street, eating with his bare hands food bought in the local store, walking in the neighborhood with his mouth open, and using different bathrooms in the home and office and even dirty public bathrooms. Additionally, C was asked to touch his genitals, to open and close the apartment door by himself, to touch homeless and ill-looking individuals, and finally to visit an infectious-disease department in a large hospital. During exposures, C was instructed to refrain from hand-washing following the touching of each item in the hierarchy, although he was allowed a 5-second washing whenever he accidentally came into contact with an item higher in the hierarchy. He was instructed, however, that as soon as he finished washing he was to "recontaminate" himself, usually by using a napkin contaminated with that item. He also agreed to take showers only every 3 days, after which he was to "recontaminate" himself with the item being practiced at the time. Throughout exposures, C was to touch each item and then contaminate his clothing, skin, face, hair, and all objects he possessed. These items were practiced in the remainder of the sessions and resulted in the gradual but steady reduction of anxiety throughout that portion of the treatment.

The application of this treatment requires a great degree of skill, empathy, and encouragement on the part of the therapist. Agreeing to the involvement of C's sister was an important treatment component. His sister was educated about OCD and the rationale for BT, and was assigned the role of reporting prohibited rituals. The therapist encouraged her to be firm but supportive. After the sixteenth session, C was seen only twice monthly for two additional months. He resumed taking one shower a day and hand-washed only twice daily. He actively interviewed for employment and received two job offers, which he declined because they did not meet his requirements.

Case 2

B, a 25-year-old woman living with her boyfriend in a metropolitan area, was referred to one of the authors for BT following a refusal to use medication and expressing the desire to deal with OCD in a "natural" way. She is an extremely intelligent woman who is gifted in the arts and languages. However, she was employed as a part-time receptionist at a business firm, despite her college education and abilities.

B was extremely secretive about her symptoms, expressed frank fear, and doubted whether she suffered sufficient symptom severity to undertake a behavioral program. This stance is frequently observed in OCD patients when the possibility of exposure becomes a reality. B's apprehension was approached as being understandable, and she was informed that this experience is common in OCD patients at the outset of treatment.

B had a 4-year history of OCD, with her primary complaint being sensory doubt—the inability to trust her own eyes or believe in her own judgment. In response, she checked objects both at home and at work many times, e.g., boyfriend's car doors, addresses on envelopes, and whether envelopes were indeed empty prior to their disposal. She checked to ensure that light switches and other appliances were turned off, and at work checked whether messages were placed in their correct boxes and reread phrases and paragraphs. In addition, B was plagued by repetitive hand-washing, continually checked for dirt and germs under her fingernails, and took 40-minute showers. She checked that water faucets were turned off completely and that the alarm clock was set correctly. Checking took up approximately 7 hours a day both at home and at work. Compulsions and perfectionism resulted in procrastination and lateness. B's primary obsessions were fears of provoking a catastrophe such as fire or gas leak, causing the deaths of her boyfriend and herself, being robbed in the car or at home, bills and deposits being credited to the wrong accounts, causing harm to others by leaving a knife sticking out in the kitchen, and oversleeping, resulting in being late to work and getting fired.

Treatment consisted of 16 twice-weekly 1-hour BT sessions with exposure to these feared situations and the prevention of checking and washing. A more intensive program was impossible in the context of the patient's life and her overall functioning was considered good. Thus, instead of a higher frequency of sessions, phone sessions supplemented weekly therapy for a portion of the treatment and B's boyfriend became involved. Following the initial interview and establishment of a sound therapeutic alliance, an anxiety hierarchy (Table 2) was developed and BT begun. B received both in vivo and imaginal exposure.

B was initially instructed to purposely leave her bathroom faucets dripping while she left the house for an hour. Fears that she would be responsible for causing a flood and harming neighbors were included in a script of imaginal exposure and taped for repeated listening. After turning on all faucets just enough to drip, B listened to the 35-minute tape under the supervision of her boyfriend, who accompanied her but offered no reassurance outside the home. He was, however, instructed to be understanding and supportive to B while away from the home and to inquire into her SUDS levels. B was successful in homework exposures, which resulted in increased self-esteem, competence, and motivation. However, she complained that her boyfriend was too pushy and critical. In a conjoint session it was decided that the therapist would pay a home visit, the goals of which were 1) to use modeling to demonstrate to B's boyfriend

Table 2   Case 2: Anxiety Hierarchy

Situation (checking compulsions)	SUDS level
Using faucets	40
Using deodorant, juice can, milk bottle	45
Turning light switches on and off	45
Rinsing toothbrush	50
Placing messages in boxes	55
Taking eyeglasses off	60
Placing knives on top of kitchen counter	60
Sending bills	65
Locking office doors	70
Closing gas jets/turning off stove	80
Reading	80
Locking apartment door	90
Closing and locking boyfriend's car door	95
Setting alarm clock	100

how to offer firm yet gentle support and 2) to further assess the extent of ritualistic behaviors. In response, B agreed to increase the pressure of the faucet's running water and to leave light switches on, thereby increasing the severity of feared consequences. Outside the home she listened to the tape on a Walkman and noted SUDS levels every 5 minutes. After 1 hour, SUDS levels were reduced from 70 to 40. Unexpectedly, B's anxiety level increased from her initial rating but she agreed to proceed with exposure.

As homework, B practiced this item with the aid of her boyfriend in addition to leaving faucets dripping in bathrooms at work. On her first practice, B felt compelled to check once prior to leaving the office, but reported no further urges to check faucets following an additional four-session exposure. This success motivated her to proceed to the next items on her hierarchy, such as double-checking that caps had been replaced on containers of deodorant, juice, etc. Sessions 9–14 included the intentional leaving off of caps for a day and imaging feared consequences of beverages spoiling and causing illness, deodorant losing strength, etc. In addition, B was instructed to leave her eyeglasses on top of scratchy surfaces, to leave knives on tables around the apartment, and to send bills to the therapist's office without return addresses or account numbers and with the checks signed imperfectly. After her SUDS levels were reduced to 30, she was instructed about how most people pay bills by mail. Finally, B confronted the most difficult items on her hierarchy, including leaving the apartment and car doors unchecked while simultaneously listening to the tape that focused on her being fired because of her irresponsible behavior. Her last exposure was to set the alarm clock once without checking and then to image arriving late to work and being fired.

At termination, B reported an 80% improvement and spent less than 30 minutes daily in obsessions and compulsions. In addition, she initiated a diet about which she had been procrastinating.

Case 3

R is a 25-year-old single religious woman working as a clerk and living with her parents and sibling in New York City. She was referred by her psychiatrist, who treated her with clomipramine and fluoxetine. She had derived benefit from these medications for 6 months prior to her entry into BT but then experienced a relapse of OCD symptoms. She expressed concern regarding the continuation of her medication and wished to attempt BT in order to ultimately discontinue pharmacotherapy if she was a positive BT responder.

R had an 8-year history of OCD and scrupulosity precipitated by the death of a family friend through suicide. Presenting obsessions were fear of an impulsive suicide attempt, disturbing sexual imagery, fear of overcharging fees to clients at work, and guilt during religious holidays due to a childhood incident of her stealing candy. Obsessions were continuous, and an average of 4 hours per day were spent in the performance of rituals. Compulsions involved seeking reassurance, the need to confess to significant others that she read about suicide or had sexual feelings during reading, and checking whether windows were locked or curtains securely closed. R feared that she would, using these objects, accidentally commit suicide, which is sinful. Because this would result in damage to her family name, she experienced extreme guilt for harboring these thoughts. R also avoided plastic bags, strings, and being close to windows, and blocked images of committing suicide. R strove to avoid the suicidal obsession by eye-blinking to remove the thought from consciousness.

The initial treatment phase involved the creation of an anxiety hierarchy of both suicidal thoughts and actions potentially resulting in suicide (Table 3). R agreed to undergo ERP to all items, with the exception of her sexual obsessions, but to later use the same technique in self-exposure without discussion of content in treatment.

Twelve sessions consisted of exposure to carrying plastic bags in R's purse, sleeping with plastic bags underneath her pillow, and carrying strings and rope with her and having them available in her bedroom. R initially practiced nearing office windows, followed by windows at home and in tall buildings, and left windows open. She was exposed to pointing a knife at her heart—first when accompanied, then while alone—and was asked to read articles on suicide completers. She wrote an imaginal scene in which she described the most probable method used in her own suicide. Treatment regarding the suicidal obsession consisted of exposure to the thought and response prevention of the covert ritual, i.e., eye-blinking to remove the obsession from consciousness. R was instructed to listen to a previously developed detailed script of imagined suicide and feared consequences to both herself and her family. This audiotape procedure is described elsewhere (45,73). Accordingly, R recorded her suicidal obsession in her own voice on a standard "looped" cassette that continuously played the suicidal obsession, during which she resisted eye-blinking or avoidance behaviors. An excerpt from the taped script follows:

Table 3   Case 3: Anxiety Hierarchy

Situation	SUDS level
Carrying plastic bags in purse	40
Sleeping with plastic bag underneath pillow	50
Carrying string or rope	55
Sleeping with string under pillow	60
Being close to windows	60
Opening window	65
Leaning out of open window	70
Reading literature on suicide	75
Holding knife pointed against chest in office	80
Holding sharp knife while alone	90
Holding knife to heart and holding rope, prepared to hang self while facing mirror	100

Today is the day that I chose to commit suicide. I am now wrapping my face in plastic and tying a rope around my neck. I am then tying the other end to a nail and I stand on a chair. As I stand on the chair, I can distinctly feel my last breath, and suddenly I realize I am jumping, my face is turning blue, my tongue is hanging out, and so I am soon dead and found in my doorway by my mother, who is becoming hysterical as she immediately phones my father. I am being buried in a nonreligious cemetery. As I am being buried, I can hear people making comments: "How could she commit suicide? What kind of religious person is she?"

During the last sessions, R was instructed to challenge her scrupulosity by exposing herself to crossing on red lights, overcharging clients 10 cents on sales tax, taking milk at a store without paying until the following day, taking and eating fruit at the fruit stand, using deodorant or perfume in a store and placing them back on the shelf, bending the cover of a book at a bookstore, moving shoe polish to the candy section of the supermarket, poking bread and other plastic packages, and owing money for a long time. Tapes were also made for imaginal exposure in which R was caught cheating a store owner and being identified as a robber, responsible for damage of food and the poisoning of others.

R was significantly improved at termination and reported minimal ideation related to hanging herself with rope. Obsessions occurred once or twice daily, but their intensity was greatly reduced and R could typically control them by labeling them as obsessive thoughts. In general, she reported feeling 70% improved and throughout the following year was seen for two booster sessions when she feared that thoughts were returning to obsessional intensity. Overall, however, R successfully maintained treatment gains.

CONCLUSIONS

Working with OCD sufferers requires flexibility and a great deal of patience, despite the straightforward appearance of standard behavior therapy. Exposure and response prevention are the hallmarks of behavioral treatment of OCD, and other therapeutic techniques are typically implemented with this basic approach as a foundation. As clinicians, we are simultaneously grateful for advances in the treatment of this disorder once considered intractable and cautious about a tendency toward overconfidence regarding our novel technology.

OCD patients presenting to private practice exhibit an array of symptoms, developmental histories, and as well as many comorbid personality disorders, cultural and socioeconomic diversity. In addition, they may represent a more severe subgroup, possibly with axis II comorbidity, than those in controlled trials because of the selection bias in favor of higher-functioning patients able to complete clinical trials. Therefore, OCD patients in private practice require a particularly empathic therapeutic relationship as much as they require effective and intensive treatment. Moreover, private-practice OCD patients have a great deal of embarrassment about their symptomatology and are overly concerned with confidentiality and the maintenance of secrecy regarding their disorder. It is through the empathic immersion in the patient's experience that BT achieves its maximal efficacy.

Assessment of the comparative efficacy of different treatment types requires further investigation. In addition, when treatment combinations are undertaken in the OCD patient, the relative contribution of each treatment to OCD symptom reduction should be ascertained by the use of appropriate controls. There remains a lack of long-term, systematic, controlled-outcome assessments of sequential pharmacotherapies, behavior therapies, and simultaneous treatments. Further investigations are required to determine the necessary and sufficient treatments for potential subgroups of refractory patients in this heterogeneous disorder. The intensive investigation of patient and informant lifetime phenomenological accounts should add to the identification of predictors of treatment outcome. Future research should assess the comparative efficacy of BT in controlled trials vs. private-practice settings, with comparable outcome measures.

REFERENCES

1. Clomipramine Collaborative Study Group. Clomipramine in the treatment of patients with obsessive-compulsive disorder. Arch Gen Psychiatry 1991; 48:730–738.
2. Hollander E, DeCaria CM, Gulley R, Nitescu A, Suckow RF, Gorman JG, Klein DF, Liebowitz MR. Effects of chronic fluoxetine treatment on behavioral and neuroendocrine response to metachlorophenylpiperazine in obsessive-compulsive disorder. Psychiatry Res 1991; 36:1–17.
3. Pigott TA, Pato MT, Bernstein SE, Grover GN, Hill JN, Tolliver TJ, Murphy DL. Controlled comparisons of clomipramine and fluoxetine in the treatment of obsessive-compulsive disorder. Arch Gen Psychiatry 1990; 47:926–932.
4. Rasmussen S, Eisen JL, Pato M. Current issues in the pharmacologic management of obsessive-compulsive disorder. J Clin Psychiatry 1993; 54(suppl):6.
5. Greist JH, Jefferson JW, Kabak KA, Chouinard G, DuBoff E, Halaris A, Kim SW, Koran L, Liebowitz MR, Lydiard B, et al. A one year double-blind

placebo-controlled fixed dose study of sertraline in the treatment of obsessive compulsive disorder. Int Clin Psychopharm 1995; 10:2:57–65.

6. Foa EB, Steketee GS, Ozarow BJ. Behavior therapy with obsessive-compulsives. In: Mavissakalian M, Turner SM, Michelson L, eds. Obsessive-Compulsive Disorder: Psychological and Pharmacological Treatment. New York: Plenum, 1985:49–120.

7. Mowrer O. A stimulus-response analysis of anxiety and its role as a reinforcing agent. Psych Rev 1939; 46:553–565.

8. Rachman S, Wilson GT. The effects of psychological therapy. Oxford: Pergamon Press, 1980.

9. Foa EB, Tillmanns A. The treatment of obsessive-compulsive neurosis. In: Goldstein A, Foa EB, eds. Handbook of Behavioral Interventions: A Clinical Guide. New York: Wiley, 1980.

10. Foa EB, Steketee GS, Grayson JB. Imaginal and in vivo exposure: a comparison with obsessive-compulsive checkers. Behav Ther 1985; 16:292–302.

11. Steketee GS, Foa EB, Grayson JB. Recent advances in the behavioral treatment of obsessive-compulsives. Arch Gen Psychiatry 1982; 39(12):1365–1371.

12. Steketee GS. Treatment of Obsessive Compulsive Disorder. New York: Guilford Press, 1993.

13. Foa EB, Kozak MJ, Steketee GS, McCarthy PR. Treatment of depressive and obsessive-compulsive symptoms in OCD by imipramine and behavior therapy. Br J Clin Psychiatry 1992; 31:279–292.

14. Steketee GS, Cleere L. Obsessional-Compulsive Disorders. In: Bellack AS, Hersen M, Kazdin AE, eds. International Handbook of Behavior Modification and Therapy. 2nd ed. New York: Plenum, 1990:307–332.

15. Emmelkamp PMG, Beens H. Cognitive therapy with obsessive-compulsive disorder: a comparative evaluation. Behav Res Ther 1991;29:293–300.

16. Riggs DS, Hiss H, Foa EB. Marital distress and the treatment of obsessive compulsive disorder. Behav Ther 1992; 23:585–597.

17. Jenike MA, Rauch, SL. Managing the patient with treatment resistant obsessive-compulsive disorder: current strategies. J Clin Psychiatry 1994; 55:3(suppl):11–17.

18. Meyer V. Modification of expectations in cases with obsessional rituals. Behav Res Ther 1966; 4:273–280.

19. Marks IM. Review of behavioral psychotherapy. I. Obsessive-compulsive disorders. Am J Psychiatry 1981; 138:584–592.

20. Rachman S, Hodgson R, Marks IM. The treatment of chronic obsessive-compulsive neurosis. Behav Res Ther 1971; 9:237–247.

21. Hodgson R, Rachman S, Marks IM. The treatment of chronic obsessive compulsive neurosis: follow-up and further findings. Behav Res Ther 1972; 10:181–189.

22. Rachman S, Marks IM, Hodgson R. The treatment of obsessive compulsive neurotics by modeling and flooding in vivo. Behav Res Ther 1973; 11:463–471.

23. Marks IM, Hodgson R, Rachman S. Treatment of chronic obsessive compulsive neurosis in vivo exposure: a two year follow up and issues in treatment. Br J Psychiatry 1975; 127:349–364.
24. Pato MT, Zohar-Kadouch R, Zohar J, Murphy D. Return of symptoms after discontinuation of clomipramine in patients with obsessive-compulsive disorder. Am J Psychiatry 1988; 145:1521–1527.
25. Stanley MA, Turner SM. Current status of pharmacological and behavioral treatment of obsessive-compulsive disorder. Behav Ther 1995; 153–186.
26. Beck JG, Bourg W. Obsessive-compulsive disorder in adults. In: Ammerman RT, Hersen M, eds. Handbook of Behavior Therapy With Children and Adults: A Developmental Perspective. Boston: Allyn and Bacon, 1963:167–185.
27. Rachman S, Hodgson R. Obsessions and Compulsions. Englewood Cliffs, NJ: Prentice-Hall, 1980.
28. Foa EB, Goldstein A. Continuous exposure and complete response prevention of obsessive-compulsive disorder. Behav Ther 1978; 9:821–829.
29. Hoogduin K, DeHaan E, Schaap C, et al. Exposure and response prevention in patients with obsessions. Acta Psychiatr Belg 1987; 87:640–653.
30. Fals-Stewart W, Lucente S. An MCMI cluster typology of obsessive-compulsives: a measure of personality characteristics and its relationship to treatment participation, compliance and outcome in behavior therapy. J Psych Res 1993; 27:139–154.
31. Foa EB, Fals-Stewart W, Lucente S. Failure in treating obsessive compulsives. Behav Res Ther 1979; 17:169–179.
32. Rasmussen S, Eisen JL. Phenomenology of OCD: clinical subtypes, heterogeneity and coexistence. In: Zohar J, Insel T, Rasmussen S, eds. The Psychobiology of Obsessive-Compulsive Disorder. New York: Springer, 1990:13–43.
33. Hoodgduin K, Duivenvoorden HJ. A decision model in the treatment of obsessive-compulsive neuroses. Br J Psychiatry 1988; 152:516–521.
34. Kozak MJ, Foa EB. Obsessive, overvalued ideas and delusions in obsessive-compulsive disorder. Behav Res Ther 1994; 32:343–353.
35. Baer L, Minchiello WE. Behavior therapy for obsessive-compulsive disorder. In: Jenike MA, Baer L, Minchiello WE, eds. Obsessive Compulsive Disorders: Theory and Management. Littleton, MA: PSG, 1986.
36. Jenike MA, Baer L, Minichiello WE, Schwartz CE, Carey RJ. Concomitant obsessive-compulsive disorder and schizotypal personality disorder. Am J Psychiatry 1986; 143:530–532.
37. Minichiello WE, Baer L, Jenike MA. Schizotypal personality disorder: a poor prognostic indicator for behavior therapy in the treatment of obsessive compulsive disorder. J Anxiety Dis 1987; 1:273–276.
38. Walker WR, Freeman RF, Christensen DK. Restricting environmental stimulation (REST) to enhance cognitive behavioral treatment for obsessive-compulsive disorder with schizotypal personality disorder. Behav Ther 1994; 25:709–719.

39. Emmelkamp PMG, Van der Helm M, Van Zanten BL et al. Contributions of self-instructional rational training to the effectiveness of exposure in vivo: a comparison with obsessive compulsive patients. Behav Res Ther 1980; 18:61–66.

40. Reed GF. Obsessional Experience and Compulsive Behavior. Orlando, FL: Academic Press, 1985.

41. Emmelkamp PMG, Visser S, Hoekstra R. Cognitive therapy versus exposure treatment in the treatment of obsessive compulsives. Cognitive Ther Res 1988; 2:103–114.

42. Van Oppen P, DeHaan E, Van Balkom AJLM, Spinhoven P, et al. Cognitive therapy and exposure in vivo in the treatment of obsessive compulsive disorder. Behav Res Ther 1995; 33(4):379–390.

43. James IA, Blackburn IM. Cognitive therapy with obsessive compulsive disorder. Br J Psychiatry 1995; 166:4:444–450.

44. Salkovskis PM. Cognitive Techniques to Limit Non-Compliance [abstr]. First International Obsessive-Compulsive Disorder Congress, Capri, Italy, March 12–13, 1993.

45. Salkovskis PM, Westbrook D. Behavior therapy and obsessional ruminations: can failure be turned into success? Behav Res Ther 1989; 27:149–169.

46. Guidano VL, Liotti G. Cognitive Processes and Emotional Disorders. New York: Guilford Press, 1983.

47. Foa EB, Steketee GS. Behavioral treatment of phobics and obsessive-compulsives. In: Jacobson NS, ed. Psychotherapists in Clinical Practice. New York: Guilford Press, 1987.

48. Zohar J, Zohar-Kadouch RC, Kindler S. Current concepts in the pharmacological treatment of obsessive-compulsive disorder. Drugs 1992; 43(2):210–218.

49. Marks IM, Stern RS, Mawson D, Cobb J, McDonald R. Clomipramine and exposure for obsessive-compulsive rituals. Br J Psychiatry 1980; 136:1–25.

50. Marks IM, Lelliot P, Basoglu M, Norshirvani H, Monteiro W, Cohen D, Kasvikis Y. Clomipramine: self-exposure and therapist-aided exposure for obsessive compulsive rituals. Br J Psychiatry 1988; 152:522–534.

51. Cottraux J, Mollard E, Bouvard M, Marks I, Sluys M, Nury AM, Douge R, Cialdella P. A controlled study of fluvoxamine and exposure in obsessive compulsive disorder. Int Clin Psychopharm 1990; 5:17–30.

52. Neziroglu F. Behavior Therapy in Obsessive-Compulsive Disorder. Presented at the Second International Obsessive-Compulsive Disorder Conference, Point-à-Pitre, Guadeloupe. 1996.

53. Baxter LR, Schwartz JM, Bergman KS, Szuba MP, et al. Caudate glucose metabolic rate changes with both drug and behavior therapy for obsessive-compulsive disorder. Arch Gen Psychiatry 1992; 49:681–689.

54. Insel TR, Winslow JT. Neurobiology of obsessive-compulsive disorder. In: Jenike MA, Baer L, Minichiello WE, eds. Obsessive-Compulsive Disorders:

Theory and Management. Chicago: Year Book Medical Publishers, 1990:118–131.

55. Steketee GS. Social support and treatment outcome of obsessive-compulsive disorder at 9 month follow-up. Behav Psychother 1993; 21(2):81–95.

56. Marks IM. Fears, Phobias and Rituals: Panic, Anxiety and Their Disorders. New York: Oxford University Press, 1987.

57. Neziroglu F, Yaryura-Tobias JA. Over and Over Again: Understanding Obsessive-Compulsive Disorder. Lexington, MA: Lexington Books, 1991.

58. Hollander E. The Quality of Life in OCD [abstr]. Presented at the American Psychiatric Association Meeting, 1996.

59. Aronowitz BR, Hollander E, DeCaria C, Cohen L, Saoud JB, Stein D, Liebowitz MR, Rosen WG. Neuropsychology of obsessive compulsive disorder: preliminary findings. Neuropsychiatry Neuropsychol Behav Neurol 1994; 7(2):81–86.

60. Head D, Bolton D, Hymas N. Deficit in cognitive shifting ability in patients with obsessive-compulsive disorder. Biol Psychiatry 1989; 25:929–937.

61. Zielinski CM, Taylor MA, Juzwin KR. Neuropsychological deficits in obsessive-compulsive disorder. Neuropsychiatry Neuropsychol Behav Neurol 1991; 4:110–126.

62. Christiansen KJ, Kim SW, Dysken MW, Hoover KM. Neuropsychological performance in obsessive-compulsive disorder. Biol Psychiatry 1991; 31:4–18.

63. Truax CB, Carkuff RR. Toward Effective Counseling in Psychotherapy: Training and Practice. Chicago: Aldine, 1967.

64. Goodman WK, Price L, Rasmussen SA, et al. The Yale-Brown Obsessive Compulsive Scale. I. Development, use and reliability. II. Validity. Arch Gen Psychiatry 1989; 46:1006–1016.

65. Goodman WK, Price LH, Rasmussen SA, Heninger GR, Charney DS. Efficacy of fluvoxamine in obsessive-compulsive disorder: a double-blind comparison with placebo. Arch Gen Psychiatry 1989; 46:36–43.

66. Hodgson RJ, Rachman S. Obsessional-compulsive complaints. Behav Res Ther 1977; 15:389–395.

67. Cooper JE. The Leyton Obsessional Inventory. Psycholog Med 1970; 1:48–64.

68. Steketee GS, Kozak MJ, Foa EB. Predictors of outcome for obsessive-compulsives treated with exposure and response prevention. Paper presented at the 15th Annual Meeting of the European Association for Behavior Therapy, Munich, West Germany, 1985.

69. Emmelkamp PMG, Kraanen J. Therapist controlled exposure in vivo versus self-controlled exposure in vivo: a comparison with obsessive-compulsive patients. Behav Res Ther 1977; 15:491–495.

70. Emmelkamp PMG, Wessels H. Flooding in imagination versus flooding in vivo: a comparison with agoraphobics. Behav Res Ther 1975; 13:7–16.

71. Kirk JW. Behavioral treatment of obsessional-compulsive patients in routine clinical practice. Behav Res Ther 1983; 21(1):57–62.

72. Emmelkamp PMG, de Haan E, Hoogduin CA. Marital adjustment and obsessive-compulsive disorder. Br J Psychiatry 1990; 156:55–60.
73. Salkovskis PM, Kirk J. Obsessional disorders. In: Hawton KP, Salkovskis PM, Kirk J, Clark DM, eds. Cognitive Behaviour Therapy for Psychiatric Problems: A Practical Guide. Oxford: Oxford Medical Publications, 1989.

11

Cognitive-Behavioral Self-Treatment For OCD Systematically Alters Cerebral Metabolism

A Mind–Brain Interaction Paradigm for Psychotherapists

Jeffrey M. Schwartz

UCLA School of Medicine
Los Angeles, California

INTRODUCTION

Behavioral self-treatment for obsessive-compulsive disorder (OCD) is becoming increasingly recognized as an effective and efficient method of clinical management (1,2). The behavioral therapy principle of exposure and response prevention, which has clinically proven effectiveness for OCD (3,4), can be self-administered after only modest modification of what are now well-established treatment methods. Marks, for example, has reported on the use of this method by his group in London (5). Baer (6), Foa and Wilson (7), and Steketee and White (8), among others, have published self-treatment books for the mass market that attempt to teach OCD patients how to apply exposure and response prevention treatment techniques in an independent setting.

Our OCD research group at UCLA Medical Center has been utilizing a cognitive-behavioral self-treatment technique over the past several years. We have also been simultaneously investigating the effects of behavioral treatment of OCD on the cerebral metabolism of a group of medication-free patients. Specifically, we have applied cognitive techniques, including structured patient education about biological aspects of OCD, to enhance patients' ability to control their responses to anxiety caused by OCD symptoms. This enables patients to better perform self-exposure and response prevention tasks, as a result of more effective management of the intensely uncomfortable feelings that arise during treatment.

This chapter updates a prior report on this self-treatment method (9), and presents new data we have recently acquired concerning the effects of this cognitive-behavioral treatment on cerebral glucose metabolism, studied with PET scanning (10). The chapter concludes with a discussion of these data in the context of a mind–brain interaction paradigm; i.e., what are some of the implications of the demonstration that patients with OCD can systematically alter their brain chemistry by successfully performing cognitive-behavioral treatment techniques to improve their clinical condition. [The treatment method is available in lay language in the form of a behavioral therapy manual currently being used by our group (11), and a detailed description of how to apply it in an entirely independent manner is now be available in book form (12).]

TREATMENT STRATEGY AND TECHNIQUES

Behavioral treatment of OCD involves patients' learning to tolerate the uncomfortable feeling states that arise from OCD symptoms (2). Hand used the term "exposure response management" to describe how coping strategies can be learned and applied to "manage" these intensely uncomfortable feelings when they arise during exposure and response prevention treatment (13). This resulted in improved treatment compliance (2,14). We utilize this concept within a specific cognitive-behavioral training paradigm composed of four steps: 1) relabel, 2) reattribute, 3) refocus, and 4) revalue.

Patients learn to perform these steps in response to OCD thoughts and urges. Self-treatment is thus the critical component of this method, because these steps are applied as part of an ongoing process of learning to manage one's responses to OCD during daily living. In this way the patient trains himself to alter the patterns of behavioral response, both internal and external, to the arising of intrusive OCD symptoms. These four steps are described below.

Relabel

It is of the utmost importance that the OCD patient work to consciously increase his or her mindful awareness that the bothersome intrusive thoughts and urges are *obsessive* thoughts and *compulsive* urges, i.e., symptoms of a medical disorder. Mindful awareness differs from simple awareness in that it implies the conscious recognition and mental registration of the arising of an obsessive or compulsive symptom. The presence of a symptom is not just superficially acknowledged, as patients usually do, but fully recognized as an intrusive OCD symptom. While superficial awareness is essentially automatic, mindful awareness comes about only when the patient exerts effort for the purpose of focusing on the task at hand. The patient trains himself to observe the unpleasant bothersome feeling as the presence of an OCD symptom.

Mental notes are made to enhance this recognition as it is happening, e.g., "I don't *think* or *feel* my hands are dirty; rather, I'm having an *obsession* that my hands are dirty." Or, "I don't feel the *need* to check that lock; I'm having a *compulsive urge* to perform the *compulsion* of checking." While this certainly will not make the urge go away (the patient should be clearly warned that relabeling will not make the symptom magically disappear), it begins the critical process of not taking OCD thoughts and urges at face value. This sets the stage for actively resisting them.

"It's not me, it's my OCD," should become a battle cry for these patients. They must learn to recognize that OCD thoughts are false and misleading, even though it strongly *feels* as if they are true. Obviously, this step requires that the patient's reality testing be essentially intact. If it is not, appropriate treatment with medication may be necessary.

The relabel step generally results in the patient's asking, "Why does this damn thought keep bothering me? How can I make it go away?" This leads directly to step 2, reattribute.

Reattribute

Structured education about the medical basis of OCD is a foundation on which we help the patient to build a working knowledge about why the OCD thoughts and urges are so intrusive, persistent, and bothersome. Cognitive techniques that merely instruct the patient to recognize the distortions of content in OCD symptoms, when done as the sole method of cognitive restructuring, have not been impressive as adjuncts to basic exposure and response prevention (see Ref. 15 for review). Using a step of cognitive reattribution helps the patient understand that it is a *neurological imbalance* that causes OCD to be so bothersome. This improves the patient's ability to not take the OCD thoughts at face value, to view them as "false messages" that are due to a "short circuit" in the brain. These insights increase the patient's willingness to use the self-directed response prevention of step 3 as a means of resisting them.

The reattribution step is particularly helpful in directing attention away from demoralizing and stressful attempts to "get rid of" the OCD symptom. Realizing that brain biochemistry is responsible for the powerful intrusiveness of the symptoms helps increase insight into the fact that frantic attempts to "make them go away" are a useless waste of energy. Instead, training is provided to focus energy and resolve on self-directed response prevention. We explain that not only is this a useful strategy that will result in functional improvement, it will also, as we have shown in our PET scan studies (10), lead to changes in brain chemistry that can help the OCD symptoms themselves to improve. The awareness of the possibility of altering their own brain chemistry by doing behavioral therapy has been a helpful motivating factor for patients working to perform exposure and response prevention exercises.

Patients are provided with access to PET scan pictures of brains of OCD patients before and after doing cognitive-behavioral self-treatment as a material aid to this cognitive reattribution step. Many patients find this motivational as well as a reminder not to take the thought or urge at face value. We are always working to improve their ability to witness the uncomfortable feelings of OCD with an "impartial spectator" perspective. The relabel and reattribute steps work together to increase patients' mental distance from the symptoms, and this enables them to keep more clearly in mind the need to change their behavioral responses from doing compulsions to response prevention exercises. This process is enhanced by making mental notes such as "It's not me, it's the OCD. It's caused by a false message from my brain. I can't make it go away, but I *can* resist acting on it. By resisting it, I am changing how my brain works."

Advances in our knowledge of the role of the basal ganglia (16,17) in the etiology of OCD symptoms (18,19) have inspired two clinical analogies that patients find useful. First, since the basal ganglia are now recognized to serve gating (20) or "switching station"–type functions, we compare it to the automatic transmission of a car and explain to patients that, "Your brain is 'stuck in gear.' Most people have brains that can shift gears automatically. OCD patients have a sticky manual transmission, so they have to work hard to shift the gears through their own effort by doing self-directed response prevention exercises. One major advantage, though, is that when the OCD patient shifts behavioral gears, he actually changes how the brain works, literally changing the function of the 'transmission' in the brain." Similarly, we can use the analogy of a broken gate that is stuck open, allowing unwanted thoughts and urges to keep barging through. By doing the hard work of behavior therapy, we can learn how to gradually "close the gate" and decrease or even prevent the OCD symptoms from coming through.

Second, since the basal ganglia can be viewed as a modulator or filter of cerebral cortex function (21), it can get a "short circuit" and cause a "false alarm." When, for example, a car alarm goes off accidentally, it's very annoying and distracting. However, once we realize it's a false alarm, we simply try to ignore it and refocus attention on something else. We don't heed a false alarm, and we don't wait for it to go away before we refocus our attention. OCD can be thought of as an extremely annoying false alarm caused by a short circuit in the brain; just as with an external false alarm, the key to an effective response is to ignore the faulty stimulus as much as possible and refocus one's attention on something else.

A more accurate assessment by patients of OCD thoughts and urges is the goal of the relabel and reattribute steps. These steps are generally performed together in preparation for the self-directed response prevention of step 3, refocus.

Refocus

The refocus step involves actively engaging in almost any reasonable activity or task rather than doing compulsions or becoming fixated on obsessive thoughts. These activities, which the patient should find pleasant to perform, may be preselected or even assigned as homework. The patient's goal is to prevent himself from responding to the OCD symptom, while acknowledging that in the short run uncomfortable feelings will not be avoidable. Refocusing attention on another specific behavior enhances one's ability to "shift gears," and redirects effort in a useful way. While homework tasks certainly can be beneficial, we give specific instructions about using self-directed response prevention on spontaneous symptoms as they arise. The need to keep a refocus diary to record response prevention work is stressed, since this boosts confidence by reinforcing achievements (we encourage patients to reward themselves, at least with self-praise) and increases the tactical repertoire of useful behaviors to refocus on.

Increasing exposures to anxiety-evoking stimuli until habituation sets in is the key to success for behavioral treatment (22). We have developed the "15-minute rule" as a practical way to increase self-exposures: whenever an OCD thought or urge arises, the patient is to wait at least 15 minutes before doing any compulsion. This is not a passive waiting period, but a time of active performance of the first three steps. Every OCD symptom is an opportunity to refocus, "shift gears" to another behavior, and perform self-directed response prevention. For obsessive thoughts, even brief periods of refocusing are meaningful, since they demonstrate that it is not essential to get intrusive thoughts entirely out of conscious awareness before beginning to do other behaviors. Even one minute of not focusing on an annoying thought can be helpful, since it prevents the overwhelming problems that getting "stuck in gear" causes. We strongly encourage the patients to put together sequences of refocusing behaviors, which enables them to learn that OCD symptoms generally decrease in intensity over time when they are not responded to.

The refocus step takes considerable effort and ability in learning to manage uncomfortable feelings. Therapist encouragement and patient creativity play big roles here. Space limitations do not allow an adequate description here of the great variety of techniques that patients have devised in the performance of this step. (The patient who carried a small notebook with the words *caudate nucleus* on the cover to consult for his refocusing strategies when a compulsive urge arose is one memorable example; see Ref. 12 for many more.) The critical point is that, as patients learn to alter their behavioral responses to OCD symptoms, they come to realize that they have a genuine choice about what to do when the dreadful feeling arises: don't give in, allow some time to pass, refocus on another behavior, and the feeling will usually fade. What's more, changing the behavior will also change how the brain works. This combination of insights has allowed a wide range of patients to alter, and revalue, their perception of the relationship between themselves and the disease.

Revalue

Practicing self-directed response prevention for enough time to allow full habituation is, of course, the ultimate treatment goal. We have found that the utilization of graded delays that fractionate the task into manageable bits, in concert with the cognitive training steps of relabeling and reattributing, facilitates this process by enhancing the clinical utility of even partial habituation. We are currently conducting a controlled study based on the hypothesis that the cognitive steps act synergistically with self-directed response prevention, resulting in a revaluation of the OCD thoughts and urges that, prior to treatment, lead to compulsive behaviors. After being trained in the first three steps, the patient begins to place a different, much lower, value on the thoughts and feelings that arise due to OCD.

Revaluing is an accentuation of the relabel and reattribute steps. By not taking the symptoms at face value, patients come to view these bothersome feelings as, in one patient's words, "toxic waste from my brain." Continued self-treatment results in decreased symptom intensity, which enhances revaluation by decreasing the effort required to dismiss the OCD symptoms as "worthless rubbish" and refocus on another behavior. One reasonable way to conceptualize this is that self-treatment leads to brain changes, which lead to diminished symptom intensity, which enhances a process of revaluation of the symptoms, which enhances continued application of the relabel, reattribute, and refocus steps, leading to further brain changes, and so on. A therapeutic, self-enabling, feed-forward process is established.

The assertive statements of the revalue step intensify the refocus step and allow a partial habituation to become the cognitive basis for the hard work of further self-directed response prevention. The diary recording of the refocus and revalue step achievements strongly reinforce and enhance this process. Thus, partial habituation becomes an indicator of progress and a cue for further application of the four steps, rather than a demoralizing sign of failure and the "impossibility" of overcoming OCD.

EFFECTS OF COGNITIVE-BEHAVIORAL TREATMENT ON CEREBRAL FUNCTION

Neuroimaging work at UCLA has recently demonstrated that systematic changes in cerebral glucose metabolism accompany the clinical improvements achieved with the cognitive-behavioral self-treatment method described above (10). Eighteen drug-free subjects were studied with PET scans before and after 10 weeks of outpatient therapy. Twelve patients demonstrated clinically significant improvement during the study period, while six did not. Three main findings emerged from this study:

1. Responders to treatment showed bilateral decreases in caudate nucleus metabolism, divided by ipsilateral hemisphere metabolism (Cd/hem), compared to nonresponders. This finding was more robust on the right ($p = 0.003$) than the left ($p = 0.02$). See Figure 1.

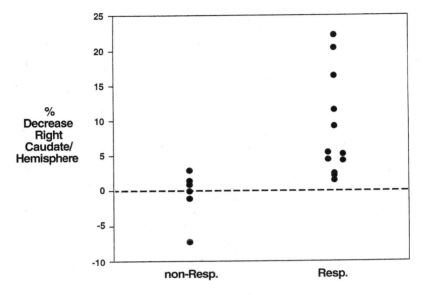

Figure 1 Plot of percent change after cognitive-behavioral treatment [(pre-
−post-/pre-) × 100] in right head of caudate nucleus metabolic rate divided by
ipsilateral hemisphere (caudate/hemisphere) for responders and nonresponders
to treatment. There is a significant difference between responders and nonresponders to treatment ($p < 0.003$).

    2.   There was a significant positive rank-order correlation between
percentage change in total Yale-Brown Obsessive Compulsive Scale (Y-
BOCS) (23) score before and after treatment and the percentage change
in orbital cortex/hem on the left ($p = 0.002$) (see Figure 2).
    3.   Before treatment, there were significant correlations of brain
activity between the orbital frontal cortex and the caudate nucleus, cingulate gyrus, and the thalamus on the right. After effective cognitive-
behavioral treatment, these correlations decreased significantly (see Table 1).

BEHAVIORAL PHYSIOLOGY OF ORBITAL CORTEX

Prior publications by our group have discussed the functional neuroanatomy of OCD in some detail (21,24). Further elaboration of the functional interaction between orbital cortex and the basal ganglia, in the
context of some interesting work on behavioral physiology in animals,
may extend our understanding of OCD. It may also help clarify the rela-

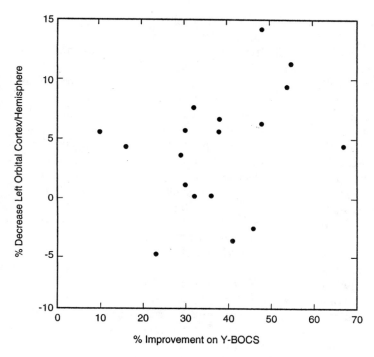

Figure 2 Plot of percentage change in Yale-Brown Obsessive-Compulsive Scale (Y-BOCS) score, a measure of OCD severity, after cognitive-behavioral treatment vs. percentage change [(pre- − post-/pre-) × 100] in left orbital cortex metabolic rate divided by ipsilateral hemisphere (orbital/hemisphere). There is a significant correlation (tau = 0.39; p = 0.002).

Table 1 Normalized Region of Interest Correlations (r) Before and After Treatment, for Behavior Treatment Responders ($n=12$)

	Before treatment	After treatment
Left orbit to left caudate	0.46	−0.01
Right orbit to right caudate	0.74[a]	0.28*
Left orbit to left cingulate	0.11	0.58[b]
Right orbit to right cingulate	0.87[c]	0.22*
Left orbit to left thalamus	0.34	0.05
Right orbit to right thalamus	0.81[d]	0.14*
Left caudate to left thalamus	0.66[b]	0.36
Right caudate to right thalamus	0.69[b]	0.41

Significance (one-tailed) of individual pre- and posttreatment correlations: [a]$p<0.01$; [b]$p<0.05$; [c]$p<0.0005$; [d]$p<0.001$.
*Significant ($p<0.05$) difference in pre- to posttreatment correlation.
Source: Modified from Ref. 10.

tionship between brain function and internal mental experience in ways that have clinical significance for psychotherapists.

Hyperactivity of metabolism and bloodflow in orbitofrontal cortex (OFC) has been a consistent finding of brain-imaging studies of OCD over the past decade (25,26). For over 30 years, problems with perseverative behaviors—the inability to stop repetitive behaviors that no longer serve a useful function—have been described and studied in monkeys with OFC lesions (27). Humans with OFC damage show personality changes (28), socially inappropriate behaviors (29), and defects in assessing the future consequences of their actions (30); monkeys show decreases in social interactiveness (31). Both monkeys and humans with damage to OFC have specific problems in the performance of go/no-go discrimination tasks; i.e., they have difficulty in suppressing inappropriate responses (32,33). They also inappropriately continue to perform behaviors that are no longer rewarded (27,34,35). C. M. Butter, the author of some classic studies on OFC function, speculated over 25 years ago that this area "contributes to motivational processes which might be involved in behavioral suppression" (34).

The work of the group of E. T. Rolls (36), recording cellular responses of neurons in alert rhesus monkeys, has contributed greatly to our understanding of OFC function. They studied how cells in OFC responded in a go/no-go behavioral task in which visual stimuli were associated with the delivery of either fruit juice or concentrated saltwater. During testing the meaning of the stimuli were frequently switched so that, for example, blue was sometimes associated with juice and other times with saltwater, and vice versa for green. Monkeys could quickly learn to change their responses so as to avoid getting saltwater and maximize getting juice. The firing rates of orbitofrontal neurons during the performance of these behaviors showed some fascinating patterns, which may be very relevant to the role of this brain area in the symptoms of OCD patients.

There were numerous neurons in the OFC that fired in distinctive patterns depending on whether the color the monkey was shown was associated with juice or saltwater. It was clearly shown that the firing pattern of these cells was related to the type of behavioral response the monkeys made in the test situation. There were also cells that fired differentially depending on whether the monkey received juice or saltwater. There was a group of cells in this category whose firing patterns were of particular interest. These cells responded very strongly, with long bursts of firing, after the monkey made an error and received saltwater because the color associated with juice had been switched by the investigators. These neurons were quiet when the monkey responded to a color and received juice, but as soon as this color became associated with saltwater, these cells would fire in a long rapid burst.

It is important to note that these cells did not respond to the taste of saltwater or other aversive stimuli outside of the test situation—what they were responding to was the fact that the monkey had made an error. After these cells fired, the monkey quickly changed responses and started receiving juice again. What's more, there were cell responses seen in this group of "error-detection" neurons that consisted of bursts of firing even when the monkey received nothing at all in response to a color that had been associated with receiving juice; i.e., a burst of neuronal firing was related to the omission of an expected reward! Thus, neuronal responses related to modification of behaviors that are no longer appropriate (e.g., alteration of behavioral responses to stimuli no longer associated with a reward) were clearly demonstrated in the OFC. Recently, Rolls has speculated that these neuronal responses could be involved in emotional responses to situations that elicit "frustration" (37).

HOW DO THESE FINDINGS RELATE TO THE CLINICAL PHENOMENA OF OCD?

The core symptom of OCD is an intrusive thought or feeling that causes problems for a person because it leads to an extremely persistent and unpleasant internal sense that something "isn't right" or that something "needs to be done" to prevent dreadful consequences. The person is plagued by terrible ideas and sensations that create an intractable feeling that something is wrong. Given the weight of data that demonstrate a hyperactive OFC in OCD (25,26), coupled with the electrophysiology data of Rolls' group (36) showing bursts of firing by orbitofrontal neurons in response to behavioral errors, it seems reasonable to consider that cellular activity in the OFC might be related to an internal sense that something is wrong or that something needs to be done to correct a problem.

The error-related bursts of firing in OFC may well generate a something-is-wrong feeling in the monkey. Working in concert with the basal ganglia (as discussed below), this can result in a functional change in behavior by the monkey. In OCD patients, the operation of this "error-detection circuit" may become inappropriately activated in a chronic fashion, perhaps because of malfunction in the basal ganglia

(18,19,21,24). The result of the overactivity of this circuit could manifest itself clinically as intrusive persistent thoughts and sensations that "something is wrong." The action of another brain region, the anterior cingulate gyrus, which closely interacts with both OFC (38) and the caudate (17,38), could greatly amplify the visceral feeling of dread that accompanies these sensations (39). Reasoning in this fashion, we can approach a clearer understanding of the mental states that lead to the functional problems seen in OCD patients. As will be elaborated on in the next section, attempting to utilize neurobiological data in ways that help clarify our understanding of the internal feeling states of our patients is an effort that can yield significant clinical benefits.

A recent study by Rauch et. al (40) helps further clarify this process. This group used PET to measure cerebral blood flow (CBF) in eight OCD subjects after exposure to a stimulus designed to provoke obsessional thoughts, as compared to a neutral stimulus. They found significant ($p < 0.01$) increases in CBF in two brain areas: bilateral orbital cortex (with more extensive changes on the left) and right caudate nucleus. Interestingly, these are the brain regions in which we found significant decreases after successful cognitive-behavioral treatment. As described above, treatment responders showed a robust decrease of metabolism in the right caudate nucleus compared to nonresponders. Figure 2 shows the data concerning changes in left orbital cortex after cognitive-behavioral treatment. The graph demonstrates that the subjects who showed the most clinical improvement in response to treatment tended to show the biggest decreases in left OFC metabolism.

These two studies complement each other in a potentially important way. When OCD thoughts and urges acutely get more intense after exposure to a provocative agent such as a dirty object, the OFC becomes activated compared to a neutral state. With treatment, decreased activity in OFC correlates with the amount of decrease in symptom severity. Given the impressive amount of data from other studies that corroborate a role for orbital cortex in OCD pathophysiology (25,26), it seems reasonable to consider that the intrusive persistent feeling that "something is wrong," a cardinal symptom of OCD, may be related to the functional role of orbital cortex neurons in "error detection" becoming inappropriately overactivated (or inadequately inactivated) and causing bothersome mental states in OCD sufferers.

The basal ganglia have also been implicated in numerous studies of OCD, and the literature on this subject has been extensively reviewed (24,41). The role of the primate basal ganglia in the integration of sensory information in preparation for motor activity is among the most elegantly researched subjects in all of behavioral neurobiology (e.g., 16,42–44). It is well known that the OFC sends a direct projection to the striatum, which includes the caudate and putamen and is the major cortical input station of the basal ganglia (45,46). Rolls (47) has pointed out that information about whether a stimulus is related to reward or punishment could readily be relayed from OFC to striatum for the purpose of switching behaviors appropriately. "The striatum would be particularly involved in the selection of behavioral responses, and in producing one coherent stream of behavioral output, with the possibility to switch if a higher priority input was received" (47).

It is the profound difficulty that OCD patients have in switching their behaviors in response to what they themselves recognize as higher-priority inputs that marks another cardinal symptom of OCD. This is why we began using the concept of being "stuck in gear" as a means of improving their understanding about *why* changing the compulsive behavior is so difficult and requires such focused effort, as explained above. The work on the behavioral neurobiology of the basal ganglia shows that the feeling of being stuck in gear may well be closely related to how a malfunction in the basal ganglia would be internally experienced.

Related examples, such as Parkinson's disease (48), could be understood in a similar way. Recent work by the group of Swedo (49) has shown that Sydenham's chorea, a variant of rheumatic fever that involves autoimmune attack on the basal ganglia, is related to the onset and exacerbation of OCD. These ongoing studies are among the best evidence we have directly implicating pathology in the basal ganglia to OCD symptoms. Indeed, Swedo has recently speculated that Sydenham's chorea might serve as a medical model of OCD (50). From the perspective of this chapter, all these data from animal and human studies can be viewed as a potential source for educating OCD patients in the reattributing step of cognitive-behavioral therapy. They can also be used by psychotherapists to more clearly understand the internal experiences related to the observable clinical phenomena of OCD symptoms.

Baxter (51) has proposed a model, based in part on the data from Table 1, that helps explain the very high correlations in activity between orbital cortex, caudate, and thalamus in terms of a "worry circuit." Because of the excitatory and inhibitory interconnections of this circuit, it could potentially become self-sustaining, and thus difficult to break. This model was initially based on data that combined treatment responders from drug and behavioral treatment (52). The model predicts that, with sucessful treatment, increases in "filtering" functions in the caudate would result in an uncoupling of this fixed "worry circuit" and allow the patient to more easily terminate OCD behaviors. New data, shown in Table 1, now allow us to demonstrate that the uncoupling of these pathological correlational relationships can be achieved by drug-free cognitive-behavioral treatment. In explaining these findings to patients for use as new information in their "reattributing armamentarium," it has been helpful to use the notion of a "brain lock." As with the stuck-in-gear and broken-gate analogies, the biological data fit patients' internal experience of the symptoms quite well, and this enhances their ability to understand and manage disturbing and anxious feelings during behavioral therapy. Thinking of the high correlations of brain activity in the "OCD circuit" as a case of "brain lock" that can almost literally be "unlocked" by the work of behavior therapy serves to motivate patients to do the difficult self-directed response prevention described in the refocus step above. Once again, the biological data can be helpful to both patients and therapists as a means of better understanding the experience of OCD. Of course, the real goal is to use that understanding as a tool to enhance performance of cognitive-behavioral strategies, since we now have data to show this can result in functional changes in the very brain structures that are most likely causing the problems.

A MIND–BRAIN INTERACTION PARADIGM FOR PSYCHOTHERAPISTS

At least three aspects of OCD make it a particularly rewarding subject to study. First, compared to many other psychiatric disorders, it has a relatively clear-cut symptom presentation. People suffering from OCD can often describe with a fair degree of precision what it feels like to have OCD symptoms, and why they cause such misery. Second, study of its pathophysiology has yielded a fairly reproducible set of findings, so the probability that symptoms involve some kind of malfunction in a brain circuit containing OFC and basal ganglia connections is now reasonably well established (24,25). Third, OCD generally does not respond significantly to placebo treatment (53), and this has facilitated the study of therapeutic responses to both behavioral (3,4) and somatic treatments (see Chapters 7–9). All these factors contributed to OCD's being the first psychiatric condition in which systematic changes in brain function have been demonstrated after successful psychotherapeutic intervention—in this case, using cognitive-behavioral therapy (10). This finding of systematic changes in a well-established brain circuit after drug-free behavioral treatment has potentially far-reaching implications. For instance, these findings may enable us to use OCD as a paradigm for better understanding the relationship between the mind and brain in the process of behavioral change.

The behavioral changes that patients make during cognitive-behavioral therapy are highly purposeful. They require profound effort. They are done in an attempt to accomplish something. OCD patients are in emotional pain. They are working to try to alleviate that pain, and to overcome the problems in functioning that the pain is causing. The cognitive part of the treatment technique described above is an attempt to have the patient better understand what might be causing the pain, i.e., a medical problem. This knowledge helps them alter the behavioral responses that the disturbing feelings elicited before treatment began. This alteration of behavioral responses, when it becomes systematic over time, can result in an alteration of the brain mechanisms that are causing the medical problem. This has been the working hypothesis of the study presented above.

Let's examine this process a little more closely. As we have discussed, malfunction in an "error-detection" circuit in the OFC may result in the sending of an intensely bothersome "false alarm" to a person with OCD. Since, before treatment, he is generally unaware that this is happening, he tends to take the false alarm at face value and does compulsive behaviors to try to make the alarm stop bothering him. This process tends to be highly repetitive, and clinical experience shows us that it usually makes the bothersome "alarm" feeling even more intense. It seems reasonable to consider that the repetitive compulsive behaviors exacerbate the condition of "brain lock" described above. (Quite a few people have referred to this as "making a groove in your brain.") When the person changes behavioral responses, even momentarily, the brain circuits being used to mediate the behavior change. When the behavioral changes become systematic, as in behavioral therapy, systematic changes occur in brain energy use, and these can be measured with PET scans.

The question arises of whether behavioral therapy with no specific cognitive component would cause essentially the same changes in brain function if it is successful. The answer is very probably in the affirmative, and in any event this is now a readily resolvable experimental issue. But whether the cognitive training is systematic or not, the fact remains that when a person with OCD systematically changes behavioral responses to OCD thoughts and urges there also occurs a change in the value and meaning that he places on the internal experience of the feeling itself. This is particularly true when there has not been a medication-induced change in the feeling. Before treatment, when an intrusive thought saying, for example, "Wash your hands or else!!!" arose, the person usually responded by repetitively washing his hands. After treatment, the response to the same OCD thought is very different (maybe something like, "Oh yeah? Go to hell!!) and he performs very different and much more adaptive behaviors. This leads to alterations in brain function that, over time, result in measurable biological changes, generally associated with a decreased intensity in the intrusive OCD symptoms themselves.

The phenomenon of a change in the value or meaning one puts on an internal feeling state is very important to see and understand clearly. This is a key element in a process that has traditionally been called insight. It is not an easy process to describe. For that reason, some of the greatest philosophical minds in human history have devised methods to enhance our ability to talk about this process, in the interest of increasing our capacity to use it. For example, the philosophers of the Scottish Enlightenment in the eighteenth century used the notion of what a "judicious spectator" would think to describe how people form opinions about issues of moral content (54,55). David Hume, in particular, was keenly aware of the need for a method whereby people could overcome the distortions that the "passions" inject into human attempts to understand and regulate their behaviors (55). His closest friend, Adam Smith, further refined this work when he developed the concept of the "impartial and well-informed spectator" (56,57). This concept is very compatable with the treatment approach described above insofar as it effectively demonstrates an applied use of mindful awareness [which is itself the foundation of Buddhist philosophy (58,59)].

In brief, the impartial spectator is "the man within" (56, p. 137) that we all have access to, and that is fully aware of our feeling states and circumstances yet capable of taking on the character of an imagined spectator. This enables us to witness our own actions and feelings not as an involved agent but as an impartial observer. As Smith describes it (56, p. 113):

> When I endeavour to examine my own conduct . . . I divide myself as it were, into two persons; and that I, the examiner and judge, represent a different character from the other I, the person whose conduct is examined into and judged of. The first is the spectator . . . The second is the agent, the person whom I properly call myself, and of whose conduct, under the character of a spectator, I was endeavouring to form some opinion.

In this manner, "we suppose ourselves the spectators of our own behavior" (56, p. 112).

When a person with OCD, after learning behavioral therapy techniques, decides to change his response to an intrusive painful thought from a pathological to a functional behavior, a profound process occurs. Great effort must be mobilized and courage must be "screwed to the sticking place" to actually carry out the decision and physically alter the behavioral response. A willful resolve arises, e.g., "I'm not going to the sink to wash my hands. I'm going to practice my violin instead." Significant fear and dread, often associated with catastrophic thoughts ("But then my violin will get contaminated . . ."), accompany the entire process, especially in the beginning stages of treatment. How does the person do it? Where are the "inner resources" coming from?

Adam Smith understood that keeping the perspective of the impartial spectator clearly in mind—a process essentially identical to mindful awareness—under painful circumstances is hard work for any person. He stressed that it requires the "utmost and most fatiguing exertions to do so" (56, p. 148). Has there ever been a better example of a mental action that specifically requires a "fatiguing exertion" than doing behavior therapy for OCD? All psychotherapists know that people get very fatigued when they do it. Reflecting on what is so exhausting about it can be very revealing.

The cognitive-behavioral method presented above is designed to enable OCD patients to apply their effort more effectively when they try to alter their behavioral responses to intrusive OCD symptoms. Getting a clearer understanding of what those bothersome thoughts and urges really are and mean is an important part of the process. This is no doubt true even in behavioral therapies without a specific cognitive component. All successful behavioral treatments of OCD have in common the fact that they result in people making different, and more functional, choices about how to behave when intrusive OCD thoughts and urges arise in conscious awareness. A critically important part of this process is the ability to see the symptom in a different cognitive context, to give it a lower value and a different meaning. A patient must come to understand that different behavioral responses to painful OCD feelings lead to very different results in terms of future functional capability, with all that this implies about the direction of one's life. Medication can make this whole process easier by decreasing the intensity of the symptoms through direct chemical action on the brain. However, the same basic choice still exists for all OCD patients: should I do the compulsion, or not?

So why is doing behavior therapy for OCD so exhausting? Because focusing your attention on a useful behavior when your brain is bombarding you with distracting doubts and disturbing mental sensations takes a lot of work. Which is not to say that repeating a compusive behavior ad nauseum is not exhausting too. Unfortunately it can take as much effort to follow a bad brain circuit as a good one. But the quality of mental attention—of whether the impartial spectator is being attended to or not, of whether the action is being done mindfully or unmindfully—turns out to make a significant difference in how the brain functions. The data presented above are consistent with the statement that when OCD patients successfully change their behavioral responses to intrusive OCD symptoms, they systematically alter the function of brain circuits that over a decade of research have consistently been implicated in OCD pathophysiology. The fact that profound changes in the valuation and meaning assigned to particular types of mental experience play a key role in this process should be kept in mind by therapists and patients alike.

John Eccles, who was awarded the Nobel Prize in 1963 for his work on the mechanism of synaptic neurotransmission, recently published a book that summarizes and updates a half century of research on the question of mind–brain interaction (60). He presents a large amount of data consistent with the hypothesis that mental events act on the cerebral cortex by increasing the probability of the release of neurotransmitter from a synaptic vesicle in response to an incoming nerve impulse. This, in the words of the book's title, is "how the self controls its brain." The book is quite precise and rigorous and could be profitably consulted by anyone interested in this subject. For our purposes, suffice it to say that the findings presented above concerning systematic changes in brain metabolism after successful cognitive-behavioral treatment are consistent in every way with the thesis of Eccles' book. Hopefully the potential role of mental events in the alteration of behavioral and cerebral function during the treatment of OCD has been at least partially clarified by this chapter. Obviously, much work remains to be done concerning all these issues.

CONCLUSION: COULD OCD BE A PARADIGM-SHIFTING ILLNESS?

Research over the past decade indicates that OCD is a neuropsychiatric illness in which symptoms involving intrusive thoughts and urges are related to a malfunction in brain circuitry involving the OFC and the basal ganglia. Certain key aspects of the behavioral physiology of these brain structures have been reasonably clarified by work in the field of neurobiology. Thus, the opportunity arises to use basic science knowledge to better understand why the clinical phenomena of OCD take the form they do. Enhanced understanding of this sort serves a variety of functions, for both patients and therapists. For example, being able to explain in a plausible and scientifically based way why the intrusive OCD symptoms are so persistent can actually help patients more effectively manage the anxiety they cause. When done within the framework of ongoing behavioral therapy, this can enhance their ability to refocus their attention away from the symptom and onto more adaptive behaviors. The growing realization that systematically altering behavioral responses to OCD symptoms over time can actually alter brain function in a therapeutic way (or at least in ways that are related to symptom improvement) can have an amplifying effect on the motivation of both patient and therapist.

Key aspects of this approach to conceptualizing illness and formulating treatment strategies are readily applicable to other psychiatric conditions. For instance, a very elegant use of the concept of a "false suffocation alarm" has been proposed by Klein (61) as a means of integrating a large amount of clinical and physiological data on panic disorder. The application of reasoning entirely consistent with Klein's model has been effectively used in the development of cognitive-behavioral techniques for the management of panic attacks (62,63). The clear analogy of these developments to those that have occurred in the study of OCD raises the possibility that behavior modification of panic disorder could lead to systematic alterations of nervous system function.

Depression is another condition in which the kind of reasoning used in the study of OCD seems readily applicable. The neuroendocrine, circadian rhythm, and appetite disturbances of depression all implicate regulatory dysfunction of the hypothalamus, and of course there is a massive literature on the biology of depression (see Ref. 64 for a recent review) that demonstrates many other changes as well. Our group at UCLA, for example, has done PET studies (65,66) demonstrating decreases in metabolism in both caudate nucleus and prefrontal cortex in depression, and we have a growing number of anecdotal reports that these changes are reversible with medication treatment. Since there are a variety of well-done studies demonstrating the effective use of cognitive-behavioral treatment for depression (67,68), it should not be long before studies are done to systematically investigate the effects of these treatments on brain function. Furthermore, to cite just two examples of biological reasoning analogous to what has been presented above for OCD treatment, Frank et al. (69) have suggested that behavioral modification aimed at systematically correcting biological disturbances in the rhythms of daily living (times of eating, sleeping, bathing, etc.) can itself have antidepressant effects. And Post and Weiss (70) recently pointed out that patterns of symptom expression in mood disorders can pro-foundly interact with underlying biological mechanisms, through alter-ations in gene expression caused by "environmental and experiential impact." This is very consistent with our patients' "groove-in-the-brain" theory of OCD. Its important to remember, however, that these "experi-ential impacts" and their associated alterations of gene expression can be for better or for worse.

Recent research has begun to elucidate possible neural mecha-nisms for the cognitive deficits seen in schizophrenia. The medial tem-poral lobe and prefrontal regions appear most clearly implicated (71). A realization that the behavioral consequences of cognitive impairment should be a key target in the treatment of schizophrenia is also clearly emerging (72). Liberman has successfully used methods of behavioral treatment for schizophrenia that have cognitive components (73), and a recent book on cognitive-behavioral therapy for schizophrenia uses techniques with intriguing similarities to those described above for treat-ing OCD (74). Studying the effects of these techniques on cerebral func-tion could potentially be of great importance.

SUMMARY

The OCD studies described in this chapter can be used to illustrate a few key points. First, improved understanding of the relationship between brain function and behavior can be used to more clearly comprehend how and why the symptoms of psychiatric diseases manifest themselves the way they do. Second, this knowledge is useful to both patients and therapists for creating strategies that enhance the behavioral manage-ment of symptoms by viewing them in different, more functional, cogni-tive contexts. Third, systematic changes in behavioral responses to the internal mental states associated with pathological brain activity can meaningfully alter both the clinical course of the condition and the function of the brain itself. It is hoped that these principles will eventu-ally be applied to the study and treatment of a wide variety of disease states.

ACKNOWLEDGMENTS

Donations from the Charles and Lelah Hilton Family made this work possible. Cindy Ehlers, Ph.D., provided helpful editorial advice. I am in-debted to the supporters, staff, and faculty of the UCLA OCD-PET Study Group for creating an environment that allowed this work to come to fruition.

REFERENCES

1. Marks IM, Lelliott P, Basoglu M, et al. Clomompramine, self-exposure and therapist-aided exposure for obsessive-compulsive rituals. Br J Psychiatry 1988; 152:522–534.
2. Munford PR, Hand I, Liberman RP. Psychosocial treatment for obsessive-compulsive disorder. Psychiatry 1994; 57:142–152.
3. Baer L, Minichiello WE. Behavior therapy for obsessive-compulsive disorder. In: Jenike MA, Baer L, Minichiello WE, eds. Obsessive-Compulsive Disorders: Theory and Management. 2nd ed. Chicago: Year Book Medical Publishers, 1990:203–232.
4. Foa EB, Steketee GS, Ozarow BJ. Behavior therapy with obsessive-compulsives: from theory to treatment. In: Mavissakalian M, Turner SM, Michelson L, eds. Obsessive-Compulsive Disorder: Psychological and Pharmacological Treatment. New York: Plenum Press, 1985:49–129.
5. Marks IM. Behavioral self-treatment for obsessive-compulsive disorder. In: Hand I, Goodman WK, Evers U, eds. Obsessive-Compulsive Disorders: New Research Results. Berlin: Springer-Verlag 1992:111–117.
6. Baer L. Getting Control: Overcoming Your Obsessions and Compulsions. Boston: Little, Brown, 1991.
7. Foa E, Wilson R. Stop Obsessing! How to Overcome Your Obsessions and Compulsions. New York: Bantam, 1991.
8. Steketee G, White K. When Once is Not Enough: Help for Obsessive Compulsives. Oakland, CA: New Harbinger, 1990.
9. Schwartz JM, Martin KM, Baxter LR. Neuroimaging and cognitive-behavioral self-treatment for obsessive-compulsive disorder: practical and philosophical considerations. In: Hand I, Goodman WK, Evers U, eds. Obsessive-Compulsive Disorders: New Reşearch Results. Berlin: Springer-Verlag, 1992:82–101.
10. Schwartz JM, Stoessel PW, Baxter LR, et al. Systematic cerebral glucose metabolic rate changes after successful behavior modification treatment of obsessive-compulsive disorder. Arch Gen Psychiatry 1996; 53:109–113.
11. Schwartz JM. Manual for cognitive-biobehavioral self-treatment for obsessive-compulsive disorder: the four step method. (Obtainable from Dr. Schwartz, $15.)
12. Schwartz JM. Brain Lock: Free Yourself from Obsessive Compulsive Behavior. New York: Harper Collins, 1996.
13. Hand I. Obsessive-compulsive patients and their families. In: Faloon IRH, ed. Handbook of Behavioral Family Therapy. New York: Guilford Press, 1988:231–256.
14. Hand I. Behavior therapy for OCD: methods of therapy and their results. In: Hand I, Goodman WK, Evers U, eds. Obsessive-Compulsive Disorders: New Research Results. Berlin: Springer-Verlag, 1992:157–180.
15. James IA, Blackburn I. Cognitive therapy with obsessive-compulsive disorder. Br J Psychiatry 1995; 166:444–450.

16. Schneider JS, Lidsky TI, eds. Basal Ganglia and Behavior: Sensory Aspects of Motor Functioning. Lewiston, NY: Hans Huber, 1987.

17. Nauta WJH. Reciprocal links of the corpus striatum with the cerebral cortex and limbic system: a common substrate for movement and thought? In: Mueller J, ed. Neurology and Psychiatry: A Meeting of Minds. New York: Karger, 1989:43–63.

18. Rapoport JL, Wise SP. Obsessive-compulsive disorder: is it a basal ganglia dysfunction? Psychopharmacol Bull 1988; 24:380–384.

19. Modell JG, Mountz JM, Curtis GC, et al. Neurophysiological dysfunction in the basal ganglia/limbic striatal and thalamocortical circuits as a pathogenic mechanism of obsessive-compulsive disorder. J Neuropsychiatry 1989; 1:27–36.

20. Swerdlow NR. Cortio-striatal substrates of cognitive, motor, and sensory gating. In: Panksepp J, ed. Advances in Biological Psychiatry. Vol 2. Greenwich, CT: JAI Press, 1996:179–207.

21. Baxter LR, Schwartz JM, Guze BH. Brain imaging: toward a neuroanatomy of OCD. In: Zohar J, Insel TR, Rasmussen SA, eds. The Psychobiology of Obsessive-Compulsive Disorder. New York: Springer-Verlag, 1991:101–125.

22. Marks IM. Fears, Phobias, and Rituals. New York: Oxford University Press, 1987.

23. Goodman WK, Price LH, Rasmussen SA, et al. The Yale-Brown Obsessive-Compulsive Scale. Arch Gen Psychiatry 1989; 46:1006–1016.

24. Baxter LR, Schwartz JM, Guze BH, et al. Neuroimaging in obsessive-compulsive disorder: seeking the mediating neuroanatomy. In: Jenike MA, Baer L, Minichiello WE, eds. Obsessive-Compulsive Disorders: Theory and Management. 2nd ed. Chicago: Year Book Medical Publishers, 1990:167–188.

25. Insel TR. Toward a neuroanatomy of obsessive-compulsive disorder. Arch Gen Psychiatry 1992; 49:739–744.

26. Hoehn-Saric R, Benkelfat C. Structural and functional brain imaging in obsessive-compulsive disorder. In: Hollander E, Zohar J, Marazziti D, Olivier B, eds. Current Insights in Obsessive-Compulsive Disorder. New York: Wiley, 1994:183–211.

27. Butter CM, Mishkin M, Rosvold HE. Conditioning and extinction of a food-rewarded response after selective ablations of frontal cortex in rhesus monkeys. Exp Neurol 1963; 7:65–75.

28. Mega MS, Cummings JL. Frontal-subcortical circuits and neuropsychiatric disorders. J Neuropsychiatry 1994; 6:358–370.

29. Damasio AR, Tranel D, Damasio H. Individuals with sociopathic behavior caused by frontal damage fail to repond autonomically to social stimuli. Behav Brain Res 1990; 41:81–94.

30. Bechara A, Damasio AR, Damasio H, Anderson SW. Insensitivity to future consequences following damage to human prefrontal cortex. Cognition 1994; 50:7–15.

31. Raleigh MJ, Steklis HD. Effects of orbitofrontal and temporal neocortical lesions on the affiliative behavior of vervet monkeys. Exp Neurol 1981; 73:378–389.

32. Iverson SD, Mishkin M. Perseverative interference in monkeys following selective lesions of the inferior prefrontal cortex. Exp Brain Res 1970; 11:376–386.

33. Drewe EA. Go-no go learning after frontal lesions in humans. Cortex 1975; 11:8–16.

34. Butter CM. Perseveration in extinction and in discrimination reversal tasks following selective frontal ablations in *Macaca mulatta*. Physiol Behav 1969; 4:163–171.

35. Rolls ET, Hornak J, Wade D, McGrath J. Emotion-related learning in patients with social and emotional changes associated with frontal lobe damage. J Neurol Neurosurg Psychiatry 1994; 57:1518–1524.

36. Thorpe SJ, Rolls ET, Maddison S. The orbitofrontal cortex: neuronal activity in the behaving monkey. Exp Brain Res 1983; 49:93–115.

37. Rolls ET. A theory of emotion and consciousness, and its application to understanding the neural basis of emotion. In: Gazzaniga MS, ed. The Cognitive Neurosciences. Cambridge, MA: MIT Press, 1995:1091–1106.

38. Van Hoesen GW, Morecraft RJ, Vogt BA. Connections of the monkey cingulate cortex. In: Vogt BA, Gabriel M, eds. Neurobiology of Cingulate Cortex and Limbic Thalamus: A Comprehensive Handbook. Boston: Birkhauser, 1993:249–284.

39. Neafsey EJ, Terreberry RR, Hurley KM, et al. Anterior cingulate cortex in rodents: connections, visceral control functions, and implications for emotion. In: Vogt BA, Gabriel M, eds. Neurobiology of Cingulate Cortex and Limbic Thalamus: A Comprehensive Handbook. Boston: Birkhauser, 1993:206–223.

40. Rauch SL, Jenike MJ, Alpert NA, et al. Regional cerebral blood flow measured during symptom provocation in obsessive-compulsive disorder using 15-O labelled CO_2 and positron emission tomography. Arch Gen Psychiatry 1994; 51:62–70.

41. Rapoport JL. Recent advances in obsessive-compulsive disorder. Neuropsychopharmacology 1991; 5:1–10.

42. Rolls ET. Information processing and basal ganglia function. In: Kennard C, Swash M, eds. Heirarchies in Neurology: A Rappraisal of a Jacksonian Concept. London: Springer-Verlag, 1989:123–142.

43. Nishino H, Hattori S, Muramoto K, Ono T. Basal ganglia neural activity during operant feeding behavior in the monkey: relation to sensory integration and motor execution. Brain Res Bull 1991; 27:463–468.

44. Graybiel AM, Aosaki T, Flaherty AW, Kimura M. The basal ganglia and adaptive motor control. Science 1994; 265:1826–1831.

45. Kemp JM, Powell TPS. The cortico-striate projections in the monkey. Brain 1970; 93:525–546.

46. Yetarian EH, Pandya DN. Prefrontostriatal connections in relation to corti-

cal architectonic organization in rhesus monkeys. J Comp Neurol 1991; 312:43–67.

47. Rolls ET. Responses of neurons in different regions of the striatum of the behaving monkey. In: McKenzie JS, Kemm RE, Wilcock LN, eds. The Basal Ganglia: Structure and Function. New York: Plenum Press, 1984:467–493.

48. Saint-Cyr JA, Taylor AE, Nicholson K. Behavior and the basal ganglia. In: Weiner WJ, Lang AE, eds. Advances in Neurology. Vol 65. Behavioral Neurology of Movement Disorders. New York: Raven Press 1995:1–28.

49. Swedo SE, Leonard HL, Schapiro MB, et al. Sydenham's chorea: physical and psychological symptoms of St. Vitus dance. Pediatrics 1993; 91:706–713.

50. Swedo SE. Sydenham's chorea: a model for childhood autoimmune neuropsychiatric disorders. JAMA 1994; 272:1788–1791.

51. Baxter LR. Neuroimaging studies of human anxiety disorders: cutting paths of knowledge through the field of neurotic phenomena. In: Bloom FE, Kupfer DJ, eds. Psychopharmacology: The Fourth Generation of Progress. New York: Raven Press, 1995:1287–1299.

52. Baxter LR, Schwartz JM, Bergman KS, et al. Caudate glucose metabolic rate changes with both drug and behavior therapy for obsessive-compulsive disorder. Arch Gen Psychiatry 1992; 49:681–689.

53. Griest JH, Jefferson JW, Kobak KA, et al. Efficacy and tolerability of serotonin transport inhibitors in obsessive-compulsive disorder. Arch Gen Psychiatry 1995; 52:53–60.

54. Rendall J. The Origins of the Scottish Enlightenment. London: Macmillan, 1978.

55. Raphael DD. British Moralists 1650–1800. London: Oxford University Press, 1969.

56. Smith A. The Theory of Moral Sentiments, or An Essay towards an Analysis of the Principles by which Men naturally judge concerning the Conduct and Character, first of their Neighbours, and afterwards of themselves. Edition 6 (1790). Raphael DD, Macfie AL, eds. Oxford: Oxford University Press, 1976.

57. Raphael DD. The impartial spectator. In: Skinner AS, Wilson T, eds. Essays on Adam Smith. London: Oxford University Press, 1975:83–99.

58. Johansson REA. The Dynamic Psychology of Early Buddhism. London: Curzon Press, 1978.

59. Silananda U. The Four Foundations of Mindfulness. Boston: Wisdom Press, 1990.

60. Eccles JC. How the Self Controls Its Brain. New York: Springer-Verlag, 1994.

61. Klein DF. False suffocation alarms, spontaneous panics, and related conditions: an integrative hypothesis. Arch Gen Psychiatry 1993; 50:306–317.

62. Salkovskis PM, Clark DM. Cognitive and physiological processes in the maintenance and treatment of panic attacks. In: Hand I, Wittchen HU, eds. Panic and Phobias: Empirical Evidence of Theoretical Models and Longterm

Effects of Behavioral Treatments. New York: Springer-Verlag, 1986:90–103.

63. Margraf J, Barlow DH, Clark DM, Telch MJ. Psychological treatment of panic: work in progress on outcome, active ingredients, and follow-up. Behav Res Ther 1993; 31:1–8.

64. Kupfer DJ, section ed. Mood disorders. In: Bloom FE, Kupfer DJ, eds. Psychopharmacology: The Fourth Generation of Progress. New York: Raven Press 1995:911–1170.

65. Schwartz JM, Baxter LR, Mazziotta JC, et al. The differential diagnosis of depression: relevance of positron emission tomography studies of cerebral glucose metabolism to the bipolar–unipolar dichotomy. JAMA 1987; 258:1368–1374.

66. Baxter LR, Schwartz JM, Phelps ME, et al. Reduction of prefrontal cortex glucose metabolism common to three types of depression. Arch Gen Psychiatry 1989; 46:243–250.

67. Rush AJ, Beck AT, section eds. Cognitive therapy. In: Frances AJ, Hales RE, eds. American Psychiatric Press Review of Psychiatry. Vol 7. Washington, DC: American Psychiatric Press, 1988:530–669.

68. Freeman A, Simon KM, Beutler LE, eds. Comprehensive Handbook of Cognitive Therapy. New York: Plenum Press, 1989.

69. Frank E, Kupfer DJ, Ehlers CL, et al. Interpersonal and social rhythm therapy for bipolar disorder: integrating interpersonal and behavioral approaches. Behav Therapist 1994; 17:143–149.

70. Post RM, Weiss SRB. The neurobiology of treatment-resistant mood disorders. In: Bloom FE, Kupfer DJ, eds. Psychopharmacology: The Fourth Generation of Progress. New York: Raven Press, 1995:1155–1170.

71. Goldberg TE, Gold JM. Neurocognitive functioning in patients with schizophrenia: an overview. In: Bloom FE, Kupfer DJ, eds. Psychopharmacology: The Fourth Generation of Progress. New York: Raven Press, 1995:1245–1257.

72. Liberman RP, Green MF. Whither cognitive-behavioral therapy for schizophrenia? Schizophr Bull 1992; 18:27–35.

73. Liberman RP, Corrigan PW. Designing new psychosocial treatments for schizophrenia. Psychiatry 1993; 56:238–253.

74. Kingdon DG, Turkington D. Cognitive-Behavioral Therapy of Schizophrenia. New York: Guilford Press, 1994.

12

Yogic Meditation Techniques Are Effective in the Treatment of OCD

David S. Shannahoff-Khalsa

University of California, San Diego
La Jolla, and
The Khalsa Foundation for Medical Science
Del Mar, California

INTRODUCTION

Obsessive-compulsive disorder (OCD) patients usually respond to medication with only a 30% to 60% reduction in symptoms, and they usually remain chronically symptomatic even after some success with pharmacological treatment (1). This improvement, however, also implies a continued use of medication, even if only at a lower maintenance dose, and the majority of patients are likely to experience some unpleasant side effects due to the drug(s). Additionally, the effects of long-term pharmacotherapy in OCD are unknown and should pose serious concerns.

The discontinuation of pharmacological treatment also poses problems, as reported in two double-blind substitution or withdrawal studies. Pato et al. (2) observed a relapse rate of 90% within 2–4 months following abrupt discontinuation of clomipramine in 18 remitted patients. In the second study, Leonard et al. (3) substituted desipramine for clomipramine in a crossover design. A high percentage of patients relapsed within 2 months of beginning desipramine. Similar results were found in an open study of 35 OCD patients who discontinued fluoxetine after having had a good initial response (4).

A recent 6-year follow-up study (the longest reported to date) that included behavior therapy (BT), as exposure and response prevention (ERP), and clomipramine (or placebo) on a 6-week inpatient basis showed that neither drug nor placebo affected long-term outcome, and that the majority of patients who were taking clomipramine or other antidepressants at follow-up were no more improved than those who were not taking antidepressants: "Clomipramine's initial short-term effect was not followed by a subsequent detectable long-term advantage" (5). Better long-term outcome was correlated with more BT (6 weeks vs. 3 weeks) and with compliance with the BT homework (5). However, the group as a whole returned to pretreatment levels of general anxiety.

Marks (6) states that BT consistently results in 60% to 70% of patients' being "much improved" after brief treatment, and improvements are maintained at 2 to 3 years of follow-up. Baer (7) summarizes studies of BT conducted mostly on an inpatient basis around the world over the last two decades. He concludes that about 75% of OCD patients "get control of their symptoms," and that "80% are able to complete BT. Of the remaining 20%, most succumb to extreme fear. Cottraux (8) claims (without specifying in- or outpatient status) that "25% of patients refuse treatment or drop out early in therapy. Of those who remain in therapy 25% will not improve. Of improved patients 20% need booster treatment for some subsequent loss of gains." He also maintains that no controlled study has demonstrated that cognitive techniques improve outcome. Also, strong belief in obsessions and severe depression interfere with progress, and patients with obsessive thoughts without rituals usually do not benefit from BT. The acute effects of ERP also lead to an immediate and increased level of fear and anxiety, affecting the patient's willingness to comply with treatment. Thus, patience is critical to success in BT.

These results suggest that much more research is needed to improve treatment outcome in what was once thought to be an intractable disorder. Efficacy needs to be extended to the drug-refractory patient and those unable to use BT because of fears or pharmacotherapy due to disturbing side effects. This chapter is about clinically tested meditation techniques and how they can be used independently or as adjuncts to pharmacotherapy and BT.

BACKGROUND

A common perception of meditation is that the practitioner sits quietly and tries to think about nothing, or to remember and repeat a mantra (or word) silently, or to observe one's own "automatic" thoughts as they stream by while maintaining an objective, detached, and distanced mental reaction. This understanding of the meditation process, and of meditation techniques in general, is incomplete and originates primarily from the longstanding use in the West of the Transcendental Meditation technique (9,10), the Relaxation Response (RR) (11), and the Mindfulness Meditation (MM) (12,13), also called the Vipassana or insight meditation technique. All three techniques are late offshoots of yoga. In the original yogic system, known as Kundalini Yoga (KY), literally thousands of different meditation techniques exist; the vast majority include specific patterns of controlled respiration with a varied range of complexity and difficulty (see examples) (14). As the system of yoga evolved over thousands of years, many techniques were discovered that were found to be particularly effective for treating specific diseases and conditions. An uncontrolled study (31) and the preliminary results of a controlled study, both employing techniques from KY, are discussed here—these are the only systematic efforts this author is aware of to test the clinical efficacy of meditation techniques in OCD.

Although the earliest reported description of OCD symptomatology in the West was in a 15th-century religious document on demonology and possession (15), this disorder was recognized in India thousands of years ago. In fact, yogis had discovered a specific technique for treating this disorder (14). Besides the promising clinical studies reported here, other recent related scientific achievements have come from exploring the uniqueness of yogic concepts and breath-control techniques.

The yogic technique prescribed for treating OCD (14) involves unilateral forced nostril breathing (UFNB) through the left nostril in a specific pattern (see "Methods" below). The number of scientific studies on UFNB has been increasing over the past 15 years and have shown nostril-specific effects on the central nervous system (CNS) and autonomic nervous system (ANS). Right or left UFNB, a method for selectively stimulating one cerebral hemisphere (16–19), has been shown to have differential effects on several peripheral autonomic dependent events: heart rate (20), blood glucose levels (21), eyeblink rates (22), intraocular pressure (23), oxygen consumption (24), and galvanic skin resistance (24). Studies on UFNB have demonstrated its use to selectively stimulate the contralateral cerebral hemisphere, altering cognitive performance (17,18), mood (19), and EEG (16). Yogis also discovered a wide range of useful variations on the patterns of UFNB and alternate-nostril breathing (combinations of right and left respiratory patterns), all of which are likely to have unique CNS-ANS effects.

Yogis also found that the nasal cycle (a marker of lateralized autonomic function manifested by alternating and asynchronous nasal congestion and decongestion) was an indicator of rhythmic alternations of cerebral hemispheric activity. This claim (41) was demonstrated in 1983 by Werntz et al. (25), using continuous EEG and nasal-cycle monitoring to show a tightly coupled relationship between the lateralized ultradian rhythms of alternating cerebral hemispheric activity (26,27) and the nasal cycle (28,29). This cerebral rhythm is also likely to play an important role in the expression of severity of OCD symptoms as well as in the symptoms of other psychiatric disorders. In anecdotal feedback to this author, several patients report greater OCD severity during right-nostril dominance. Positive and negative moods are also characterized by similar ultradian cycles. Hall et al. (30) studied nine normals and nine depressed patients over 12 hours while conducting mood assessment every hour from 8:00 AM to 8:00 PM. There was a much greater amplitude in mood variability with patients compared to normals but no significant difference between groups in periodicity (depressed, mean = 4.7 h; normals, mean = 5.3 h). Two patients had 3-hour rhythms in which the mood variability was much greater than the amplitude of the circadian component. This variable-period range is also characteristic of the nasal cycle (28,29) and cerebral rhythm (25,26).

The lateralized cerebral dominance rhythm plays an important role in verbal and spatial skills, sleep processes, memory processes, visual perception, arousal, performance, and both individual and social behavior (reviewed in Ref. 26). Putative rhythms of OCD symptoms have never been reported, and the likely chronobiological features (especially the "hourly" ultradian domain) of this disorder deserve special attention. Findings with chronobiological features are likely to provide a better understanding of the lateralized cerebral deficits of OCD (reviewed in Ref. 31) that have been discovered using both brain-imaging and psychological measures.

I have designed a protocol to help facilitate the use of and compliance with the otherwise difficult yogic technique specific for treating OCD. Besides the clinical results, preliminary observations using magnetoencephalography (MEG) and impedance cardiography are also reported here for studying the effects of this unique left-nostril breathing pattern.

All the techniques (see Appendix) included here (with the exception of the RR and the MM techniques) are from the system of KY as taught by Yogi Bhajan. This protocol was also used in the first experiment (31) without a control population.

In the second study (unpublished; coauthors: J. Sidorowich, L. E. Ray, B. J. Schwartz, J. Wright, S. Levine, C. C. Gallen, H. D. I. Abarbanel, and F. E. Bloom), a comparison protocol using two other meditation techniques (RR and MM; see last section of Appendix) was employed as a control therapy to compare with the protocol employed in study 1. The comparison-control group is referred to here as group 2, and the group using the original KY protocol is referred to as group 1. The RR and MM techniques were chosen to be combined as comparison therapies since both are quite different from the KY techniques, they are popular, and they have been well studied and are frequently cited in the medical literature.

METHODS

Procedures for Studies 1 and 2

Two-hour meetings were held once a week for 1 year in study 1 and for 9 months to date in study 2. Only preliminary results are provided here for study 2. Groups 1 and 2 of study 2 met separately but on the same day and time. Weekly meetings were held to ensure compliance and proper use of the techniques, which required about 1 hour a day.

Study 1 subjects volunteered to participate knowing that they would employ yogic breathing techniques in a therapeutic trial. Study 2 subjects were instructed prior to signing consent forms that the study would be a controlled study comparing two meditation protocols. They were also told prior to testing that the two comparison groups would be determined by the flip of a coin once they were equally matched for age, sex, and use of medication. They were aware that one protocol had been tested in a pilot study and that the researchers had no idea, or any reason to believe, that one protocol would be more effective than the other. And this in fact was the purpose of the study, to test the relative efficacies of the two protocols. They were informed that if a significant difference in efficacy was observed at any one of the 3-month testing intervals, the two groups would be merged into the more efficacious group and the group to later merge would then also receive 12 months of the more efficacious protocol. Only I was aware of the content of the two protocols. Coauthor Leslie Ray, the therapist for group 2, was not aware of the contents or nature of the KY protocol. Each group was kept from knowing what techniques were employed by the other group or their responses to the protocols.

Subjects in both studies were also informed that if they were not using medication at the beginning of the study they could not begin any pharmacotherapy for OCD or any other psychiatric disorder during the course of the study. If they were on medication, they had to be stabilized at that dose for a minimum of 3 months. They were also not allowed to participate in BT, group therapy for OCD, or individual psychotherapy for OCD while in the study. In addition, they were told that they could reduce or eliminate their medication(s). Study 2 subjects were also informed that if they were medication-free at the beginning of the study they would have to undergo an MEG scan prior to therapy and again 1 year later after use of the more efficacious protocol if one protocol proved to be more effective.

Psychological Testing

All testing for both studies was held at near 3-month intervals after initial baselines. The baseline tests in study 2 were taken before the subjects were divided into the two matched groups.

Study 1 employed the Yale-Brown Obsessive Compulsive Scale (Y-BOCS) (32), the Y-BOCS symptom checklist, the Symptoms Checklist-90-Revised (SCL-90-R) (30), and the Perceived Stress Test (PSS) (34). The SCL-90-R was given only at baseline, 9, and 12 months. The Y-BOCS symptom checklist was given only at 0 and 12 months.

In study 2, the Y-BOCS, SCL-90-R, PSS, Profile of Moods Scale (35), and Purpose-in-Life (36) tests have been administered at 0, 3, 6, and 9 months. The Y-BOCS symptom checklist was given only at baseline and will be administered at 12 months with the others. Because study 2 is not complete, only the Y-BOCS results are reported here; the other tests have not been scored.

Meditation Techniques

The techniques taught to the study subjects are described in the Appendix.

Subjects: Study 1

Eight adults (seven women, one man) entered the study with a mean age of 39.4 years (range 29–55 years). All patients had met the DSM-III-R criteria for OCD and had previously received at least one other form of therapy (medication, BT, individual psychotherapy). The subjects' initial obsessions and contaminations are listed in Table 1 as identified from the Y-BOCS symptom checklist, with the number of symptoms listed per subtype for obsessions and compulsions. Table 3 includes the demographics for these eight subjects; they are discussed in greater detail elsewhere (31).

Table 1 Study 1 Subjects' Initial Obsessions and Compulsions

Subject no.	Obsessions								Compulsions						
	Aggressive	Contamination	Sexual	Hoarding	Religious	Symmetry/exactness	Somatic	Misc.	Cleaning/washing	Checking	Repeating	Counting	Ordering/arranging	Hoarding	Misc.
1								2		1	2				1
2		1						1	2	1					
3	1	1		1		1				1	1	1			6
4		1		1		1	1	6				1	1		2
5			1			1	1	2			2				1
6	1				1		1			1	1				4
7						1	1	2		1	2		1		2
8	1	1		1		1	1	10	1	1	1	1		1	8

Subjects: Study 2, Groups 1 and 2

The subjects' obsessions and compulsions are listed in Table 2. The letter T identifies subjects with tricotillomania. All patients met the DSM-III-R criteria for OCD, and all (except patient 22) had previously received at least one other form of therapy (medication, BT, individual psychotherapy). Group 1 includes subjects 1–11, and adolescent subjects 24 and 25. Group 2 includes subjects 12–21. Female adolescent subject 24 entered at the beginning of the study and was put into group 1 since it required more physical activity. Male adolescent subject 25 and female subjects 22 and 23 entered at 3 months. Table 4 includes the demographics for subjects 1–25. All subjects (except subjects 3, 6, 9, 11, 13, 16, 19, and 20) are discussed as representative cases.

Group 1: Sample Case Studies

Subject 1 is a married housewife (age 37) with three children. Her mother had OCD. When she was 3, her parents went through a bitter divorce and custody agreements were violated, leading to long-term isolation from parents. She believes her OCD started at age 3. She was sexually molested by two male relatives. She developed depression in 1987. She started 20 mg of Paxil in September 1993 after a 10-day hospital stay for depression. She had 2 months of BT in late 1993.

Subject 2 is a single female (age 38) with one child and grandchild, and has limited part-time employment. She developed severe trichotillomania at age 7 during turbulent years with her alcoholic, adulterous father, who also gambled. She was taken to the father's adulterous interludes and kept outside; upon returning home to her angry mother, she felt responsible and internalized the blame. She and her brothers were verbally abused by the father and her brothers were also physically abused. She came close to being shot when her father was in a dispute. The fear of being shot through her bedroom window while she was asleep remained for years. She tried Anafranil and had severe side effects. Her mother is a compulsive cleaner.

Subject 4 is a single unmarried male (age 36) born and raised on military bases. He, his older brother, and his mother had been psychologically abused by his alcoholic Marine father, who during his stupors would regularly terrorize and occasionally physically abuse them. When the subject was 8, and for the 11 following years, his father would "come to our room—it would be lights on, stand at attention, room inspection, maybe a few war stories or lessons on how to fight or even kill." By the time he had finished high school, he had moved nine times and attended 12 schools. He could "never quite relax," between the frequent moves and his father's rampages—or, as the father called it, his "kill program: burn the town and kill the people." His OCD symptoms started at 13 on one occasion of moving to a new school. He became terrified by some of the "punks" in his remedial math class, who verbally abused him in front of the

Table 2 Study 2 Subjects' Initial Obsessions and Compulsions

Subject no.	Obsessions								Compulsions						
	Aggressive	Contamination	Sexual	Hoarding	Religious	Symmetry/exactness	Somatic	Misc.	Cleaning/washing	Checking	Repeating	Counting	Ordering/arranging	Hoarding	Misc.
1	2	5				2	1	7	2	2	2		1	1	1
2	2						T	1		2					T,1
3	1	5				1	2	7	1	1	2	1	1		3
4	5		1		1	1	3	5		2					2
5	3	4	1	1		1	1	7	3	3	1	2			6
6	2	3					2	4	1	2	1				1
7	2		2		1		1	4		2	2				4
8		5				2			5				2		
9	1	2					T	6	2						T
10	3	8	2	1	1		2	6	3	4	2			1	4
11		3		1	1	2	2	1		3	2		1	1	3
12	3	2					1	7		3	2		1		
13	1			1			T	7							
14	1	6	1	1	1		2	4	1	1	1			1	T,2
15	1					2	2	1		3				1	2
16	4				1						2				T,1
17							T,1								
18	1	4		1		2		6	2	1	3	1	2	1	T,1
19	2	3	1	1		2	2	4	1	1	2		1	1	3
20				1	1			6	1		3			1	3
21							1	3	1	1					5
22				1		1									1
23	5	4		1		1	2	2		2	2		1	1	3
24	2	6		1		2	2	8	3	4	2	1	2	1	4
25	4	5		1		2	2	8	3	1	2	1		1	4

Table 3 Study 1 Demographics

| Subject no. | Sex | Age (yr) | Age at onset | History | | | Employed | Marital status | Psych. history | Physical disease | Relatives with OCD | Trauma |
				BT	Meds	Psych.						
1	M	44	Teens	+	+	+	+	M				+
2	F	29	20			+		M				
3	F	40	5	+	+	+	+	D				+
4	F	31	Ch	+	+	+	+	S	Anr/Dep; Anr/Bul; SAD	TMJ, IF, O, PMV	+	+
5	F	34	Ch		+			M				+
6	F	38	18	+	+	+	+	M				+
7	F	55	14	+	+	+		M		BP	?	+
8	F	45	Ch	+	+	+	+	D		BP		+

Ch = childhood onset; Anr = anorexia nervosa; Dep = depression; Bul = bulemia; SAD = seasonal affective disorder; TMJ = temporlo mandibular joint syndrome; IF = ideopathic fibromyalgia; O = osteoporosis; PMV = prolapsed mitral valve; BP = back problems.

Table 4 Study 2 Demographics

Subject no.	Sex	Age (yr)	Age at onset	History			Employed	Marital status	Psych. history	Physical disease	Relatives with	
				BT	Meds	Psych.					OCD	Trauma
1	F	37	3	+	+	+		M	Dep	BP	+	+
2	F	38	7	+	+	+	PT	D		BP	+	+
3	F	25	13			+	St	S				
4	M	36	13		+	+	+	S				+
5	F	22	Ch		+	+	St	S	Dep/Anr/Bul			+
6	F	62	30s		+	+		M				+
7	M	24	8		+	+	St	S			+	+
8	F	38	18	+	+	+	+	M				?
9	F	36	5	+		+	+	M		BP		+
10	M	46	11	+	+	+		S	Sp, Dep, ADD	CFS	?	+
11	F	60	24		+	+	PT	D				+
12	F	40	14		+	+	+	M	Dep	BP	?	+
13	M	67	?		+	+	PT	D	BD			+
14	F	49	Teens		+	+		M		SD		+
15	M	29	8		+	+	+	S				
16	M	30	19	+	+	+	+	M			+	+
17	F	46	20			+	+	M	Dep		+	+
18	M	29	5		+	+	+	M	Dep		+	+
19	F	28	Ch		+	+	St	S	Dep		+	+
20	F	57	Ch			+		D				
21	F	26	19		+	+		S	Anr/Bul			+
22	F	30	Ch		+	+	St	S	Dep			+
23	F	62	16			+	PT	M			+	+
24	F	14	Ch		+	+	St	S	Dep/ADHD			+
25	M	14	11		+	+	St	S	ADHD/Dep/TS			+

Dep = depression; BP = back problems; PT = part-time employment; St = student; Anr = anorexia; Bul = bulemia; Ch = childhood onset; SP = social phobias; ADD = attention deficit disorders; CFS = chronic fatigue syndrome; BD = bipolar disorder; SD = sleep disorder; ADHD = attention deficit hyperactive disorder; TS = Tourettes Syndrome.

"neurotic lady teacher who had absolutely no control over them." To get out of the class, he had to enter a higher-level one. Although he had excellent grades in the new class, he lived with the constant fear of falling back; getting good grades was "the condition of his freedom." In the new class he developed the OC symptoms. For a short time his symptoms diminished until, at age 15, his father took him drinking and to a house of prostitution. In his later teen years and into his early 30s, he used alcohol and illicit drugs extensively "in part to try and fix his head." His early attempts with medication (Nardil, Zoloft) failed and he experienced numerous side effects.

Subject 5 was a female college student (age 22) with a childhood onset of OCD symptoms and depression in early teens. She was physically abused as a child, and at age 7 her parents "demanded accountability and productivity and a strong work ethic," leading to an "unhappy family life." When she was 15, her family moved across the country, at which point she developed anorexia; she was hospitalized three times for her eating disorder by the age of 18. She had exposure to a "sexually deviant" grandfather with whom her family lived for several months upon arriving in California. She tried Anafranil, Busbar, and Prozac for her OCD without success and started taking 200 mg of Zoloft 7 months prior to the study, with a final increase to 250 mg 6 weeks before entry. She elected to drop out of KY therapy after the first 2 weeks because she did not believe that it could help her. At 250 mg of Zoloft she complained of headaches, drowsiness, and fatigue.

Subject 7 was a single male (age 24) living with his family. His OCD symptoms started at age 8 with fears and thoughts of hurting his mother, which still occurred at the time of entry to the study. He said his mother made him sleep with garbage in his bed if he did not clean his room. His mother also had OCD. He had tried 80 mg of Prozac for a period of 1.5 years ending 6 months prior to the study, without success. He also had fears of being around people and being alone in his room. After 2 months he elected to leave the study, finding that he could not use the meditation practices at home. He also developed a personal relationship with subject 3 after she left the study. She further encouraged him to leave and to try Prozac again after her own initial but short-lived success.

Subject 8 is a part-time-employed married woman (age 39) with two children. Her OCD symptoms started after her marriage at age 18, when she and her husband emigrated to South Africa from England. She was the oldest child of four, with a later stepsister and stepbrother. Her parents divorced when she was 12. Her stepfather was manic-depressive and two sisters have a "mild compulsive personality." She had "tried Prozac without much of an effect," and BT with limited success.

Subject 10 is a single male (age 46) living on Social Security disability. His father was in the military. Constant moves, different schools, and living in a war zone all caused "a lot of anxiety and insecurity." His family was emotionally and physically abusive. The father was an alcoholic (suspected OCD); his mothered, angered by this, was "overcontrolling and demanding." His parents were both "withdrawn, depressive people and emotionally distant." He never felt that he bonded with his father or that he belonged in the family. His younger brother became an alcoholic and drug abuser. He also suffers from chronic fatigue immune dysfunction syndrome, attention deficit disorder, learning disabilities, social phobias, and depression exacerbated by seasonal changes. His OCD symptoms started during his preteen years. He tried Prozac, Zoloft, and Anafranil, three 11-week sessions of BT, and biofeedback.

Group 2: Sample Case Studies

Subject 12 is a married female (age 40) employed as a systems analyst, has one sister 15 years older, and "grew up basically as an only child." When she was 4, her sister, who had been the primary caregiver, married and left the house. Her parents both worked—her vivid memories of them were that they "drank and fought a lot." "I was afraid and in emotional pain most of the time, and I felt obligated to try to make things better. My job was to keep my dad from getting drunk. I never succeeded. I also tried to defend my dad from my mother's vicious words." Her mother had a preoccupation with getting killed and a fear of fire because her own mother died in a fire when she was 13. Her mother was also very concerned about hurting others. "I was in pain, even [from fear of hurting others], though I was careful and determined not to do or say anything wrong." Her mother was always depressed (possible OCD), and her father was an alcoholic. Between the ages of 17 and 31, she abused drugs and alcohol, and at age 31 checked herself into a 30-day drug and alcohol rehabilitation program. Her OCD may have started in childhood, but clearly by age 14, and it is exacerbated by her depression. She also has body dysmorphophobia. She has been prescribed Elavil, Desyrel, Tofranil, Sinequan, Nardil, Xanax, Parnate, Librium, Tranxene, and Zoloft, and eventually got relief from 80 mg of Prozac for depression.

Subject 14 is an unemployed married female (age 49) and mother of two. She is the youngest of three children. Her father was ill most of her life and died when she was 13. The mother struggled to support the family. She had a lonely, unhappy childhood. Her OCD began in her adolescence. She has marital difficulties and is "a constant worrier and procrastinator" with chronic insomnia. She was prescribed Klonopin in June 1993 after a one-night sleep clinic evaluation with a suspected myoclonus.

Subject 15 is a single male (age 29) employed as an engineer. When he was 19, his alcoholic father died of liver cancer. He is the third of four children. The oldest sister drinks heavily and has a "compulsive personality," the second oldest sister has panic attacks and mild agoraphobia, and the youngest has had an eating disorder and depression. His OCD started at age 8 and he developed trichotillomania at 11. He tried Anafranil (300 mg) in 1990; after 6 months he stopped due to lack of relief and major side effects. He also tried Prozac and group therapy.

Subject 17 is married (age 46) with one child employed as a counselor. She is the youngest of three sisters, and her oldest sister was "many times the caregiver" because her mother worked. Her father rejected her emotionally and died when she was 27. Her OCD and trichotillomania started at age 20, and on occasion she has insomnia related to work stress. She complains of "feeling tense" and has "a lot of anger." She entered group therapy (1 year) for depression 4 years prior to the study.

Subject 18 is a married employed male (age 29) with two children. He came from a "chaotic and dysfunctional" family with an alcoholic father with OCD. His alcoholic brother was hyperactive, and possibly has OCD. His OCD started when he was 5. He tried Anafranil and Prozac in 1991, and both exacerbated his OCD. At age 20 he attempted suicide, as a result of depression, poor grades, and drug abuse. Between the ages of 18 and 24 he drank heavily, and he used cocaine and amphetamines between 20 and 23.

Subject 21 was a single female (age 26) on disability raised in a dysfunctional family and abused and beaten by a sister and raped at 14. Her OCD began at age 19. She has anorexia nervosa and bulimia. She tried group 2 for 2 of the first 3 weeks and quit because she was not getting relief. She later joined the KY group after the merging of the groups and attended two of the first four meetings accompanied by a driver who was no longer able to bring her to therapy.

Subject 22 is a remarried woman (age 62) with one child and one stepchild, with part-time self-employment. She was raised in an impovrished home and says her mother was emotionally abusive and never willing to help her, showed her no affection, and denied sex to her father. Her mother was continually insulting toward her, "like her worst enemy." Her mother had OC symptoms of cleaning, hoarding, and eating rituals. When she left for school in the morning, her mother would regularly say "you should get killed by a car" or "you shouldn't live to come home." She eloped at 16 and was kicked in the stomach by her mother when she found out that she was pregnant. Her memories of her OCD symptoms go back to when she first moved out of the house, when she began to acquire things of her own to hoard.

Subject 23 (age 30) was a single female college student born to 16-year-old parents and immediately placed into foster-care homes. At age 6 months, she was adopted into a home where she suffered psychological and physical abuse. She "always felt that something was wrong." She hated herself by age 5, and her OCD symptoms "go back as far as I can remember." At age 12 she developed the fear of hurting herself that has continued, and she has been in and out of depression her entire life. She has tried Prozac, Zoloft, and Anafranil for her OCD and was taking Effexor 375 mg for the 5 months prior to the study. She attended three of the first 10 sessions and dropped out because she "did not believe that it could work" for her and that her roommates "would not approve of her odd yoga practices."

Subject 24 was a female adolescent (age 14) with one younger brother; her father is a therapist and her mother a housewife. Her OCD symptoms started after the family made a major relocation. She has always had a phobia of her parents' leaving her. She was diagnosed with OCD at age 8 and has depression and attention deficit hyperactive disorder. She was taking 200 mg of Zoloft for

14 months prior to the study. Anafranil and Prozac gave no relief for her OCD or depression. She left the group after participating in seven of the first eight sessions even though she began to achieve results. She refused to do the therapy at home. Her parents approved of her decision.

Subject 25 was a male adolescent (age 14). His parents divorced when he was 18 months old. The mother psychologically abused him with increasing negativity, criticism, and unusually high expectations. His older brother was the "model son." The subject developed both OCD and Tourette's syndrome at age 11. Just before he turned 14, his mother decided she no longer wanted him and he was forced to move in with his father and stepmother. He believes his OCD started when his wealthy mother forced him to wear used clothes from garage sales. He has attention deficit hyperactive disorder, depression, learning disabilities, and Tourette's syndrome, for which he is taking Haldol 2 mg with minimal relief. He has taken imipramine, ritalin, and Anafranil. He was stabilized on 40 mg of Prozac for 9 months prior to the study. After one session, he told his stepmother he no longer wished to participate in the group.

MEG Equipment and Methods

The multichannel biomagnetometer is located at the Scripps Clinic and Research Foundation in La Jolla, California. Neuromagnetic field patterns were recorded in a circular area with a diameter of 144 mm using two Magnes 37-Biomagnetometers (Biomagnetic Technologies, Inc., San Diego). One probe recorded from the left hemisphere and the other from the matching region of the right hemisphere. Both probes together provide 74 channels of data recorded here at 231.5 Hz. Each probe was initially centered on a position 7 cm rostral to the external auditory meatus at the inferior part of the parietal lobe, approximately at the central sulcus (for details see Refs. 42,43).

The 10 unmedicated OCD subjects (2, 3, 4, 7, 9, 15, 17, 18, 21, and 22) and nine age- and sex-matched control subjects without psychiatric histories or health problems were comfortably positioned in a right recumbent position and 30 minutes of resting baseline activity was recorded from both the right and left hemispheres with 74 channels of data. Eyes remained closed, and the subjects were instructed not to sleep or think about anything specific but to let their minds go on "automatic." Only control subjects without medications and meditation practices were included. The pre- and posttherapy MEG scans for OCD subjects, along with those of a pre- and post- no-therapy 12-month period for controls, await analysis.

Reported below are the preliminary data on one normal, well-trained subject performing the OCD breathing (OCDB) for 31 minutes with 10-minute resting baseline periods immediately before and after the OCDB. This subject was also in a right recumber position, but with eyes open during all three periods. A small red light positioned on the wall at eye level was flashed for 5 milliseconds at 15-second intervals to provide a time marker at the four 15-second phases of the OCDB pattern.

Impedance Cardiography Monitoring and Methods

The BoMed NCCOMR7 Noninvasive Cardiac Monitor (Cardio-Dynamic International Corp., Irvine, CA) was used to measure: 1) heart rate (HR) in beats/min; 2) stroke volume (SV) = volume of electrically participating tissue $\times$ ventricular ejection time $\times$ $(dZ/dT)_{max}$/Thoracic Fluid Index in milliseconds; and cardiac output in liters/min. The Sleeptrace Program (International Biomedical Inc., Austin, TX) collected the cardiac data online using a 386 PC. The cardiac measures were collected as beat-to-beat data.

The same subject who participated in the MEG scan sat with a straight spine in a chair while observing a digital timer on a desk. The subject was acclimated to the environment and rested. The OCDB was then performed after collecting 10 minutes of additional resting baseline measures followed immediately by the OCDB exercise period lasting 31 minutes with a second 10-minute baseline.

CLINICAL RESULTS OF STUDIES 1 AND 2

Study 1: Clinical Results of 1 Year of KY Therapy

The mean Y-BOCS score for the totals for the eight patients at baseline was 21.125 (STD = 4.32). Table 5 includes the baseline and 3-month intervals for the Y-BOCS scores (obessions and compulsions) for subjects 1–8.

For those who completed the program, the group results showed a mean improvement of 54% using the Y-BOCS (totals) as based on the individual improvements of 83%, 79%, 65%, 61%, and −18% for subjects 6, 5, 7, 1, and 8, respectively. Subjects 2, 3, and 4 withdrew at 3 months with respective improvements of 26%, 32%, and −14%. A one-way repeated-measures ANOVA was performed to test the hypothesis that the Y-BOCS means were the same at each of the different time periods, i.e., baseline, 3-, 6-, 9-, and 12-month periods. Table 5 includes the means, N values, and standard deviations for the Y-BOCS totals at each time period. The hypothesis of equality of means for the different 3-month Y-BOCS scores may be rejected, $F(4,12) = 3.343$; $p \leq 0.046$. Pairwise differences were investigated using Newman-Keuls multiple

Table 5 Study 1 Y-BOCS Results (obsessions + compulsions = totals)

Subject no.	0 Months	3 Months	6 Months	9 Months	12 Months
1	14+14=28	7+8=15	5+5=10	8+8=16	6+5=11
2	14+13=27	10+10=20			
3	11+11=22	6+9=15			
4	11+10=21	12+12=24			
5	9+10=19	7+8=15	5+5=10	3+5=8	0+4=4
6	10+8=18	7+3=10	7+5=12	4+0=4	3+0=3
7	9+8=17	5+5=10	0+6=6		
8	8+9=17	10+11=21	10+10=20	11+11=22	10+10=20

Repeated-measures ANOVA for Y-BOCS scores (obsessions + compulsions; SD), for baseline ($N=8$) 21.125 (4.32), 3 months ($N=8$) 16.25 (5.06), 6 months ($N=5$) 11.60 (5.17), 9 months ($N=4$) 12.50 (8.06), and 12 months ($N=5$) 8.80 (6.98). $F(4,12)=3.343$; $p \leq 0.046$.

range test (0.05 level). The results are as follows: 12 month <> 6 month = 9 month <> 3 month <> baseline.

The results of the SCL-90-R are presented in Table 6 for 4 subjects (1, 5, 6, and 8) at baseline and 12-month intervals for the OC symptoms, anxiety, and global severity index (GSI). The SCL-90-R showed significant results comparing baseline and 12 months using two-tailed paired T-tests with three degrees of freedom for OCD ($t = 13.856$; $p < 0.001$) and GSI ($t = 7.314$; $p = 0.005$), and a marginal result for anxiety ($t = 3.167$; $p < 0.051$).

PSS scores for the eight subjects are presented individually in Table 7. A one-way repeated-measures ANOVA was performed to test the hypothesis that the PSS scores were the same at each of the different 3-month periods. The baseline and 3-month group means (+SD) for the five tests are 21.375 (7.44), 16.50 (5.9), 14.20 (6.14), 13.50 (6.56), and

Table 6 Study 1: Symptoms Checklist-90-R

Subject no.	OCD-0	OCD-12	ANX-0	ANX-12	GSI-0	GSI-12
1	1.30	0.40	0.60	0.30	0.44	0.16
5	1.0	0.10	1.0	0.20	0.78	0.21
6	0.80	0.10	1.10	0.0	0.60	0.10
8	2.90	2.20	1.30	1.0	1.71	1.20

OCD-0=baseline results; OCD-12=12-month results; ANX-0=baseline anxiety results; ANX-12=anxiety results at 12 months; GSI-0=general severity index at baseline; GSI-12=general severity index at 12 months. The scale for each measure ranges from 0.0 to 3.0.

Table 7 Study 1: Perceived Stress Scale Scores (all eight subjects at 3-month intervals)

Subject no.	0 Months	3 Months	6 Months	9 Months	12 Months
1	20	15	13	15	13
2	35	15			
3	22	12			
4	18	20			
5	15	9	6	7	4
6	12	13	13	10	8
7	20	20	16		
8	29	28	23	22	22
Mean =	21.38	16.50	14.20	13.5	11.75

Subjects 2, 3, and 4 dropped out after 3 months. Subject 7 completed the study at 6 months.

11.75 (7.76), respectively. The hypothesis of equality of means for the different 3-month PSS scores may be rejected, $F(4,12) = 9.114$; $p \leq 0.001$. Pairwise differences were investigated using the Newman-Keuls multiple range test (0.05 level). The results are as follows: 12 months <> 9 months = 6 months <> 3 months <> baseline.

Of the initial group of eight, five subjects (subject 1 = 20 mg; subject 5 = 40 mg; subject 6 = 40 mg; subject 7 = 20 mg; and subject 8 = 40 mg) had been stabilized with Prozac for a minimum of 3 months prior to the start of the study. Of these, three (60%) had been completely free of medication for at least 5 months (subject 1 for 7 months, subject 6 for 5 months, and subject 7 for 8 months) by the end of the study (May 13, 1993). The other two (40%) had reduced their doses by 25% and 50%, respectively, for at least 4 months in the case of subject 8 and 2 months in the case of subject 5.

As of April 6, 1994, four of the five subjects (subjects 1, 6, 7, and 8) have been off medication for 18, 16, 19, and 9 months, respectively. As of April 6, 1994, all these subjects report lasting improvement. No further testing has been administered to these subjects at the time of preparation of this chapter.

Study 2: Preliminary Clinical Results

The preliminary results for the Y-BOCS are presented in Table 8 for the baseline and 3-, 6-, and 9-month test periods of the study for all subjects. The SCL-90-R, PSS, POMS, and PIL await scoring for all periods. Group 1 initially included adult subjects 1–11 (eight females, three

Table 8 Study 2: Y-BOCS Obsessions + Compulsions = Totals

Subject no.	0 Months	3 Months	6 Months	9 Months
1	10+12=23	10+ 7=17	9+ 6=15	9+ 6=15
2	11+13=24	2+ 3= 5	0+ 4= 4	0+ 2= 2
3	6+12=18			
4	12+15=27	8+11=19	10+11=21	5+ 6=11
5	13+13=26			
6	14+11=25	16+15=31		
7	12+ 6=18			
8	8+10=18	8+ 9=17	8+10=18	4+ 7=11
9	10+10=20	6+ 8=14	9+ 9=18	9+ 7=16
10	15+15=30	11+13=24	13+13=26	11+ 9=20
11	14+16=30	5+ 5=10	5+ 5=10	5+ 5=10
12	11+ 8=19	11+10=21	7+ 5=12	4+ 0= 4
13	8+15=23			
14	12+ 7=19	9+ 7=16	8+ 5=13	6+ 5=11
15	11+14=25	6+12=18	4+10=14	6+13=19
16	11+ 5=16	8+ 4=12	6+ 5=11	
17	12+ 9=21	10+10=20	0+ 0= 0	0+ 0= 0
18	12+13=25	10+ 9=19	6+ 8=14	5+ 5=10
19	9+10=19	8+10=18	7+ 6=13	
20	13+13=26			
21	17+18=35	19+19=38		
22		10+ 9=19	2+ 1= 3	0+ 0= 0
23		14+13=27		
24	7+ 7=14			
25		15+17=32		

males) and adolescent female subject 24. Group 2 initially included subjects 11–21 (six females and four males). Each group had six medicated adult subjects. The mean age for (adult subjects) group 1 was 38.55 (STD = 13.25; N = 11) and for group 2 40.00 (STD = 14.3; N = 10). (Note: subjects 22, 23, and 25 entered the study after the two groups merged at the 3-month period.)

The mean baseline Y-BOCS score for the totals (obsessions + compulsions) for group 1 was 22.75 (STD=5.15; N = 12) and for group 2 22.80 (STD = 5.39; N = 10). The mean baseline Y-BOCS obsessions score for group 1 was 11.0 (STD = 2.89; N = 12) and for group 2 11.6 (STD = 2.41; N = 10). The mean baseline Y-BOCS compulsions score for group 1 was 11.75 (STD = 3.11; N = 12) and for group 2 11.20 (STD = 4.05; N = 10). There were no significant differences at baseline

302   Shannahoff-Khalsa

between mean scores for the Y-BOCS totals, obsessions, or compulsions for the two groups. This result also indicates that the groups were also matched for the severity of symptoms.

During the first 3-month period, each group had three adult subjects voluntarily withdraw: group 1—subjects 3, 5, and 7; group 2—subjects 13, 20, and 21. Subject 6 in group 1 was excused from the study due to her medication complications with Ativan. If the researchers had known of her problems earlier, she would not have been admitted to the study. The adolescent subject in group 1 also voluntarily withdrew. This left each group with seven adults, changing the baseline group means for the Y-BOCS totals to 24.57 (STD = 4.68; N = 7) and 20.57 (STD = 3.36; N = 7) for groups 1 and 2, respectively. Determining whether the two group baseline means were significantly different after the respective subjects withdrew was carried out using a two-tailed independent groups T-test. Even though the mean for group 1 increased and that for group 2 decreased, these changes were not statistically significant: t = 1.836; P = 0.091.

A two-way mixed-model ANOVA was performed to investigate group differences, pre- vs. post-differences, and the group interaction. The interaction term of the ANOVA model was of particular interest to us, since it reflects the potential differential effects of each therapy over time. This term was statistically significant, $P(f1,12 = 4.89) \leq 0.0471$, indicating that the change in the KY group from baseline to 3 months was significantly more dramatic. The 3-month Y-BOCS totals for groups 1 and 2 are 15.14 (STD = 6.2; N = 7) and 17.71 (STD = 2.98; N = 7), respectively. This result suggested that the KY therapy was significantly more efficacious than the RRMM therapy.

The RRMM therapy also proved not to be significantly effective when comparing the Y-BOCS totals for the baseline (mean = 20.57; STD = 3.36) and 3-month (mean = 17.71; STD = 2.98) test periods using a two-tailed paired T-test (t = 2.414; p = 0.052) even with a minimal improvement of 13.9%. A two-tailed paired T-test on the baseline (mean = 24.57; STD 4.68) to 3-month (mean = 15.14; STD 6.20) change for the KY therapy for Y-BOCS totals showed a statistically significant improvement of 38.36% (t = 3.461; p = 0.013). The mean group change in Y-BOCS totals from 0 to 3 months was 9.43 and 2.86 for groups 1 and 2, respectively. Since the comparison therapy (RRMM) proved to be less effective than the KY therapy, the two groups were merged so as not to withhold the more efficacious therapy.

There was also a significant difference in the attendance rate for the two groups during the first 3 months. Group 1's attendance rate was 73.91%; group 2's was 60.16%. The subjects in both groups were asked independently to state whether they thought they had improved in their OCD symptomatology. The response was written down before they were informed of their individual or group changes and before they were told that the two groups would be merged. All subjects (except subject 6, who was having medication problems) in group 1 responded that they were experiencing improvements with their OCD symptoms, while no subject in group 2 reported perceived improvement. This may be the reason for the differences in attendance rates between the two groups. Group 1 was apparently achieving greater relief from the therapy.

The number of subjects remaining in the study after the merging of the groups at 3 months was 14, or 64% of the original 22. Added to this total of 14 was one of the originals from group 2 (subject 21), who had withdrawn earlier but elected to re-enter and attempt therapy with the more efficacious protocol. She also took the Y-BOCS again and re-entered with a total score of 38. Additionally, three new candidates (adult subjects 22 and 23 and adolescent subject 25) entered at this time. The total number of subjects starting the second 3-month period was 18, but subjects 21, 23, and 25 eventually dropped out, leaving a total of 15 subjects at 6 months.

The mean Y-BOCS totals (obsessions + compulsions) at the 0-, 3-, and 6-month points for the subjects from group 1 were, respectively, 24.57 (STD = 4.68; $N = 7$), 15.14 (STD = 6.20; $N = 7$), and 16.00 (STD = 7.23; $N = 7$). For Group 2 they were 20.57 (3.36; $N = 7$), 17.87 (STD = 2.8; $N = 8$), and 10.00 (STD = 5.39; $N = 8$). Subject 22, who entered at 3 months, was included with group 2 since it was her first 3-month session with KY therapy. A repeated-measures ANOVA for 0, 3, and 6 months for group 1 showed a $p \leq 0.004$, indicating a significant improvement for the 6 months of therapy. However, the 3- to 6-month scores for group 1 were not significantly different. Pairwise differences were investigated using the Newman-Keuls multiple-range test (0.05 level), showing 0 months <> 3 months = 6 months. Group 2 showed a $p \leq 0.001$ for the 6 months of therapy, with a large improvement during the first phase of KY therapy: a Y-BOCS decrease of 17.87 to 10.00. The Newman-Keuls multiple-range tests results (0.05 level) showed 0 months <> 3 months <> 6 months. This repeated-measures ANOVA, which now includes subject 22, shows a 0- to 3-month difference in Y-BOCS total mean scores whereas the two-tailed paired T-test did not show significance for the seven original subjects of group 2 from 0 to 3 months.

During the 6- to 9-month period of the study, subjects 16 and 19 dropped out because of religious conflicts and school-related problems, respectively. This left a total of 13 subjects at the 9-month testing. The

0-, 3-, 6-, and 9-month results for groups 1 and 2 combined with the Y-BOCS totals for the remaining 13 subjects (of which 12 started the study at its inception) are: 0-month = 23.42 (STD = 4.166; N = 12), 3-month = 16.85 (STD = 4.91; N = 13), 6-month = 12.92 (STD = 7.35; N = 13), and 9-month = 9.92 (STD 6.74; N = 13). A repeated-measures ANOVA shows that when testing the hypothesis of equality of means, it can be rejected at $p \leq 0.001$. The Newman-Keuls multiple-range test results (0.05 level) are 0 months <> 3 months <> 6 months <> 9 months.

Table 9 presents the medication profiles of all medicated subjects entering the study. Of the original 13 medicated adult subjects (1, 5, 6, 8, 10, 11, 12, 13, 14, 16, 19, 20, and 23) to enter the study, six subjects remain at 9 months (subjects 1, 8, 10, 11, 12, and 14). Of these six, three subjects (8, 10, and 11) are no longer on medication after 11 months (time of preparation of this chapter). Therefore, of the subjects

Table 9   Medication Profiles (adults = 13; adolescents = 2)

Subject no.	Medication	Dose (mg)	Month ended/reduced
Adults			
1	Paxil	20	At 9.5 mo 50% reduced
5[a]	Zoloft	250	
6[a]	Ativan	1 mg b.i.d.	
8	Anafranil	150	Off at 7.5 mo
	Zoloft	200	Off at 9 mo
10	Paxil	10	Off at 8.5 mo
11	Paxil	20	Off at 5 mo
12	Prozac	80	At 5 mo reduced 25%
13[a]	Lithium	300	
14	Klonopin	0.5	
	Trazadone	50	Off at 1 mo
16[a]	Zoloft	100	
19[a]	Prozac	80	
20[a]	Paxil	40	
23[a]	Effexor	375	
Adolescents			
1[a]	Zoloft	200	
2[a]	Prozac	40	
	Haldol	2	

[a] Withdrew from study, voluntarily or otherwise.

remaining in the study, 50% have eliminated medications and the other 50% have significantly reduced their levels.

Figure 1 shows the Y-BOCS results for the 13 subjects as they progressed in groups 1 ($N = 7$) and 2 ($N = 6$) independently, and Figure 2 shows the means of all subjects in groups 1 and 2. Group 2 is calculated with $N = 5$ at baseline and $N = 6$ at 3, 6, and 9 months. Subject 22 entered at 3 months.

PHYSIOLOGICAL EFFECTS OF THE OCDB: PRELIMINARY RESULTS

MEG Results: Analysis of Subjects and the OCDB

Ten unmedicated subjects entered the study and had baseline scans; seven remain and await follow-up scans after a 1-year course of KY therapy. Four of the subjects (15, 17, 18, and 21) who participated in

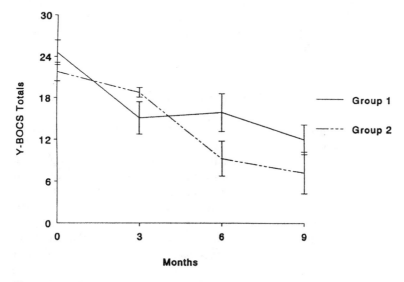

Figure 1 Mean Y-BOCS totals scores for the 13 remaining subjects over the 9-month period, with their respective changes noted at 3-month intervals after their baseline Y-BOCS score. Group 1 (solid line) consists of seven subjects who initiated treatment with KY; group 2 (broken line) consists of five remaining subjects who initiated treatment with RRMM therapy and at 3 months began treatment with the KY therapy after one subject, 22, was added. Vertical bars represent the standard errors for each group at the respective test periods.

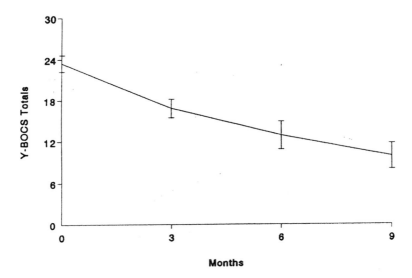

Figure 2 Mean Y-BOCS totals scores for all 13 subjects independent of the first 3 months when different therapies were employed for the two groups. After 3 months all subjects were in the KY therapy group. The mean at each 3-month interval is plotted including the standard error bars.

study 2–group 2 for the initial 3 months also had a second baseline scan at 3 months prior to entry into the KY therapy. The scans on these four subjects also allow for intrasubject variability with a nonsignificant change in symptom status.

Preliminary data are presented here (Figures 3–5), utilizing channel 1 of both the left and right hemispheres to measure the dynamic effects of the OCDB on the magnetic-field strength of the brain. This channel records from homologous regions of both hemispheres over the inferior part of the parietal lobe approximately at the central sulcus, a region related to the motor and somatosensory cortex and also to attentional and arousal mechanisms. Phase-space plots are presented here that are constructed from 15 seconds of data per state. The time series of channel 1 at any one point $n(t)$ on the x-axis is plotted against itself lagged by eight measures $n(t + 8)$ on the y-axis. This plot is only one way to compare the activities of the two homologous channels over time. Here it elucidates the variability of the signal at one location and demonstrates the relative magnitude of the magnetic-field strength in fempto-tesla at this location. These phase-space plots also help to eluci-

date any recurring patterns that emerge and the nature of the oscilla-
tions.

Figure 3 compares the left and right homologous locations in both
the pre- and post-OCDB periods. Each period has a 15-second segment,
with a 10-point moving average, extracted from the beginning of the
resting recordings. A considerable asymmetry is observed where the left
hemisphere shows a much greater variability in the signal of the magnetic-field strength in the pre-OCDB period. Figures 4 (inspiration and
breath-retention phases) and 5 (expiration and holdout phases) compares all four phases of both hemispheres. The 31 minutes of the OCDB
is separated into the four specific phases: a slow (15 seconds) inspiration
period, a 15-second breath-retention period, a slow (15 seconds) expiration period, and a final 15-second period of holding the breath out. This
one-breath-a-minute pattern was repeated for 31 minutes. The data for
each of the four phases were averaged separately for the entire 31 minutes; i.e., 31 segments of inspiration were first averaged, etc. The data
were then smoothed using a 10-point moving average and then plotted
as $n(t)$ vs. $n(8 + t)$. The original left- $>$ right-hemisphere variability
shifted to a right- $>$ left-hemisphere variability. All four phases of the
right hemisphere exhibit patterns different from one another. The variations of activities of the left hemisphere are much less discernible. Figure
3 also shows the post-OCDB phase, in which the activities in the respective 15-second segments extracted from the beginning of the 10-minute
postexercise period show a normalization of activities of both hemispheres. A comparison of the other recording locations for the dynamic
interactions during these four respective phases and comparisons of
other trained subjects await analysis.

Cardiovascular Results: Analysis of the Effects of the OCDB

Figure 6 illustrates the beat-to-beat measures of SV for a 10-minute resting period, followed by 31 minutes of the OCDB, and a final 10-minute
resting period. Figure 7 shows the corresponding beat-to-beat measures
for HR. A doubling of SV occurs during the one-breath-per-minute cycle
of the OCDB and a consistent 40-beats-per-minute shift occurs for HR.
Figure 8 illustrates this in more detail, and also shows that in most of
the cycle SV and HR are inversely related. During the first phase, the
slow inspiration period, both SV and HR approximate 80 ml/beat and
80 beats/minute, respectively. Also in the first stage of the holdout
phase, both SV and HR again approximate each other. Figure 9 shows
the inverse relation of both SV and HR in a 2-minute sample of the first
resting phase.

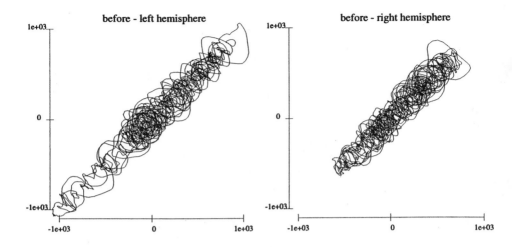

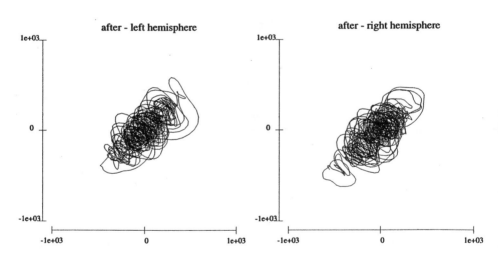

Figure 3   MEG phase-space plots for channel 1 of both the left and right hemispheres. The top pair are from the beginning of the resting period before the 31 minutes of the OCDB exercise period. The bottom pair show the same channels of data from the first 15 seconds of the postexercise period. Each plot represents 15 seconds of data with the time series of the magnetic field strength in femptotesla measured at 231.5 Hz and plotted as $n(t)$ vs. $n(t+8)$; i.e., each data point is plotted against the same series of measures 8 time steps or 0.0345 seconds later. A moving average of 10 was run on each series before plotting.

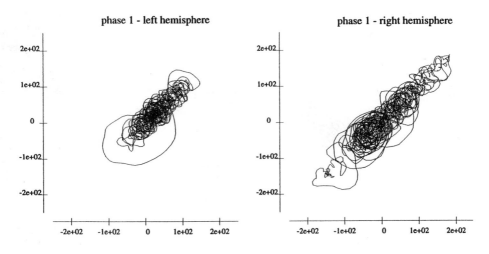

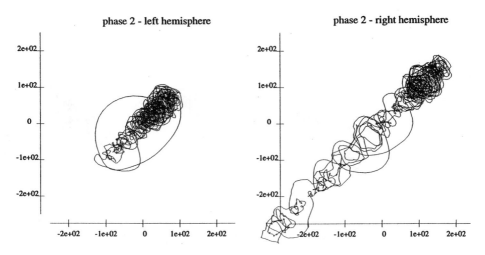

Figure 4   MEG phase-space plots for channel 1 of both the left and right hemispheres. The top pair are from the first phase, the 15-second inspiration phases, of the 31 minutes of the OCDB exercise period. The bottom pair are from the second phase, the 15-second breath-retention phases, of the 31 breath cycles. Each plot represents 15 seconds of data, with the time series of the magnetic field strength in fempto-tesla measured at 231.5 Hz and plotted as $n(t)$ vs. $n(t+8)$; i.e., each data point is plotted against the same series of measures eight time steps or 0.0345 seconds later after the averaging of all 31 similar phases of the breath cycle, e.g., 31 inspiration phases were first averaged.

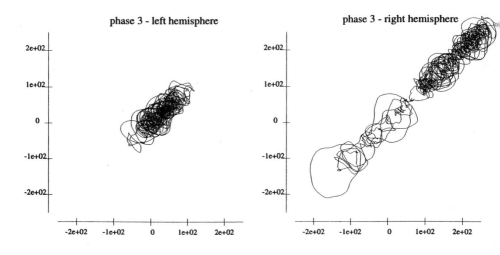

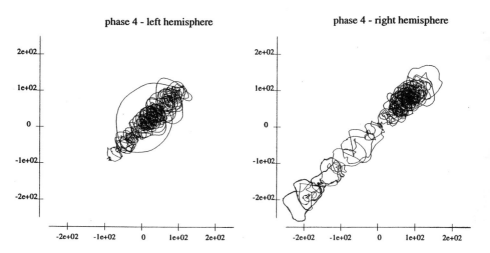

Figure 5 MEG phase-space plots for channel 1 of both the left and right hemispheres. The top pair are from the third phase, the 15-second expiration phase, of the 31 minutes of the OCDB exercise period. The bottom pair are from the fourth phase, the 15 seconds of holding the breath out during the 31 breath cycles. Each plot represents 15 seconds of data, with the time series of the magnetic field strength in fempto-tesla measured at 231.5 Hz and plotted as $n(t)$ vs. $n(t+8)$. This is plotted after the averaging of all 31 similar phases of the breath cycle; e.g., 31 expiration phases were first averaged.

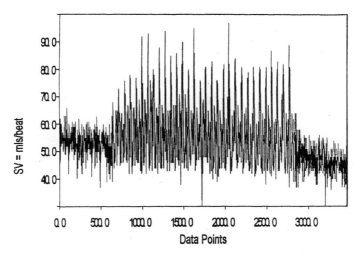

Figure 6 Beat-to-beat measures of SV for one subject from the three respective periods of the recording: 10 minutes of resting baseline, 31 minutes of the OCDB exercise, and 10 minutes of postexercise rest. The *y*-axis is SV in ml/beat and the *x*-axis represents the measures of consecutive data points, or each beat-to-beat measure during the 51 minutes of the experiment. The subject in this figure is the same subject as in the MEG recording but on a different day.

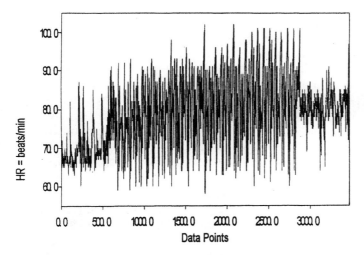

Figure 7 Beat-to-beat measures of HR for the same subject as in Figure 6 from the three respective periods of the recording: 10 minutes of resting baseline, 31 minutes of the OCDB exercise, and 10 minutes of postexercise rest. The *y*-axis is HR in beats/min and the *x*-axis represents the measures of consecutive data points, or each beat-to-beat measure during the 51 minutes of the experiment.

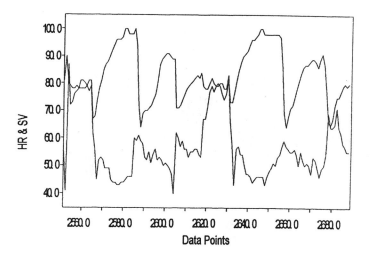

Figure 8 Beat-to-beat measures of both HR and SV for the subject's data in Figures 6 and 7 for 2 consecutive minutes of the OCDB exercise period—minutes 27 and 28. The measures are captured at each heartbeat and are extracted from Figures 6 and 7 for the same 2 minutes, data points 2552–2690. The *y*-axis scale includes values for both HR in beats/min and SV in ml/beat. The *x*-axis represents the measures of consecutive data points, or each beat-to-beat measure during these 2 minutes of the experiment.

Figures 6–8 demonstrate the dramatic beat-to-beat effects on the cardiovascular system as a linear time series during the performance of the OCDB. Figure 10 illustrates three separate phase-space plots for the three respective periods of the recording. The corresponding beat-to-beat measures of SV and HR are plotted versus each other and provide a description of how the dynamic interaction of SV and HR covary as they both contribute to cardiac output. The mean cardiac output values during the three respective periods of the recording are 3.725 L/minute (STD 0.3047), 4.572 L/minute (STD 0.8033), and 3.838 L/minute (STD 0.3803). In Figure 10 a difference in the pre- and post-OCDB patterns of HR vs. SV is also discernible, showing the displacement of the mean locus of points to a lower SV value and a higher HR value. The phase-space plot of the OCDB exercise period in Figure 10 also indicates a strong inverse relationship between SV and HR as expected, but a significant portion of the representation is displaced, further indicating the convergence in magnitude of the two parameters during the inspiration phase of the cycle. The OCDB induces a 22.7% increase in CO compared to the first resting period. This overall increase in CO is fairly dramatic

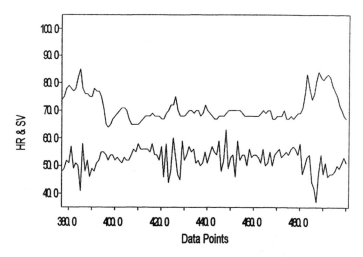

Figure 9 Beat-to-beat measures of both HR and SV for the subject's data in Figures 6 and 7 for 2 consecutive minutes of the first 10-minute resting period—minutes 6 and 7. The measures are captured at each heartbeat and are extracted from Figures 6 and 7 for the same 2 minutes, data points 378–502. The *y*-axis scale includes values for both HR in beats/min and SV in ml/beat. The *x*-axis represents the measures of consecutive data points, or each beat-to-beat measure during these 2 minutes of the experiment.

and probably signifies a much greater need for oxygen during this slow respiratory process. The shift in the main locus of points between pre- and post-OCDB periods suggests that, due to increase in HR, the OCDB increases the activities of the sympathetic nervous system.

DISCUSSION

Study 1

The eight subjects in study 1 had all previously received some form of therapy (medication, BT, individual insight-oriented psychotherapy, group therapy) and had longstanding histories of OCD. The mean Y-BOCS totals score went from a baseline value of 21.13 for all eight subjects (or 19.8 for the five completing the study) to 8.8 for the five subjects completing at their respective final timepoint. This is a 55.5% improvement in mean scores for these five subjects. The three subjects (2, 3, and 4) who had dropped out at 3 months had all done so because of uncontrollable circumstances (pregnancy, work-schedule conflicts,

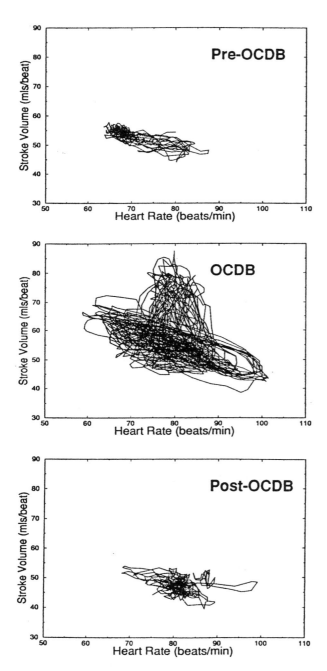

Figure 10   Three phase-space plots: the top = the first 10-minute resting period, the middle = the 31 minutes of the OCDB exercise period, and the bottom =

and fibromyalgia, respectively). These three subjects were unmedicated and had a mean improvement in 3 months of 15%, with individual improvements of 26%, 32%, and −14%, respectively. Of the five initially medicated subjects, three (subjects 1, 5, and 7) were able to eliminate medication for considerable periods prior to the end of the study (7, 5, and 8 months, respectively). All five subjects had failed earlier to respond successfully to other forms of therapy.

Even though this is a small number of subjects, their improvements here are unlikely to be due to placebo effects or time since it is known that patients with this recalcitrant disorder do not respond to placebo. Their improvements on the Y-BOCS are also paralleled by almost identical improvements on the SCL-90-R OCD scale (mean improvement = 53.3%). (Note: only subjects 1, 5, 6, and 8 have SCL-90-R scores for 12 months.) Their improvements on the two other SCL-90-R scales (Anxiety Scale = mean of 62.5%; Global Severity Scale = mean of 53.25%) and the PSS scores (mean of 39% for subjects 1, 5, 6, 7, and 8) from baseline to 12 months are similar. In sum, these results are remarkable considering the earlier controlled and double-blind studies in which improved or remitted patients who eliminated or substituted medications failed to maintain improvement (2–4). At the 1-year follow-up, four of the five subjects (subjects 1, 6, 7, and 8) had been off medication for 18, 16, 19, and 9 months, respectively, and continued to report (without psychological testing) lasting improvement. Further testing with 4–6-year follow-ups are necessary to determine the long-term success with these subjects. It should also be noted that three (subjects 5, 6, and 7) of the five subjects to complete the study had scored a zero for either their obsession or compulsion scores at their final timepoint.

Study 2

Study 2 is a controlled study; however, the results presented here are preliminary and include only one (Y-BOCS) of five psychological scales employed to determine the efficacy of treatment. However, the Y-BOCS

---

the 10 minutes of the final resting, or post-OCDB exercise, period. The x-axis represents values of the time series for HR measures plotted against the corresponding SV measures taken at the same beat on the y-axis. Each of the serial measures is represented by one point. These points are connected with lines and describe a locus of points showing how SV and HR covary over time for the three respective periods. Each plot describes the respective hemodynamic state changes during the experiment.

is generally considered the most reliable measure of treatment outcome for OCD.

Using two treatment protocols in matched groups in which both the subjects and the therapists are unaware of which protocol will prove to yield better results meets the rigorous standards necessary to control for the factors of time and placebo. Both groups were very closely matched (for age, sex, medicated/unmedicated, and severity of symptoms) at baseline, especially given the population sizes. While each group lost three adult subjects prior to the 3-month test, a two-tailed T-test failed to reveal a significant difference in baseline Y-BOCS totals for the two groups even though group 1's mean score increased and group 2's mean score decreased. This insignificant ($t = 1.836$; $p = 0.091$) 4-point difference in baseline Y-BOCS totals between the two groups nonetheless could be interpreted to indicate that group 2 was less severe at baseline. One might expect that a group of subjects whose symptoms are less severe may more readily comply and benefit from treatment. However, the mean changes in Y-BOCS totals (group 1 = -9.43; group 2 = -2.86) for the first 3 months clearly indicate that the KY therapy was far more efficacious (two-way mixed-model ANOVA; $p \leq 0.047$), with an improvement of 38.36% vs. a 13.9%. The second 3-month period, in which group 2 first utilizes the KY therapy and shows a 44% improvement, is also a good indication that this population derived substantially more benefit from the KY therapy than from the RRMM therapy. Group 1 in the second quarter regressed about 5%. However, overall, from 0 to 9 months both groups (1 and 2) improved 51% and 66%, respectively, or 57.6% for all 13 subjects. This preliminary 9-month result is similar to the 12-month result for study 1. One could assume that since group 1 has improved less overall, initial severity may play a role in the rate and degree of improvement.

In addition, female subjects 2, 12, 17, and 22 all scored 0 for the obsessions and/or compulsions by the 9-month timepoint. However, this was only 6 months of KY therapy for subject 22, who entered the study at 3 months. Subject 17 scored 0 for both obsessions and compulsions at both her first 3-month and 6-month KY timepoints. She initiated treatment with the RRMM therapy and went from a 21 to 20 for those 3 months. Of these four subjects, only subject 12 started on medication. She initially went from 19 to 21 for Y-BOCS totals with the first 3 months of RRMM, and with the KY therapy she went to 12 and 4 for the first and second quarters.

At the beginning of the study, most OCD subjects see the OCDB as being very difficult if not impossible to perform. However, informing them that other patients have achieved this ability is mildly reassuring.

In study 1, three of the five subjects to complete the study, (subjects 1, male age 44; 5, female age 34; and 6, female age 38) managed to perform the OCDB for one breath per minute for the entire 31 minutes on a regular basis by the first 8 months of therapy. These three subjects were medicated at the beginning of the study. In study 2, to date, only subject 2 (unmedicated female age 38) has been able to complete the OCDB for 31 minutes at one breath per minute. However, this is not something she can perform at every occasion unlike the three subjects in study 1. Perhaps the closer contact achieved between therapist and subject (smaller population) in study 1 made a difference.

In summary, subjects in study 2 seem to be doing equally well or slightly better than subjects in study 1 according to the Y-BOCS. For the respective 9-month periods, study 1 subjects ($N = 5$) reduced Y-BOCS totals from 19.8 to 12.5, or 7.3 points, and study 2 subjects ($N = 12$ at baseline; $N = 13$ at 9 months) reduced totals from 23.42 to 9.92, or 13.49 points. At the 9-month timepoint, three of the four initially medicated subjects (8, 10, and 11) in group 1 are off medication. Subject 1 (group 1) has reduced her medication by 50% and subjects 12 and 14 (group 2) have substantially reduced their medications. This result is another promising parallel to study 1 subjects. The early results of study 2 are encouraging.

MEG and Cardiac Impedance Results of the OCDB

This is the first study that we are aware of to use MEG to analyze OCD patients. The effects of the KY therapy may induce changes in brain dynamics that compare with clinical improvements. The control subjects will give indications about the possible changes that may occur within normals over a similar 1-year period. Intraindividual and group differences may result.

The MEG results for the OCDB are compelling for several reasons. They show dramatic shifts in the relative strength of the magnetic-field patterns in the two hemispheres compared to baseline, and that these large lateral effects support the contralateral effects found with other UFNB studies. In one study on EEG and UFNB, a greater amplitude of EEG activity was found in the contralateral hemisphere (16). The two studies on cognitive performance (17,18) and mood (19) also show contralateral activation. The magnitude of activity in the MEG study also shows a greater amplitude of activity (and variability) in the contralateral hemisphere. The pre- vs. post-comparisons indicate that the OCDB induced an equalization of hemispherical activity. Also, the differences of the four 15-second phases of the respiratory cycle show that the

OCDB has unique and phase-specific effects on the right hemisphere that are not exhibited in the left hemisphere during the use of the technique. These results suggest that the OCDB has unique lateral effects that predominantly affect the activities of the right hemisphere. It is not surprising that a respiratory rate of one breath per minute for 31 minutes has unique cortical effects. However, it may be surprising that the use of this therapeutic technique through the left nostril has unique lateral and phase-specific effects.

The OCDB also has dramatic effects on the cardiovascular system. Figures 6, 7, 8, and 10 clearly illustrate large hemodynamic shifts. A doubling in the range of SV and a 40-point range in HR (see Figure 8) regularly occur during the performance of the OCDB. The shift in hemodynamic state for the periods before and after the exercise period clearly show that there is also a latent effect for at least the first 10 minutes following the 31 minutes of exercise. We are currently studying the differential effects of various breathing patterns at one breath per minute for 31 minutes and find that altering the patterns of the breath cycle affects the hemodynamic state both during and after the exercises.

Etiological Issues

Jenike (39) states that "there are currently more than 20 different ideas of what might be the cause of OCD, and the only statement we can make with certainty is that we still have no idea of the cause of this mysterious but treatable disorder." However, "a growing consensus favors a multilayered biological basis for this complex and intriguing disorder" (40). A psychogenic or traumatic experience is one of the earliest and longest-prevailing theories of causation (40). Nearly all the subjects from these two studies (identified in seven of eight in study 1 and in 22 of 25 in study 2) have had reasons for developing substantial insecurities and fears based on incidence of trauma. Sometimes the trauma is single and acute, but more frequently it is prolonged. The concordance of OCD and traumatic experience with these subjects is unquestionably very high. While these subjects may not represent the typical OCD patient presenting, perhaps because the vast majority have already attempted other forms of therapy without significant success, the role of trauma and other significant developmental incidences may play an etiological role here.

Compliance with Therapy

The critical element in treatments employing yogic meditation techniques is compliance. Attendance at weekly meetings has been a clear indication of commitment and compliance with daily homework therapy. While it is not strictly a one-to-one relationship, the results from both studies reinforce this idea. Of course, this is not a surprising relationship. Compliance with meditation techniques is ultimately the only real test of the therapy. We have not analyzed the data to assess whether results are related to OCD subtypes, nor have subjects been treated differently. The cross-section of subjects has not been compared with similar geographic populations.

If the KY therapy was employed on an inpatient basis and the subjects guided through the protocol two or three times per day, the success rate would very likely be higher. However, the cost-effectiveness of a 40–90-day program may be considered prohibitive in the new arena of managed care. As employed, this group approach to treatment, independent of symptomatologies, is highly cost-effective and it appears that 1 year is a suitable course of therapy if the subjects attend regularly.

The key to the KY therapy is the immediate results that can be obtained from one treatment. The bold experience of the therapy is enough to convince subjects that they are at least able to achieve acute relief when guided through the therapy by a trained practitioner. This experience keeps them coming back, and eventually they begin to employ the protocol, or portions of it, on their own. They also begin to recognize the changes in other subjects over time and how they have responded to treatment. The positive experience of the KY protocol is something that all patients enjoy. Employing it on their own is more of a challenge.

Requirements and Role of the Therapist

The most important role of the therapist is primarily that of a coach. While the therapist must clearly understand the nature of the disorder, the job of inspiring and guiding the subjects with the techniques is of paramount importance. Negative thoughts, doubts about the therapy or oneself, anger, fear, and all the negative emotions that are the baggage of the subject must be dealt with, but primarily through employment of the techniques. The subjects must learn through experience that the techniques can provide immediate and ultimately lasting results. Therefore, the personality of the therapist is important to the outcome. Confidence and conviction must be communicated to the subject. Personal experience with the techniques is the best source of this conviction. Time-tested personal experience with the techniques is probably more important than the usual talents of a compassionate and understanding therapist who has not had the experience. Subjects need to see the techniques employed. I have practiced the techniques along with the subjects during these studies. Subjects prefer to see that the therapist is also doing what they are instructed to do, because of the degree of difficulty. The only caveat is that the therapist must ensure that the subjects are doing the techniques correctly. Therefore, a training/learning phase with the therapy must come first.

The therapist (L. Ray) for the RRMM group had 12 years of daily experience using the RR and MM techniques. She also employed them in her private practice. She had confidence in their general clinical efficacy and was very able to inspire the subjects in group 2 to employ them. I have had 20 years of personal daily experience with KY techniques and have been teaching them for as long. Prior to study 1 I had no clinical experience with OCD patients.

Issues of Age, Sex, Medication, and Group Size

The subjects of study 1 were more homogeneous in age, and therefore suitability based on age was not a parameter that could be tested. However, subject 7 (female age 55) was the oldest subject, and she was the first to begin (at 3 months) to employ the OCDB for 31 minutes per day on a regular basis. However, this was not at one breath per minute.

Study 2 included two adolescents. One dropped out after 8 weeks and the other after 1 week. (They were not in the group at the same time.) While this small number is not conclusive, it may be that the structure of the therapeutic setting could be improved, especially by including a significant number of peers or running a group specifically for younger subjects. The commitment of a child or adolescent is clearly different from that of an adult who has lived with the disorder for years. If a child wants to overcome the disorder, his youth and vitality could be advantages. These elements require further study. Additionally, other KY techniques may also be more suited to children for the beginning stages of therapy. However, subject 24 (female age 14) began to make significant strides during the therapy session as the only adolescent at that time in the group. Unfortunately, her parents allowed her to quit, in the belief that she was mature enough to make this decision for herself. Interaction with the other family members, especially the parents in the case of adolescents, is vital to the subjects' compliance and ultimate success. A supportive relationship, or at least one of noninterference, is important.

Study 2 had nine of 23 adult subjects (3, 5, 7, 13, 16, 19–21, and 23) withdraw voluntarily. Their respective ages were 25, 22, 24, 67, 30, 28, 57, 26, and 30. Therefore, age appears to play a role in who is likely to remain. However, subjects 11 and 22 (ages 60 and 62) have been very successful in the study, indicating that older age is not necessarily a handicap. The mean age of the younger subjects to drop out is 26.4, clearly lower than the group mean of 39. Maturity appears to be an important element, not surprisingly, with compliance. It may also be that if this protocol becomes officially recognized as a successful therapy compliance will be less problematic for younger people. Potentially, they have fewer physical handicaps to limit them in practice.

The role of gender here is difficult to clearly assess. However, all the subjects in both studies who have achieved a 0 score for Y-BOCS obsessions or compulsions have been female. The final results may help clarify this question.

The question about medication is not clear. In study 1, the three subjects to drop out were unmedicated, but their reasons included pregnancy, work-schedule conflicts, and fibromyalgia. In study 2, six of the nine adults to drop out were medicated. Of the medicated adult subjects, three withdrew because of doubts in the therapy (subject 20 never entered the KY therapy). Larger numbers are required to determine whether medicated patients are more likely to withdraw from or succeed in therapy. In study 1, three of three subjects to achieve 0 for either Y-BOCS score were initially medicated; in study 2, to date, three of the four subjects were not.

The ideal group size is also not clear. Too few would likely make most subjects in an experimental study feel insecure. They are also aware that the group outcome, which is based in part on their compliance, can affect the opportunity for others. On the other hand, too many subjects may make it seem too impersonal and lessen personal contact with the therapist. However, when these techniques are practiced among experienced individuals in groups, the "group energy" is directly proportional to size. Subjects tend to ask questions that others also have. Time for anecdotal feedback is a great source of inspiration to others; from this perspective, therefore, a large group is beneficial. It is not inconceivable to run a therapy group with 30–50 subjects, or even more. However, a study would obviously be more difficult. Subjects differ in the amount of personal interaction that they want with the therapist. They must know that they can have the opportunity for one-to-one conversation.

Other Alternative Modalities and Other KY Techniques

I am unaware of any other official or unofficial studies in which monitoring of patients' progress is conducted using alternative techniques such as biofeedback, meditation techniques, acupuncture, and relaxation therapies.

While this protocol appears to be successful, there are many other KY meditation techniques that could be substituted to complement the OCDB (see Appendix, technique h). However, it is not clear if other techniques would necessarily be more effective. The fear technique (g) is very helpful and does not have a counterpart that is as simple, short, and easy to perform. The victory (i) and anger (k) techniques are also without equivalent counterparts in KY. Technique f, for mental tension, requires 1 minute to perform once it is learned; this isometric-like technique is very powerful when applied correctly, making it especially useful when subjects are not able to practice the routine at length. Technique e, for reducing emotional stress, is particularly helpful since it involves long breath-retention phases. This is excellent training for the OCDB. However, many other KY techniques for treating nervous disorders, breaking habits, and altering mental patterns also deserve study.

Potential Therapeutic Value for Other Anxiety Disorders and Impulse-Control Disorders

This protocol could easily be implemented in the treatment of other anxiety-related disorders. The OCDB could be eliminated for the purpose of simplifying the rigor of the protocol. However, it could also be beneficial. But, because of its level of difficulty, other techniques are more likely to facilitate compliance and success. The primary techniques (a–g) may constitute an effective protocol for treating generalized anxiety, phobic, or panic disorders. Techniques i, j, and k would be useful supplements.

The use of these techniques may be helpful in the treatment of other impulse-control disorders—the classic addictive disorders or other behavioral disorders. The results of these two OCD studies suggest that such trials are warranted.

ACKNOWLEDGMENTS

This work was supported in part by the National Institutes of Health, the Office of Alternative Medicine, grant 1 R21 RR09677-01, the Waletzky Charitable Lead Trust, and Mr. John DeBeer. We thank Paul Shragg for biostatistical assistance supported in part by a grant from the General Clinical Research Centers Program, M01 RR00827, N.I.H. We also thank Patti Quint, Lacey Kurelowech, and Joslene Foley for technical assistance with the MEG studies at The Scripps Research Institute.

APPENDIX: MEDITATION TECHNIQUES

Techniques for Study 1 and Study 2–Group 1 (the Kundalini Yoga Protocol)

This protocol includes eight primary techniques (a–h) to be used on a daily basis and three additional techniques (i–k) to be used at personal discretion.

a. To Induce a Meditative State, "Tuning In"

Description of technique: Sit with a straight spine and with the feet flat on the floor if sitting in a chair. Put the hands together at the chest in "prayer pose"—the palms are pressed together with 10–15 pounds of pressure between the hands. The area where the sides of the thumbs touch rests on the sternum with the thumbs pointing up (along the sternum), and the fingers are together and point up and out at a 60-degree angle to the ground. The eyes are closed and focused at the "third eye" (imagine a sun rising on the horizon). A mantra is chanted out loud in a 1 1/2-breath cycle. Inhale first through the nose and chant "Ong Namo" with an equal emphasis on the Ong and the Namo. Immediately follow with a half-breath inhalation through the mouth and chant "Guru Dev Namo" with approximately equal emphasis on each word. The practitioner should experience the vibrations that these sounds create on the upper palate and throughout the cranium while letting the mind be carried by the sounds. This should be repeated at least three times; it was employed here in therapy about 10–12 times. This technique helps to create a "meditative state of mind" and is highly recommended as a precursor to the other techniques.

b. Spine Flexing for Vitality (37)

Description of technique: This technique can be practiced while sitting either in a chair or cross-legged on the floor. If you are in a chair, hold the knees with both hands for support and leverage. If you are sitting cross-legged, grasp the ankles in front with both hands. Begin by pulling the chest up and forward, inhaling deeply at the same time. Then exhale as you relax the spine down into a slouching position. Keep the head up straight without allowing it to move much with the flexing action of the spine. This will help prevent a whip action of the cervical vertebrae. Breathe only through the nose for both the inhale and the exhale. Close your eyes and imagine you are looking at a central point on the horizon, the "third eye." Mental focus is kept on the sound of the breath while listening to the fluid movement of the inhalation and exhalation. Begin the technique slowly while loosening up the spine. Eventually, a very rapid movement can be achieved with practice, reaching a rate of 1–2 times per second for the entire movement. A few minutes are sufficient in the beginning. Later, there is no time limit. Eating should be avoided just prior to this exercise. If a feeling of light-headedness develops, it could be an indication of hypocapnia and the technique should be stopped momentarily. Be careful and flex the spine slowly in the beginning. Relax for 1–2 minutes when finished.

c. Shoulder Shrugs for Vitality (37)

Description of technique: While keeping the spine straight, rest the hands on the knees if sitting in a cross-legged position or with hands on the thighs if on a chair. Inhale and raise the shoulders toward the ears; then exhale, letting them down. All breathing is only through the nose. Eyes should be kept closed and focused at the third eye. Mentally listen to the sound of the inhalation and exhalation. Continue this action rapidly, building to three times per second for a maximum of 2 minutes. This technique should not be practiced by individuals who are hyperactive.

d. Technique for Reducing Anxiety, Stress, and Mental Tension

Description of technique (14): Sit and maintain a straight spine. Relax the arms and the hands in the lap. Focus the eyes toward the tip of the nose. (You cannot see the end, just the sides of the nose, because they appear blurred while you try to focus on the tip.) Open the mouth as wide as possible, slightly stressing the temporomandibular joint; touch the tongue tip to the upper palate where it is hard and smooth in the center. Breathe continuously through the nose only, making the respiration slow and deep. Let the mental focus be on the sound of the breath; listen to the sound of the inhale and exhale. Maintain this pattern for at least 3–5 minutes or for a maximum of 8 minutes on the first trial. With practice it can be built up to 31 minutes maximum. This technique was originally taught as a meditation for insanity, and to curb a restless mind and bring stillness and mental quiet.

e. Technique for Reducing Anxiety, Stress, and Mental Tension

Description of technique: Sit and maintain a straight spine. The hands are in front of the chest at heart level. The left hand is 2 inches from the chest and the right is about 2 inches beyond the left (4 inches from the chest). The fingers on the left hand point to the right; the right palm faces the back of the left hand with fingers pointing to the left. The thumbs of both hands point straight up. The eyes are open and focused on the tip of the nose. Breathing is through the nose only. Inhale, keep the breath in as long as possible; then exhale and keep the breath out as long as possible, without causing undue discomfort at any stage. When finished, inhale—maintaining the eye and hand posture—and then tense every muscle in the body for about 10 seconds; exhale and repeat two times. Build the capacity for this technique to a maximum time of 15 minutes. Avoid this exercise if you have high blood pressure or are pregnant.

f. Technique for Reducing Anxiety, Stress, and Mental Tension

Description of technique: Sit as above. Eyes are open and focused on the tip of the nose during the entire exercise. Attempt to pull the nose down toward the upper lip by actually pulling the upper lip down over the upper front teeth using the muscles of the upper lip. The mouth is left open during this exercise with constant tension on the upper lip. There are three steps to this exercise. Step 1: start with the hands and arms up 45–60 degrees from the side of the body, inhale deeply, and tightly clench the fists and pull them down toward the abdomen. Step 2: Keeping the breath in, eyes focused, and lip pulled, and maintaining tension in the fists, bring the shoulders up toward the ears, tensing the shoulders while raising them. Step 3: exhale and relax (but keep the lip pulled down and the eyes focused on the tip of the nose). Repeat the entire exercise six times. Avoid this exercise if you have high blood pressure or are pregnant. It has been claimed that this short exercise is so effective that if done correctly it can relax even the tensest person.

g. Technique for Managing Fears

Description of technique: Sit with a straight spine. Close the eyes. With the four fingertips and thumb of the left hand grouped, press very lightly into the navel point. Place the right hand with the four fingers pointing left over the third eye point (on the forehead just above the root of the nose) as if feeling your temperature. Play the tape of Chattra Chakra Varti (Golden Temple Enterprises, Espanola, New Mexico) for 3 minutes while assessing your fears and consciously relating to the mental experience of your fears. This technique is claimed to help manage acute states of fear or help eliminate fearful images and negative emotions that have developed due to fearful experiences. The effect is that the negative emotions related to specific fears are replaced with positive emotions, thereby slowly creating a new and different mental association with the stimulus.

h. Technique for Obsessive Compulsive Disorders (OCDB)(14)

Description of technique: Sit with a straight spine in a comfortable position, either with the legs crossed while sitting on the floor or in a straight-backed chair with both feet flat on the floor. Close the eyes. Use the tip of the right thumb to block the right nostril, with the other fingers pointing straight up; allow the arm to relax (the elbow should not be sticking up and out to the side, creating unnecessary tension). A secure plug can also be used for the right nostril. Inhale very slowly and deeply through the left nostril, hold in long; exhale out slowly and completely through the same (left) nostril only, hold out long. The mental focus should be on the sound of the breath. Continue this pattern with a maximum time of 31 minutes for each sitting. Begin with a comfortable rate and time, but the effort should be enough to present a fair challenge for each phase of the breath. The length of time for holding the breath in or out varies from person to person. The ideal time per complete breath cycle is 1 minute, with each section of the cycle lasting exactly 15 seconds. This rate of respiration can be achieved within 5–6 months for the full 31 minutes with daily discipline. It has been claimed that 90 days of 31 minutes per day using the perfected rate of one breath per minute with 15 seconds per phase will completely eliminate all OCDs (Yogi Bhajan, personal communication).

i.   Meeting Challenges: the "Victory Breath"

Description of technique: This technique can be used at any time. It does not require that the practitioner be sitting, and it can be employed while driving a car,
during a conversation, while taking a test, etc. The eyes can be open or closed,
depending on the situation. Take a deep breath through the nose and hold this
breath over 3–4 seconds. During the hold phase only, mentally hear the three
sounds "vic" "to," and "ry," then exhale. Mentally creating the three sounds
should take 3–4 seconds, not longer and not less. The entire time of each repetition should be about 10 seconds. It can be employed multiple times until the
patient achieves the desired relief. When employed in the therapy sessions, it
was usually done for 3 minutes with the eyes closed and while sitting with a
straight spine to maximize the effects. This technique is very helpful as a
"thought-stopping" technique for a patient "on the go." There is no time limit
to its practice. Hypertensive patients should be careful not to hold the breath
too deeply, creating pressure with the abdominal muscles. The technique can be
used to help resist obsessive thoughts and performing compulsive rituals.

j.   Chant to Turn Negative Thoughts into Positive Thoughts

Description of technique: Sit with a straight spine and the eyes closed in a peaceful
environment. The mantra "Ek Ong Kar Sat Gurprasad Sat Gurprasad Ek Ong
Kar," repeated a minimum of five times, can be practiced for up to 5 minutes
while chanting it rapidly with up to five repetitions per breath. Eventually one
no longer thinks about the order of the sounds; they come automatically. The
mental focus should be on the vibration created against the upper palate and
throughout the cranium. If performed correctly, a very peaceful and "healed"
state of mind is achieved.

k.   Technique for Anger (37)

Description of technique: Sit with a straight spine and close the eyes. Simply chant
out loud "Jeeo, Jeeo, Jeeo, Jeeo" continuously and rapidly for 11 minutes without stopping (pronounced like the letters *G* and *O*). During continuous chanting
do not stop to take long breaths, but continue with just enough short breaths to
keep the sound going. Eleven minutes is all that is needed.

Techniques for Study 2–Group 2 (the RR and MM Techniques—the RRMM Protocol)

The details for the RR (38) and MM techniques (13) have been previously published. The practice time in group therapy, and recommended at home, was 30
minutes for each technique to compare with the techniques for group 1.

REFERENCES

1. White K, Cole J. Pharmacotherapy. In: Bellack AS, Hersen M, eds. Handbook of Comparative Treatments. New York: John Wiley & Sons, 1990:266–284.
2. Pato MT, Zohar-Kadouch R, Zohar J, et al. Return of symptoms after discontinuation of clomipramine in patients with obsessive-compulsive disorder. Am J Psychiatry 1988; 145:1521–1525.
3. Leonard HL, Swedo SE, Lenane MC, et al. A double-blind substitution during long-term clomipramine treatment in children and adolescents. Arch Gen Psychiatry 1991; 48:922–927.
4. Fontaine R, Chouinard G. Fluoxetine in the long-term treatment of obsessive compulsive disorder. Psychiatric Ann 1989; 19:88–91.
5. O'Sullivan G, Noshirvani H, Marks I, et al. Six-year follow-up after exposure and clomipramine therapy for obsessive compulsive disorder. J Clin Psychiatry 1991; 52:150–155.
6. Marks IM. Review of behavioral psychotherapy: obsessive-compulsive disorders. Am J Psychiatry 1981; 138:584–592.
7. Baer L. Getting Control: Overcoming Your Obsessions and Compulsions. Boston: Little, Brown, 1991:36.
8. Cottraux J. Behavioural psychotherapy for obsessive-compulsive disorder. Int Rev Psychiatry 1989; 1:227–234.
9. Dillbeck MC. Meditation and flexibility of visual perception and verbal problem solving. Memory Cogn 1982; 10:207–215.
10. Orme-Johnson DW. Transcendental meditation and reduced health care. Psychosoma Med 1987; 49:493–507.
11. Benson H. The Relaxation Response. New York: Morrow, 1975.
12. Kabat-Zinn J. An outpatient program in behavioral medicine for chronic pain patients based on the practice of mindfulness meditation: theoretical considerations and preliminary results. Gen Hosp Psychiatry 1982; 4:37–47.
13. Kabat-Zinn, J. Full Catastrophe Living: Using the Wisdom of Your Body and Mind to Face Stress, Pain, and Illness. New York: Delacorte Press, 1990.
14. Shannahoff-Khalsa DS. Stress technology medicine: a new paradigm for stress and considerations for self-regulation. In: Brown MR, Koob G, Rivier C, eds. Stress: Neurobiology and Neuroendocrinology. New York: Marcel Dekker, 1991:647–686.
15. Sprenger J, Kramer H. Malleus Maleficarum. London: Rotker, 1928.
16. Werntz DA, Bickford RG, Shannahoff-Khalsa DS. Selective hemispheric stimulation by unilateral forced nostril breathing. Hum Neurobiol 1987; 6:165–171.
17. Shannahoff-Khalsa DS, Boyle MR, Buebel M. The effects of unilateral forced nostril breathing on cognition. Int J Neurosci 1991; 57:239–249.
18. Jella SA, Shannahoff-Khalsa DS. The effects of unilateral forced nostril breathing on cognitive performance. Int J Neurosci 1993; 73:61–68.

19. Schiff BB, Rump SA. Asymmetrical hemispheric activation and emotion: the effects of unilateral forced nostril breathing. Brain Cogn 1995; 29:217–231.

20. Shannahoff-Khalsa DS, Kennedy B. The effects of unilateral forced nostril breathing on the heart. Int J Neurosci 1993; 73:47–60.

21. Backon J. Changes in blood glucose levels induced by differential forced unilateral nostril breathing, a technique which affects both brain hemisphericity and autonomic activity. Med Sci Res 1988; 16:1197–1199.

22. Backon J, Kullock S. Effect of forced unilateral nostril breathing on blink rates: relevance to hemispheric lateralization of dopamine. Int J Neurosci 1989; 46:53–59.

23. Backon J, Matamoros N, Ticho U. Changes in intraocular pressure induced by differential forced nostril breathing, a technique that affects both brain hemisphericity and autonomic activity. Graefe's Arch Clin Exp Ophthalmol 1989; 227:575–577.

24. Telles S, Nagarathna R, Nagendra HR. Breathing through a particular nostril can alter metabolism and autonomic activities. Indian J Physiol Pharmacol 1994; 38:133–137.

25. Werntz DA, Bickford RG, Bloom FE, Shannahoff-Khalsa DS. Alternating cerebral hemispheric activity and lateralization of autonomic nervous function. Hum Neurobiol 1983; 2:39–43.

26. Shannahoff-Khalsa DS. The ultradian rhythm of alternating cerebral hemispheric activity. Int J Neurosci 1993; 70:285–298.

27. Shannahoff-Khalsa DS. Lateralized rhythms of the central and autonomic nervous systems. Int J Psychophysiol 1991; 11:225–251.

28. Keuning J. On the nasal cycle. J Int Rhinol 1968; 6:99–136.

29. Hasegawa M, Kern EB. The human nasal cycle. Mayo Clin Proc 1977; 52:28–34.

30. Hall DP, Sing HC, Romanoski AJ. Identification and characterization of greater mood variance in depression. Am J Psychiatry 1991; 148:1341–1345.

31. Shannahoff-Khalsa DS, Beckett LR. Clinical case reports: efficacy of yogic techniques in the treatment of obsessive compulsive disorders. Int J Neurosci 1996; 85:1–17.

32. Goodman WK, Price LH, Rasmussen SA, Mazure C, Fleishmann RL, Hill CL, Heninger GR, Charney DS. The Yale-Brown Obsessive Compulsive Scale. Revised ed. Sept 1989. Part 1. Development, use and reliability. Arch Gen Psychiatry 1989; 46:1006–1011.

33. Derogatis LR. Symptom Checklist-90–Revised. Minneapolis: National Computer Systems, 1993.

34. Cohen S, Kamarck T, Mermelstein R. A global measure of perceived stress: Perceived Stress Scale. J Health Hum Behav 1983; 24:386–396.

35. Profile of Moods Scale. San Diego: Educational and Industrial Testing Service, 1971.

36. Crumbaugh JC, Maholick LT. Purpose in Life Test. Test 168, Form A. Murfreesboro, TN: Psychometric Affiliates, 1976.

37. Shannahoff-Khalsa DS, Bhajan Y. The healing power of sound: techniques from yogic medicine. In: Droh R, Spintge R, eds. Music Medicine. St. Louis: MMB Music, 1991:179–193.
38. Benson H. The Relaxation Response. New York: Avon Books, 1975:27.
39. Jenike MA. Theories of etiology. In: Jenike MJ, Baer L, Minichiello WE, eds. Obsessive-Compulsive Disorders: Theory and Management. St. Louis: Year Book Medical Publishers, 1990:99.
40. Alarcon RD, Libb JW, Boll TJ. Neuropsychological testing in obsessive-compulsive disorder: a clinical review. J Neuropsychiatry Clin Neurosci 1994; 6:217–228.
41. Bhajan Y. The rhythm of the breath. In: Healing: Ten Lectures. Pomona, CA: Kundalini Research Institute Publications, 1976.
42. Gallen CC, Sobel DF, Waltz T, Aung M, Copeland B, Schwartz BJ, Hirschkoff EC, Bloom FE. Noninvasive presurgical neuromagnetic mapping of somatosensory cortex. Neurosurgery 1993; 33:260–268.
43. Gallen CC, Schwartz B, Rieke K, Pantev C, Sobel D, Hirschkoff E, Bloom FE. Intrasubject reliability and validity of somatosensory source localization using a large array biomagnetometer. Electroencephal Clin Neurophysiol 1994; 90:145–156.

13

Group and Multifamily Behavioral Treatments for OCD

Barbara Van Noppen
Butler Hospital
and Brown University
Providence, Rhode Island

Gail Steketee
Boston University School of Social Work
Boston, Massachusetts

Michele Pato
State University of New York at Buffalo
Buffalo, New York

INTRODUCTION

The psychosocial treatment for obsessive-compulsive disorder (OCD) that has become considered the "gold standard" is behavioral therapy that includes exposure for obsessions and prevention of rituals or response prevention. The treatment has been conducted mainly in an individual format. Exposure and response prevention (ERP) is based on early findings that obsessions increase anxiety and compulsions reduce it, observations that have now been incorporated into the diagnostic criteria for OCD. It is widely accepted that obsessions "cause marked anxiety or distress" and compulsions are "aimed at preventing or reducing distress" provoked by obsessions (1). Not surprisingly, behavioral therapy based on this model has proven very effective for those patients who receive adequate treatment, which includes procedures to reduce anxiety associated with obsessions, as well as to prevent or curtail ritual-istic behavior.

In spite of this progress, 25% of the patients who initially present to our clinic refuse behavioral therapy and another 15–20% do not wish to take medication. An additional group of approximately 20% of pa-tients are willing to engage in pharmacotherapy or behavioral therapy but are "nonresponders." Although ERP can moderately to significantly improve the symptoms of the remaining 80%, a large group of patients are still left with chronic symptoms that interfere with their daily activi-ties and family functioning. Our clinical experience suggests that the family support system ("family" refers to all significant others), particu-larly family responses to obsessive-compulsive symptoms, may play a critical role in the prognosis and outcome of treatment. This may be relevant for those patients who fail to respond to standard individual behavioral treatment and pharmacological interventions and have sig-nificant others who are overly involved in or critical of the obsessive-compulsive symptoms. Treatment in a group context, with or without family members, may offer therapeutic benefits for living with family members or those not engaged in supportive interpersonal relationships.

The role of psychosocial factors in the pathogenesis and treatment of OCD has been overshadowed by advances in our understanding of the neurobiology of the disorder, as well as by newly developed phar-macological and behavioral treatment strategies. In addition, as the costs of health care spiral upward, there is a call to clinical researchers to explore alternative methods of applying ERP. We have developed two types of behavioral treatments modeled after individual behavioral treat-ment (IBT), both time-limited and using a group modality. Group be-havioral treatment (GBT) is for patients only and multifamily behavioral treatment (MFBT) includes patients and their significant others. Prelimi-nary findings reveal comparable efficacy after 12 weeks of treatment for both group treatments relative to standard individual behavioral ther-apy. Furthermore, reductions in OC symptoms for the patients who completed GBT and MFBT have been maintained at 1-year follow-up.

In this chapter we briefly review the group and family literature in OCD and present descriptions of both our group and multifamily behav-ioral treatments through case examples.

GROUP BEHAVIORAL TREATMENT

Group behavioral treatments have proven effective for several other anxiety-disordered patient populations, and a handful of studies have investigated group treatments for OCD. In this era of growing concern with health care expenditures, the use of a group treatment modality holds considerable interest because of its potential for reducing costs without sacrificing benefits. In addition, the group context offers additional benefits for OCD patients who report prominent feelings of social isolation. A supportive treatment group may provide a motivational boost for those sufferers who feel they can't carry out the homework without the accountability of the group and compassion of other OCD patients. In his landmark writings on interpersonal group therapy, Yalom (2) identified "curative factors" common in groups. Some of these are clearly present and powerful forces in behavioral treatment groups for OCD patients: instillation of hope, imitative behavior, imparting of information, universality, development of socializing techniques, group cohesiveness, catharsis, altruism. In addition, Budman (3) recognized the pragmatic, economic, and motivation-enhancing reasons to develop more time-limited models in group therapy.

In one of the early uncontrolled studies on GBT in OCD, Hand and Tichatzky (4) treated 17 OCD patients in three groups, targeting OC symptoms, social interaction problems, and problem-solving ability. The format of the group was based on a minimum of 25 sessions, held twice weekly, which included in vivo exercises, homework assignments, attention to communication skills, and separate support group meetings for spouses. As therapist involvement was gradually withdrawn, therapy eventually continued in an entirely self-help model. The treatment was fairly labor-intensive, and the decrease observed in OCD symptoms and anxiety was variable across groups of patients. Two reports, also uncontrolled on smaller samples, described a similar but shorter group treatment (five or six patients per group) with 10 to 14 sessions of education, goal-setting, behavioral skills training, exposure, response prevention, homework logs, and, in one case, cognitive restructuring (5,6). Both of these studies reported benefits at the end of treatment and at follow-up, and the results were comparable to those reported for individual behavioral treatment studies.

There are reports of four larger uncontrolled trials using GBT in an OCD population. In a program similar to that described above, with the addition of assertiveness-training, Enright (7) used nine weekly 90-minute sessions to structure the group. There were some statistically significant findings of decreases in OCD symptoms, depressed and anxious mood, and improvement in functioning posttest and at 6-month follow-up. However, only 17% made clinically significant improvement. This study did not focus on ERP during sessions as much as the other group clinical trials did. In a second uncontrolled study, Krone et al. (8) treated 36 OCD patients with a short 7-week group program that included education, instruction in cognitive and behavioral self-treatment, and therapist-directed ERP. As in the Enright (7) study, significant improvement was evident in reductions of Yale-Brown Obsessive Compulsive Scale (Y-BOCS) scores from moderately severe before therapy to below clinical levels at 3-month follow-up. Depression also decreased, particularly in medicated patients, and improvement was independent of medication use. Van Noppen et al. (9) provided GBT to 73 OCD outpatients that included eight to 10 sessions of in-group ERP, cognitive exercises, and homework assignments with self-monitoring. This produced average reductions in Y-BOCS scores of 5–6 points at a follow-up of at least 6 months. In a more recent trial by our group using an identical but longer intervention of 10 to 12 group sessions, Y-BOCS scores improved an average of 9 points at 1-year follow-up, with 43% of patients showing clinically significant improvement (10). These OCD patients who received group behavioral treatment also showed substantial improvement in general functioning capacity (work, social, family). A clinical example of GBT procedures from Van Noppen and colleagues' latter project is described below.

The only controlled trial for OCD was conducted by Fals-Stewart et al. (11). They compared group imagined and/or in vivo ERP ($N = 30$) to individual behavioral treatment ($N = 31$) and to an individual relaxation control treatment ($N = 32$) using 24 twice-weekly sessions. Subjects in both group and individual treatment conditions showed significant improvement in OCD symptoms, depression, and anxiety at posttest and follow-up, whereas the control group changed only on anxiety. Reductions of 10 points in posttest Y-BOCS scores and 8 at follow-up were recorded for the group treatment subjects. Although these score changes are substantial, the generalizability of these findings are limited by the exclusion of patients with major depression and axis II diagnoses.

Thus, it is apparent from the above case series and controlled trial that behavioral treatment can readily be applied using a group modality, with results that are generally equivalent to those of individual treatment. This is particularly true when the number of sessions is comparable to that usually provided to individual patients in other controlled research studies (12–20 sessions). GBT for OCD is clearly a cost-effective and efficacious alternative to standard individual treatment. This mode of therapy may be particularly suited clinical settings where there are few trained therapists and a sufficient patient flow to permit running of groups for patients with OCD.

Clinical Example

Eight OCD patients were referred for GBT. They were initially screened by an experienced clinician, then evaluated by the group therapist to ensure appropriateness for group treatment. Following this, each patient met with the therapist in two 90-minute information-gathering sessions prior to starting the group. During those meetings, the therapist collected general information, history of OCD, other symptoms, and mental health treatment, along with general history about family and social relationships. The detailed information about the OCD symptoms was used to generate a hierarchy that each patient brought to the first group session. The goals of the GBT were outlined, OCD and behavior therapy were defined, and family members were invited to accompany the patient to the first half of the second information-gathering session, although they were not involved in the treatment. The behavioral treatment group ran for 12 consecutive weeks, with each session lasting 2 hours. The first sessions consisted of introductions and psychoeducation about phenomenology, etiology, and behavioral and cognitive techniques. Simultaneously, in-group ERP was demonstrated and practiced, and group modeling took place. Patients were required to select homework assignments and record daily distress levels between group sessions. After completing the active treatment, the group continued to meet for six monthly sessions for the purpose of consolidating treatment gains and discussing relapse prevention. No active therapy occurred during the 6-month follow-up period.

GBT Session 1

The therapist welcomed the patients, asked them to introduce themselves, and then outlined the agenda for all 12 sessions, reviewing dates and times. The therapist discussed confidentiality, coverage between groups and a crisis plan, and the importance of consistent attendance. "What do you hope to get out of this group? What do you expect to gain from this group?" were questions posed by the therapist to the group members. A handout entitled "Obsessive Compulsive Disorder: What Is OCD?" was distributed, and each patient took turns reading aloud from this psychoeducational handout. The booklet covered the definition of OCD; its phenomenology, course, and comorbidity; and OCPD; and provided an overview of treatments, introducing the concepts of exposure and response prevention. Likewise, each patient was given the self-rated version of the Y-BOCS Symptom Checklist to review, with members volunteering to read. Allowing patients to draw from their experience of OCD to provide examples for each symptom type promoted disclosure. Jan, a single 34-year-old computer programmer, spoke about her extensive repeating rituals to prevent "bad things from happening." Relieved to hear this, Dan, a married 52 year-old-salesman, told the group about his fear of the number 4 and how he "couldn't say that number" in the same sentence as one of his kid's names because they might get hurt and it would be his fault. "Oh, everything's always my fault!" chuckled Jan. The group laughed along with her at this common trait, underscoring a general theme of excessive responsibility. Chuck, a married 40-year-old attorney, talked about his "need to have everything in order," while Anne, a single 20-year-old college student, said her life was full of clutter that she couldn't get rid of. Mark, another college student, returning to school after a leave of absence, told the group about his "superstitions" and rituals to ward off "bad luck."

Sue, a 38-year-old homemaker, reported that ever since she had her son, she had "terrible thoughts" about him that made her feel like an awful person. Cheryl, a married 27-year-old nurse, identified with Sue, saying that she stopped cooking because she was afraid of poisoning her kids: "What good mother thinks that?!" Peter, a divorced, 60-year-old retired fireman, told the group that he had been "struggling" with OCD for "as long as I can remember," and that the one thing he has learned is that "OCD is not a personal or moral issue, that no one wants to have these thoughts, and they are not a reflection of the kind of person you are." Peter shared his belief that his wife left him after 20 years of marriage because of his contamination obsessions, washing rituals, avoidance, and "stubbornness," and said he realized that he could make his life better. Others felt inspired by Peter, and his story generated much discussion about the effect of OCD on people's lives. The group "curative factors" as described by Yalom (2) were evident in this first group session. The group process appeared effective in decreasing feelings of isolation, stigma, and shame while universalizing problems, instilling feelings of hope, and utilizing imitative behavior to promote change.

During the disclosure of symptoms, the therapist sensed a growing atmosphere of group cohesion and trust. This paved the way for the use of ERP and modeling in the group. In addition, the heterogeneity of symptoms seemed to promote insight into OCD by facilitating greater participation in the in vivo exersises that led to group consensus on normative behavior and beliefs. For example, it would be difficult to get a group of eight patients with contamination fears to agree that people should be able to touch the flusher of a toilet and resist washing their hands without feeling significantly anxious. Patients had learned to appreciate the various forms of symptoms that allowed them to depersonalize the obsessive content.

After disclosing their situation, patients were asked to select an item in the 35–45 discomfort range from their personal hierarchy for ERP homework. Homework forms were distributed and explained. The therapist instructed the group members to record their distress levels through the week, while practicing their homework task. Everyone was reminded of the time-limited nature of the group and that there was a lot to cover in a relatively short period of time.

GBT Session 2

At the second session, patients reported on their homework, receiving praise for the accomplishments and problem-solving feedback when they experienced difficulties achieving habituation. The group input was intended to expand behavioral alternatives and offer consensual validation on normative beliefs and behaviors. Mark said it was helpful to talk with other OCD patients and "hear that no one else gets upset when they hear the words I do. Yet Dan has trouble with the number 4 which doesn't bother me . . . so that tells me it is just my OCD. Although other people tell me the same thing, it is different because I feel that they don't really understand what I'm going through. When I'm here I feel at home because everybody has their weird worries and strange behaviors. We can laugh at ourselves without feeling like freaks that no one else can relate to. We know we aren't alone!" During this psychoeducational phase, the therapist also introduced the concept that although patients "feel" or "think" thay have to perform their rituals, most everyone spoke in absolutes: "I *have* to check," "I *have* to straighten the magazines."

After the therapist gave a detailed 15-minute overview of in vivo and imaginal exposure, examples of these techniques were practiced in the group. Chuck and other members were asked to take out their wallets, shuffle the money and credit cards, report on their distress, put the wallet away, continue to monitor the distress, then repeat the task. The therapist asked how other patients could tailor the challenge to make it an appropriate exposure task for their particular symptoms. Peter said it would help him to pass around his wallet, allowing other group members to "contaminate" it. Jan's task was to open her wallet then close it once, allowing herself to think about "something bad happening" to her sister. Mark's wallet was so full he carried it in his coat pocket because it wouldn't fit in his pants. His in vivo challenge was to take out an item and discard it. Dan carried pictures of his children in his wallet that he took out to look at while he said "4" aloud. All of the patients rehearsed their exposure tasks and rated their discomfort levels. The exercises were repeated until discomfort reduced. This in vivo exposure was very lively, as is typical in GBT.

During this time, some patients displayed tremendous discomfort and seemed to benefit from the other patients' support, feedback, and encouragement to stay in the dreaded situation. Most patients reported that it was invaluable to observe others expose themselves, experience mounting anxiety, and, after repeated and prolonged exposure, watch the discomfort recede. Thus, although therapist modeling has not been shown empirically to improve outcome, patients have reported that participant modeling was beneficial to them. Often for homework, the patients continued their in-group challenges and added items from their hierarchies. The exposure homework practice and discomfort ratings were recorded on the homework forms.

GBT Session 3

Patients began with a check-in and go-round, reporting on homework tasks. A 15-minute videotape that discussed the neurobiology of OCD and medications was viewed in the group, followed by a brief discussion of this material. The remainder of the 2-hour session was devoted to in vivo and imagined exposure. At this session, patients selected items with discomfort ratings between 50 and 60 on their hierarchies. Again, in-group exposure exercises were modified to address individual symptoms. Dan read a creative script about his son and daughter playing baseball wearing uniforms with numbers 4 and 44. The whole scene repeatedly introduced the number 4. Others listened intently as Dan read, watched him experience discomfort and repeat the task until his anxiety decreased. Mark, who had superstitious concerns, threw salt over his shoulder and talked about having "bad luck." Cheryl took out her bottle of medication, opened it, poured juice for all the group members, and spoke about her fears of poisoning everyone: "What if I put medication in the juice and don't remember it?" Other patients started to give her reassurance but were instructed by the therapist not to do so. After this exposure task was repeated a few times, Cheryl reported that she knew she hadn't put anything in the juice, she "just gave in to the anxiety." Sue made a joke about "keeling over from the arsenic in the juice" and Cheryl was able to laugh at the absurdity.

All patients selected homework assignments, receiving feedback from the group to ensure that the tasks chosen were reasonable but challenging. This process was intended to increase individual patients' problem-solving options and promote the use of various behavioral techniques. Imparting information and learning from other patients appeared to be beneficial because patients respected the advice that came from someone "in the same boat" who had had success.

GBT Sessions 4–11

These sessions proceeded in a fashion similar to that outlined in session 3. After a check-in and go-round report from each patient on his or her homework successes and obstacles, the therapist quickly addressed any problems patients encountered in carrying out their homework assignments. For patients who had not experienced any progress, it was often in this phase that dropout occurred. Although the sense of competition observed in GBT was a powerful motivator ("If Cheryl can do that, so can I"), a patient who had selected inappropriate challenges, or who had not utilized exposure for long enough to allow habituation, felt discouraged as others progressed. Other non-ERP obstacles may also hamper treatment. To prevent dropout, which can discourage other group members, the therapist looked for signs that a patient was repeatedly unsuccessful in employing ERP and used in vivo group exercises to provide an opportunity for a corrective experience. Often, group cohesion had become so developed that patients took more risks to avoid disappointing other group members.

As each session progressed, patients selected items from their hierarchies that evoked increasing levels of distress. By session 8, the most distressing stimulus was introduced to allow time for habituation. The group experience became more interactive and patients pressed one another to tolerate anxiety. The therapist asked that patients change the way they talk about the OCD to help change the way they thought and felt about it. When group members, in describing a scenario, used the phrase "I have to . . . ," the therapist corrected them, asking them to insert "I feel I have to" or "I think I have to." Over time, group members began to catch each other doing this and took on the role of the therapist, asking each other to correct how they spoke about the OC symptoms. This promoted self-help stategies intended to encourage independent skills after the formal treatment ended. Often a positive group experience convinced otherwise shy patients to become interested in joining self-help groups for people with OCD. After her experience in the GBT, Sue went on to run for president of her local OC Foundation chapter, spoke at public awareness-raising functions, and served as liaison to the national organization. Many patients have reported that they felt a sense of pride and self-worth when they could help fellow OCD patients. This may be another active ingredient of GBT.

Examples of in vivo and imaginal exposure in the later sessions included the following. When the entire group went for a walk throughout the hospital and on the grounds, Mark stepped on sidewalk cracks while saying, "I have bad luck." He was not allowed to go back over the cracks or seek reassurance. Peter touched the doornobs of all the bathrooms they passed, then ate small candies without washing his hands. Mark looked at all the literature and magazines in the various waiting rooms and resisted his urge to take things with him. Jan walked through doorways, down stairs, and on changing surfaces (rug to cement to grass) without repeating while talking about her mother getting into a car accident. Several patients performed each exposure task to provide participant modeling.

GBT Session 12

The final session was conducted in the same way as those described above, except the therapist left ample time to address concerns and questions regarding the end of active treatment. Jan expressed her fear that she "wouldn't be able to do it" on her own without the support of the group. Peter reminded her that she had come so far due to her independent use of the behavioral techniques in her homework and that she had become a primary inspiration for others. As a "veteran" of OCD, he went on to thank everyone for giving so much of themselves to make the group so comfortable that he could share the "embarrassment of OCD" that he felt troubled by for so many years. Sue spoke about her new ability to help other people with OCD, since she had learned to help herself. She attributed her "commitment" to improving her life and "the lives of other sufferers" to her experiences in the group and became tearful as she spoke: "I will never forget any of you and how much this group has made a difference in my life . . . no one else really understood my OCD and how it made me feel." Mark remarked that he appreciated everyone's gratitude to the group but he said he worried that they were forgetting that they "needed to get on" with their lives and not become an "OCD cult." He said he felt "kind of relieved" that the 12 weeks were over so he "didn't have to continue to lie" to his classmates about where he was going each week. Thus, the responses to termination were varied. The therapist allowed individual expression of parting but did not let the group stray too far off the track. The task of putting closure on the weekly treatment sessions needed attention to manage the high level of intimacy in the group. The main focus was on fostering self-instruction and self-efficacy. Group members were asked to comment on the enormous changes they had observed in others while identifying the most helpful elements of the group treatment. Six monthly meeting dates were scheduled, and patients were encouraged to call for help troubleshooting between sessions as needed.

FAMILY TREATMENT INTERVENTIONS

Rationale

OCD rarely leaves the family system unaffected. Often unknowingly, the social support system is brought directly into the patient's symptoms. Marital discord, divorce, and separation, alcohol abuse, and poor school performance are common results of the stress that OCD puts on the patient and family members. In addition, guilt, blame, and social stigma affect patients and relatives. It is not unusual for family members to blame themselves for their child's or spouse's illness. Relatives fear that early childhood traumas or child-rearing pratices were causative.

Advice from friends and relatives may further reinforce the family's sense of guilt and shame. They are often told that the patient is "not ill, just going through a phase" or are given suggestions that more discipline or more attention is the solution. The family is uncertain whether the prolonged rituals and constant need for reassurance are really part of an illness or reflect willful rebelliousness and demands for attention and control. OCD patients may try to hide their rituals and their thoughts out of shame. Preoccupied with the needs of the patient and feeling blamed and burdened, family members may pull away from their usual social contacts and become increasingly socially isolated themselves.

Resarch Findings and Relevant Literature

Recent research by Calvocoressi and collegues (12) has demonstrated that OCD symptoms can engender extensive family involvement in patients' OCD symptoms, and that 88% of family members participated in some way in OCD symptoms. Greater family participation in symptoms was significantly correlated with family dysfunction and negative attitudes toward the patient. Other clinical researchers have reported that OCD symptoms have adverse effects on family functioning (13,14). Thus, these difficulties might be involved in the maintenance of OC symptoms, and interventions to address these family factors might be helpful in overall recovery. To date, however, most of the research reported on family treatment for OCD has not directly addressed family involvement in symptoms or family stress and associated costs.

Support groups with psychoeducational foci for patients and family members may provide a useful avenue for families to learn about OCD and decrease feelings of isolation (15–17). In these psychoeducational groups, the goals usually include improving self-esteem, sharing feelings and experiences, accepting patients' realistic limitations, and learning strategies for coping with OCD symptoms. Overall, good satisfaction has been reported by the participants of psychoeducational groups for OCD, but no outcome data are available regarding group effects on family variables or patient symptoms.

With regard to family involvement directly in behavioral treatment, Hafner (18) reported several cases in which poor marital relationships appeared to interfere with benefits from behavioral treatment for OCD outpatients. He noted that these patients showed improvement when spouses participated in the behavioral treatment process (19,20). Similar benefits were also evident in case studies of parental involvement in behavioral treatment of children (21), adolescents, and adults (22,23). In reports on larger samples, including family members in behavioral treatment has produced mixed results. Despite improvement in marital satisfaction, adding spouse assistance made no difference after treatment or at follow-up in two Dutch studies (24,25). However, in these studies spouses were not specifically trained in communication with patients regarding their symptoms. In a later report, Emmelkamp et al. (26) emphasized empathic communication as an important factor in outcome.

In contrast to Emmelkamp's findings, Mehta (27) reported that involving family members in behavioral treatment for 30 patients in India led to significantly greater gains in OCD symptoms, mood state, and social and occupational functioning compared with an unassisted treatment condition. At follow-up, the patients who received family treatment showed continued improvement, whereas individually treated patients lost some gains, making the outcome gap even wider. The patients with family members who were nonanxious and firm were more successful than those who had anxious and inconsistent ones, especially ones who engaged in argument and ridicule. Correspondingly, our own work with family group interventions has led us to believe that special strategies are needed to alter antagonistic or critical communication styles. The discrepancy in the findings of Emmelkamp and Mehta may be due to the less confrontational family role and greater intensity of treatment (24 sessions twice weekly versus eight sessions in 5 weeks) in the India study, as well as to cultural differences in family expectations. Also, there are differences in the "family intervention" utilized in their studies.

Two uncontrolled trials of family treatment have included efforts to reduce relatives' involvement in OCD symptoms. An inpatient treatment program in Great Britain for patients with a variety of diagnoses, including OCD, emphasized self-treatment and teaching relatives to assist in the therapy program (28). A family component that focused on training relatives to monitor patient behavior and encourage self-exposure in a noncritical manner was combined with individual behavior therapy. The relatives involved practiced under the therapist's supervision on the ward. This treatment program led to improvement in functioning, with a 45% decrease in symptoms at discharge and 60% at 6-month follow-up. Promising results from this program indicated excellent success for patients who scored in the extreme range on disability from OCD symptoms.

Multifamily behavioral treatment (MFBT), like group treatment, may be a cost-effective and efficacious alternative to individual treatment for OCD. MFBT offers the therapeutic benefits of family and group treatment and provides a nonthreatening context to effectively address family involvement in rituals. A recent pilot study ($N = 19$ patients) conducted in our center examined the outcome of 10 to 12 sessions of MFBT, conducted in groups of six to eight families, that included OCD patients and a mixture of spouses, partners, parents, and others in daily contact with the patient (10). Treatment included psychoeducation on OCD, family exchange of information about symptoms and coping strategies, group exposure with ERP, family communication skills training via family behavioral contracting, and patient and family homework assignments. Positive results were obtained following treatment and 1 year later: Y-BOCS scores improved by an average of 9–10 points, and 58% of patients were clinically significantly improved, somewhat more than occurred with group behavioral treatment (43%). Significant improvements in daily functioning scores, as measured by the Sheehan Disability Inventory, were also evident. In addition, most scales assessing family functioning showed posttest improvement. Although this study requires replication in other centers, MFBT appears quite promising and may be a particularly appropriate choice for some patients.

Family Responses to OCD

In our clinical experience with OCD patients and their significant others, responses to OC symptoms fall along a continuum of behavioral interactional patterns. This continuum, or spectrum, can be visualized as having two polar opposites of either unequivocally opposing the behavior—antagonistic—or totally giving in to and participating in the rituals—accommodating. A third type of response pattern that commonly emerges is a split family. In this case, the family members (usually parents) are divided in their reactions to the symptomatology, with one family member at the antagonistic end one at the accommodating end of the continuum of responses. Often—with children or adolescents, for example—it is the mother who may be more accommodating, e.g., going to the store to buy soap and paper towels to assist with washing rituals, whereas the father takes a firmer stance, shutting the water off in the house to put an end to washing rituals. The result is a split in the approach to the OC symptoms. The two most extreme positions are depicted in Table 1.

Another common scenario occurs when family members oscillate in their responses, swinging from one end of the spectrum to the order as the frustration and anger toward the patient and his or her symptoms escalate. Usually out of frustration that "nothing seems to work," family members become inconsistent—trying to participate in the rituals, then trying to cut them off. Despite extreme presentations of response styles in some families, the majority of family responses lie somewhere in the middle of the continuum described above. Regardless of which combination of family response patterns emerges, the message to the patient is usually inconsistent. As accommodating responses reinforce rituals and antagonistic responses fuel conflict, both patients and family members often feel confused, angry, and anxious.

Theoretical Considerations

The concept of expressed emotion (EE), based on the British studies of schizophrenia published in the 1970s, is an area of considerable interest in family research (29,30), and may be particularly applicable to families dealing with OCD. The term *expressed emotion* has come to be understood as a measure of relatives' critical, hostile, or emotionally overinvolved attitudes toward the identified patient. It is our clinical impression that these features of EE are present in the family responses to OC symptoms (see figure above). Furthermore, these characteristics are targets of change in our treatment approach with OCD patients and their families.

Numerous studies have consistently reported that high expressed emotion is significantly correlated with high rates of relapse. To date, 14 studies have reported on the association of EE with relapse, mainly for

Table 1 The Continuum of Family Response Patterns in OCD

Antagonistic---------------------------------Accommodating	
Rigid	Enmeshed
Demanding	Lack of boundaries
Intolerant	Poor limit-setting
Critical, hostile	Avoids conflict

Source: Ref. 41.

schizophrenic patients, depressed patients, bipolar manic depressives, disturbed adolescents, and weight-loss clients. EE has been found to predict outcome independent of illness severity (31), supporting the contention that criticism and/or emotional overinvolvement is not merely a response to severe symptomatology in patients.

There is little in the clinical literature that examines the impact of EE in OCD. In a pediatric population, Hibbs et al. (32) noted that high EE was more frequent among parents of children with OCD or conduct disorder than among controls. Leonard et al. (33) found that high parental EE was the second strongest predictor of long-term global functioning, superseded only by response to clomipramine at 5 weeks. This study was a 2- to 7-year follow-up study of 54 children and adolescents with OCD. In adults, Emmelkamp and colleagues (26) observed that high EE ratings were evident in three of four relapses. A self-report measure of EE combined with patient's coping style and life events accounted for a significant portion of relapse. Steketee (34) reported similar findings: negative family interactions (anger, criticism) and relatives' belief that the OCD patient was malingering predicted fewer gains at 9 months' follow-up.

In the literature on schizophrenia and depression, treatment to reduce the adverse features found in high EE homes has mainly employed psychoeducational paradigms. Patients from families whose EE levels were reduced from high to low following family psychoeducation and communication training were considerably less likely to relapse than those from families who remained high on EE (35–37). In a large multicenter treatment trial, McFarlane et al. (36) found that schizophrenic patients who received multifamily treatment had lower rates of relapse than those in single-family treatment. Despite the consistent reports of the benefits of psychoeducation and communication-skills training in multifamily groups, there has been little data on behaviorally oriented multifamily groups. One of the few to make such a report, Falloon and colleagues (38), noted a reduction in critical comments and overinvolvement among family members following 25 sessions of a behavioral multifamily group for schizophrenics.

It is our clinical experience that OCD families also benefit from a multifamily treatment. However, our MFBT utilizes interventions that are aimed specifically at reducing OC symptoms, as well as changing dysfunctional patterns of communication between family members that seem to fuel OC symptoms. This family group treatment incorporates psychoeducation, training in communication and problem-solving skills, clarification of boundaries, social learning, and in vivo rehearsal of new behaviors. The treatment also entails observing the application of ERP with therapist and participant modeling. Thus, the use of a multifamily group format is another potential strategy for reducing treatment costs and enhancing maintenance of gains. An illustration of the MFBT method is given below.

Clinical Example

Kim, a 28-year-old secretary and mother of a 2-year-old daughter, described symptoms of OCD that dated back to childhood. She sought treatment following severe exacerbation of her symptoms during her first pregnancy. Kim was referred for MFBT after a partial response to clomipramine and pimozide and 6 months of unsuccessful psychotherapy elsewhere. Kim reported that her primary fears had to do with extreme worry that she would contract cancer from various "substances," even when they could not be seen. These included detergents, chemicals (asbestos, a Chemlawn truck), gasoline, oil spills at the beach, batteries, exhaust, makeup, and the surface of cigarettes. In response to these fears, she was washing her hands more than 100 times a day, avoiding any situation or object that would trigger the worry about cancer. In addition, out of fear of "additives," Kim had restricted her diet to only one brand of "natural" ice cream and "natural" granola. Kim also spoke about feeling as if she had to sit with clenched fists to be sure that she wasn't making blasphemous gestures to God. She had given up on doing laundry, grocery shopping, and cooking because every task "took too long." Kim described "piles of clothes on the basement floor that have been there for 3 years" and said that some were "starting to mold" because of her avoidance. When asked about her husband's response, Kim said that he would "give in" to her requests in order to "keep the peace." She involved him in extensive reassurance-seeking rituals, usually more than 50 times a day, although she stated that she wanted to stop her "strange behaviors" because they were "tearing apart" her family. However, Kim "really believed" she could die from the "cancer germs." Kim had begun to involve her daughter, Lilly, by washing her hands so frequently that she had protested. Kim's husband, Joe, "gave up" trying to get Kim to cook. Sneaking food into the house created such an "uproar" that he usually resorted to taking Lilly to his mother's house for dinner.

The beginning of Kim's OC symptoms dates back to the age of 8, when she felt she "had to touch certain things" in her room to ward off fears that people close to her would die. She described a life riddled with magical thinking and ideas that she "had to" perform actions a certain way to prevent "bad things" from happening. For example, she would open and close the refrigerator in a certain way, touch the floor and then both eyes, walk up and down steps with the right foot leading, say ritualized prayers at bedtime, and get in and out of bed. She hid most of her rituals from others. Kim described herself as an average student who had friends but few real interests. Despite her worries, she was able to manage without seeming peculiar. The aggressive fears, mental rituals, and undoing behaviors became a hidden way of life for her until her pregnancy, during which she began to make "unreasonable" demands on her family, became withdrawn, and showed apparent decline in her occupational functioning.

Joe had viewed Kim's worries as just part of her personality, and their life appeared quite "normal" to others. He worked as a computer programmer and she landed a good job as a secretary at a large company. Shortly after they bought their own home, Mary—Kim's sister, to whom she was very close—was diagnosed with ovarian cancer. To make it easier for Mary to receive chemotherapy, Kim insisted that she move in with her and Joe. Kim was wonderful to Mary during this time, sharing everything she owned. Mary's cancer remitted and she moved back to live with their mother. Two years later, Kim became pregnant and began to express fears that she and the fetus would contract cancer from Mary or anything Mary had touched. Since Mary had been living in Kim's house, nearly everything seemed "contaminated."

To avoid conflict, Joe went along with all of Kim's requests, no matter how extreme. For example, he complied with the OCD rules of taking specific routes to the grocery store, so as not to drive by "asbestos-contaminated" areas; buying dairy items at the back of the case so they weren't exposed to "radiation"; not using certain dishware, spices, and foods that had been used by Mary; and not sitting on certain "clean" chairs. Once Kim insisted that they leave a store in the middle of a purchase because she saw a dead fly on the shelf and thought that was a sign of "air quality so poor it could result in death."

Much of this history and detailed description of Kim's OC symptoms was obtained during the first two 90-minute information-gathering sessions. Kim attended the first of these sessions alone, and it was clear that despite her strong conviction about her beliefs she was eager to change her behavior, which was generating conflict in her marriage and distressing her daughter. Furthermore, due to fears of contamination, Kim had not seen her mother and sisters in months. Kim was no longer fearful of contact with her sister, whose cancer had been in remission for a year. Kim avoided touching objects (makeup, mugs, clothing, books, silverware, bedding, etc.) that had been used by Mary when she was first diagnosed. This posed a big problem for Kim, both in her own house and at her mother's. In addition, because her mother lived in an area that Kim heard had "rust in the pipes," Kim viewed the water and all that it touched as being contaminated. Kim's family could not understand why she refused to bring her daughter to visit. Once again, Joe was called on to make excuses for Kim.

Kim and Joe appeared at the second information-gathering session eager to learn more about the OCD and what to do to handle it. Joe spoke about feeling as though "Kim's demands were controlling everything." He gave up trying to convince her not to be afraid because nothing seemed to work. Joe reported that recently Kim had been "going too far, by involving Lilly." He went on to report that Lilly was not allowed to go to his mother's if anyone in the neighborhood had their lawn treated with "chemicals," which involved a lengthy interrogation process. Lilly's clothes were changed at least five times a day; $25 a week was being spent on paper towels; and activities were usually abandoned because of Kim's demands to go home to wash and shower. Joe said his strategy had been to give in, but he felt that "this whole thing is getting way out of hand and I have no idea what to do!" The therapist described how MFBT offers help to family members. Besides problem-solving with other families dealing with OCD, Joe would learn a specific technique—behavioral contracting—to set some limits on his participation in the compulsions. Also, the more that Kim and Joe learned about OCD, the better they would be able to control it. The hierarchies shown in Tables 2 and 3 were established.

Kim and Joe were asked to read Chapters 1–4 in *When Once is Not Enough* by Steketee and White (39) before the group began, and were encouraged to call the therapist if they had any lingering questions.

MFBT Session 1

At the outset of this co-led MFBT group, anticipatory anxiety ran high. Kim and Joe were among a total of seven couples or families. Some families arrived very early to be certain they were not late; others, arriving late, rushed through the door with apologies, explaining that the patient had trouble getting to places on time because of obsessions and compulsions. The initial anxiety about the group was alleviated by providing structure, especially at this first session. However, the therapists also allowed room for individual expression that would collectively determine the "climate" of the group with regard to blame, responsibility, overprotection, overinvolvement, distance, impotence, and denial. Once people began talking, they appeared relieved to be with others "who know," and it was difficult to redirect the informal conversation to begin the session. We observed the level of interaction and content, as well as

Table 2   Hierarchy of Fears of Contamination: Cancer from Sister and Cigarettes

Situation	Discomfort (1–100)	Treatment session
Holding unopened cigarette pack	45	1
Stepping with shoe on cigarette butt	45	1
Touching makeup sister used	50	1
Touching mug sister used	50	1
Touching door knobs (general)	55	2
Holding opened cigarette pack	55	2
Holding "clean" ashtray	60	3
Standing near someone smoking, outside	65	3
Touching doorknobs at work	70	4
Holding clothes worn by sister	70	4
Holding unburned cigarette	75	4
Holding "dirty" ashtray	75	4
Standing near someone smoking, inside	80	5
Touching clothing that smells of smoke	80	5
Stepping with sock on cigarette butt	85	5
Touching "dirty" clothes (basement)	85	5
Touching side of dryer	85	5
Touching sand in used ashtray	90	6
Touching cigarette filter	90	6
Touching tobacco	90	6
Using cup served by a smoker	90	6
Stepping barefoot on a cigarette	95	7
Holding a "used" cigarette	95	7
Touching cigarette to lips	95	7
Rubbing cigarette on food and eating	100	8

seating choices that could reveal alliances, conflicts, and level of trust within the group.

As people arrived, the therapists distributed nametags. Once everyone was seated in the circle, the formal group began. We asked each person to introduce himself and indicate what he hoped to get out of the group. This facilitated participation and laid the foundation for trust and group cohesiveness. The themes at the beginning of this and other MFBTs were: "What should I do when my daughter is in the shower for 3 hours? Can that really be OCD?" "How do other families deal with the rituals?" "What is OCD?" "How can each of us cope with it effectively?"

Table 3   Hierarchy of Fears of Contamination: Cancer from "Chemical" Contact

Situation	Discomfort (0–100)	Treatment session
Microwaving food	30	1
Pumping gasoline	35	1
Driving behind bus, windows closed	35	1
Touching sand in sandbox	35	1
Touching White-out	40	2
Touching Sweet & Low	40	2
Holding batteries	40	2
Driving behind bus, windows opened	45	3
In car with air-conditioning on	45	3
Standing by digital clock	45	3
Touching gasoline	45	3
Touching basement doorknob	50	4
Touching rust	50	4
Passing Chem-Lawn truck	55	4
Driving by landfill	60	5
Touching sand at beach	65	5
Sleeping near digital clock	65	5
Eating food items exposed to bright light	70	5
Walking barefoot at beach	70	5
Eating food items scanned at checkout counter	75	6
Getting cleaning products on hands	75	6
Chewing sugarless gum	75	6
Walking on treated lawn	80	7
Ingesting Sweet & Low	80	7
Drinking soda	85	7
Eating unwashed apple	90	7
Eating seafood	100	8
Eating chicken	100	8
Drinking caffeinated coffee	100	8
Showering at mother's house	100	8
Using utensils at mother's house	100	8
Drinking from cups at mother's house	100	8

A quick review of the "ground rules" clarified group expectations about the time frame of the group, the meeting place, confidentiality, and notification of absence from the group. Group members were encouraged to contact the leader(s) to discuss any feelings or issues that arose as a result of their group experience. The proposed agenda for the

12 weekly sessions and six monthly check-in sessions was outlined. After this, a handout entitled "What Is OCD?" (defining obsessions and compulsions, theories of etiology, course of illness, common coexisting disorders, and treatment) and the Y-BOCS Symptom Checklist were distributed. The information was reviewed, and the checklist served as a springboard for patients and family members to disclose the OC symptoms and the behaviors that were typically hidden in shame. As usual, there was great relief that others had had similar thoughts and experiences. Kim said, "Wow, you do that too! I thought I was the only one who won't let anyone else sit in *my* chair!"

As family members listened to many others describing the identical symptoms and feelings they had struggled with for many years, some began to consider that OCD was a real disorder beyond the patient's control. They seemed to attend to what the patients said with more objectivity. The notions of displaced agression ("They're just trying to spite me") and faulty parenting ("Was I too strict?") were deliberately challenged in the multifamily context. The group provided the first real opportunity for several family members to learn about the content of the patient's obsessions and the extent of the rituals.

A stress diathesis model of OCD's pathogenesis was presented. In addition to genetic factors, the following familial and cultural factors were discussed as being important in the development and expression of OCD: 1) child development and parent–child interaction, 2) family functioning, and 3) overall levels of stress. Patients and their families often attempted to understand the patient's symptoms in psychodynamic terms as a result of prior therapy. Attempts to explain causation by analyzing the content of the obsessions were shown to be speculative at best and unhelpful in deciding how to effectively manage the symptoms. Some moments of silence occurred in the group as the excitement of comparing stories died down, and it appeared that many were trying to come to terms with the illness in these silences.

Families enthusiastically compared experiences. Joe was relieved to hear other spouses express their helplessness and how they ended up "just giving in to keep the peace." Families talked about the bizarre symptoms in an atmosphere with little social stigma. Fears that maybe their loved one was going crazy seemed quieted by meeting others with OCD who were "normal people."

As it often does, medication became the focus of conversation, with several members asking: "What are you on? What dosage? Any side effects? How does the doctor choose which medication is best?" The group was reminded to save these questions for a later session with a psychiatrist. This group exhibited some reluctance to address issues with direct emotional content by switching to questions about another possible "cure" for OCD. The therapists noted that most people with OCD do get better with the ERP treatment but that hoping for a complete cure was unrealistic. This was met by reports of having "suffered long enough"—"We don't deserve this, take it away!"—and incredulity that advanced medical technology could not relieve OCD symptoms.

The leaders allowed time for patients to select ERP homework challenges in a "go-round" fashion, with patients taking turns. Kim chose to begin with the items lowest on her hierarchies. After homework forms had been distributed, the session formally ended with the therapists encouraging that this first week was a trial time to begin to practice ERP. If patients did not any sense that their distress was decreasing, they were encouraged to modify the exposure challenge and stay with one item until the discomfort diminished. Family members were reminded that one of the goals of MFBT is to learn to be involved in the OCD as little as possible, except in life-threatening or dangerous situations. They were instructed to keep their involvement to a minimum but not to make any drastic changes in their responses to the demands of OCD until they learned to utilize behavioral contracting. The leader asked all patients to bring any of the items on their hierarchy to the next session so that they could be used therapeutically. All families and patients were asked to finish reading *When Once is Not Enough* (39) before the next session.

Session 2

The second session began with a review of what had been covered and accomplished in the group the previous week. The leader then asked the group, "Does anyone have any thoughts, questions, or feelings that they would like to talk about before moving on?" This provided continuity between sessions, allowed members to "warm up," and conveyed a sense of respect and appreciation for the concerns that any group member might have. However, this was kept brief and to the point. Each patient reported on the homework he or she had completed during the week and the therapist collected homework forms, verifying that patients had completed it as assigned. Therapists reinforced patients for completing the form and for doing the exposure, thereby modeling positive feedback to the group. Others were also asked to comment. Patients reported on their levels of anxiety during the exposure homework; if anxiety had declined, they discussed this and noted that prolonged exposure made this possible. If anxiety had remained high, patients were reinforced for their courage and perseverance in tolerating it. When the homework was inadequately completed or reported, therapists discussed any problems identified by the patient, but encouraged positive group feedback and empathic confrontation to promote a corrective experience. Kim said she wasn't sure if she was doing the homework "right" but that she had had "success with holding a cigarette pack, using the microwave, and pumping gas with Joe next to me." She reported that her discomfort level decreased to about 20 in all these situations. She had difficulty with some of the other exposure situations but was given credit for trying to tolerate the discomfort rather than simply avoid it. Joe said he felt Kim should do the homework alone and asked what he should do if she wants him present "for security." Some group members suggested that if his presence helped Kim to get started with the exposure, it was probably okay as long as he didn't encourage rituals.

The majority of this session was dedicated to the description of behavioral therapy and ERP techniques. The leaders asked group members to explain what they thought behavioral therapy means. After a few responses, the therapist constructed a working definition for the group: "Behavioral therapy provides tools for changing unwanted behaviors without analyzing in detail the childhood history and meaning of the behaviors." Next, the sequence of obsessions and compulsions was reviewed, explaining how a trigger or cue evoked an obsession leading to feelings of anxiety and the urge to ritualize. The techniques of direct and imagined ERP in vivo and imaginal exposure were described. Examples were given, and patients were asked to practice by choosing an exposure homework task. To initiate, one of the group leaders asked, "Who would like to begin by selecting a behavioral homework task?" Feedback and support from other group members served to develop an optimal homework assignment.

As each patient selected his or her homework, the group leader translated the task into a form that could be rehearsed in the group, and the therapist and other group members participated in the exposure challenge. Kim was asked to touch the doorknobs in the room, as were all the other group members. This was difficult for the other patients who had contamination fears but not, of course, for members with other forms of OCD. Patients with aggressive obsessions joked that they wished they had this problem instead of their own, a common remark made in such groups. Observing so many people unaffected by the task led Kim to comment that it helped to see how easy touching doorknobs was for most people because it made her question her behavior and beliefs. When someone asked Kim if this wasn't already obvious to her, especially since she could see that Joe didn't avoid doorknobs, she replied that she relied on Joe for reassurance but she "never really believed him anyway . . . he's probably just trying to appease me." Other patients spoke about feeling the same way, and how this angered family members because they would "try to help but never could." Joe spoke about all the hours wasted talking about the irrationality of Kim's beliefs to the point of desperation, when he would shout at her and call her "crazy." "Kim would end up crying, but at least it would stop the questioning."

The leader asked Kim to take out the cigarette pack, batteries, Sweet 'n Low packet, bottle of White-Out, makeup, and mugs she had been avoiding and pass them around the group. Every 10 minutes she was asked, "What is your level of anxiety or discomfort, from 0 to 100, right now as you focus on what you're doing?" Other group members were asked the same question. The unreasonableness of the fears, the anxiety associated with them, and the compulsive behavior were identified by the therapist as hallmarks of OCD. Since the content of the fear could not be reasoned with, why try? This universal problem was identified as another symptom of OCD: reassurance-seeking that, like checking or washing, leads to more of the same. As patients and families experienced this in the group, the therapist encouraged symptom identification and the rehearsal of dismissal, distraction, and redirection. Kim began to develop better insight into her OCD and how she had grown to rely on Joe to answer "the unanswerable." The strategy of ERP started to make sense as her confidence grew through education, exposure, homework, and the support and feedback of the group.

At the end of the second session, the therapists instructed patients to continue the exposure from that day's session and add any other homework items, to be practiced at least one hour a day, preferably all at one time rather than split into segments. Patients were reminded not to leave the exposure situation until their anxiety had declined noticeably and to record their distress levels on their homework form. Joe asked, "But what should I do when Kim asks me to buy her more paper towels or bathe Lilly for the third time?" The therapist acknowledged that all families were eager to have these dilemmas solved, and that they would be getting to this more specifically at the next session. Families were encouraged to try to use what they had learned so far to modify their responses and to limit involvement in rituals, while communicating an appreciation for how hard it is to "just stop."

Session 3

The group began in its usual way, with each patient reporting on his or her homework task results. The members engaged in troubleshooting for problems that patients were experiencing in completing the ERP homework and the homework forms. Kim reported that she continued to make headway, but she felt that there were so many things that bothered her she didn't know if she would "ever get over the OCD." Other patients commented on the progress she had been making and that she needed to be patient with herself. Joe added that he noticed a big improvement in Kim's outlook and that she seemed more willing to take risks. For example, they went out to eat pizza for the first time in 8 months and Kim stepped on a cigarette butt, drove behind a bus, touched the doorknobs, sat with her hands open, and didn't perform any rituals. The group was tremendously supportive of her. Despite this, she asked, "If the OCD is a neurobiological disorder, how can I change it?" Others nodded, and an insightful spouse responded that "it's as our therapist said: changing behavior can change thoughts and feelings; look, it's already happening for you!"

At this session, the therapist presented a brief videotaped lecture on the neurobiology of OCD. This tape provided information on medication and the interplay of behavioral therapy with biological processes in the treatment of OCD. Following the discussion of the tape, the therapist asked each patient to select exposure items with a discomfort level of approximately 50 to 60. For those with contamination fears like Kim, patients and family members took out an object to hold and were asked to touch the object or their "contaminated" hands directly to their face, hair, and clothing. Contact with the contaminant was continuous, with touching of face, hair, etc., repeated every few minutes throughout the session, immediately after which the patient was asked to report the discomfort level. Kim held a rusted object, a "clean" ashtray, and sand Joe had collected from the beach. As she did the exercise, she experienced an initial increase in her discomfort and wanted to seek reassurance: "What if someone who smoked touched this ashtray; now I have cancer germs on my hands and they will seep through my skin. Are other people worried they will get cancer from touching rust? Are you sure there were no oil spills on this sand?" Joe started to offer explanations but another patient interrupted him to ask what he was doing. The group laughed, and Kim responded that it was true that she was "just OCDing again."

After about 60 minutes of in vivo or imaginal exposure, the group's attention was shifted to the "Guidelines for Living with OCD" in Van Noppen and coauthors' *Learning to Live with OCD* (40). These include:

1. Learn to recognize the signals that indicate a person is having problems.
2. Modify expectations during stressful times.

3. Measure progress according to the person's level of functioning.
4. Don't make day-to-day comparisons.
5. Give recognition for "small" improvements.
6. Create a strong supportive home environment.
7. Keep communication clear and simple.
8. Stick to a behavioral contract.
9. Set limits, yet be sensitive to the person's mood.
10. Keep your family routine "normal."
11. Use humor.
12. Support the person's medication regimen.
13. Make separate time for other family members.
14. Be flexible!

As the group members took turns reading aloud, the therapist
asked the families which categories of family response style they fell
into. This promoted insight into family response patterns and the impact
of those responses on the patient. Joe said the accommodating pattern
fit him, yet he started to see that he also oscillated at times out of frustration. He spoke about the time he got so angry that Kim wouldn't get
out of the shower that he shut off the hot water. She continued to
shower anyway, in the cold water, so he turned off all the water in the
house. This resulted in a screaming battle and Lilly awoke crying, so he
turned the water back on. Other families related to Joe's story, adding
that it was hard to be consistent or to really follow through on threats.

Kim reported that she had given *Learning to Live with OCD* to her
mother and siblings to read, and that "for the first time they seemed to
understand that my fears weren't personal feelings about them." Joe
talked about this as a beginning so that they could now work on exposure to Kim's mother's house, where Kim fears the water because of
"rust contamination." He said how sad he was that they had "missed all
of the kids' birthday parties and big family events . . . . I always had to
call with some lame excuse." Both Kim and Joe acknowledged that they
started to feel that Lilly would eventually feel left out and they didn't
want this to happen. Almost everyone commented that their routine, if
they had one at this point, was anything but "normal."

Kim and the other patients reassessed their behavioral homework
task with the family guidelines in mind, and added another challenge.
Kim and Joe said they hoped to end their arguments about so many
things, and that they saw how Joe's giving in really hadn't helped
much. Other people offered support: Joe shouldn't blame himself for
"helping" because he was doing the best he could, especially since he

didn't know what he was dealing with. Now, with education and some tools, there was hope.

Session 4

The first three sessions provided patients and families with a clearer understanding of OCD. The next step was to learn how to cope more productively with the symptoms as a family using cognitive and behavioral techniques. This fourth session was designed to prepare them for the family contracting in the following sessions, which forms the essence of family collaboration in the treatment of OCD. As usual, each patient reported on his or her homework during the week, with family members commenting on their role or observations. Kim and Joe said they felt discouraged because they went away for the weekend and Kim was "afraid that the condo was sprayed with pesticide." She "stayed in the same clothes all weekend, didn't let Joe bring their suitcases out of the car, didn't allow Lilly to play on the floor, felt like the makeup was ruined," and that she was "back to base 1." Joe had brought to the session the makeup and some of the clothes, even though Kim had begged him not to do so. Knowing he had to be firmer, he insisted despite the bickering. The group gave Joe positive feedback for doing this and confronted him about his "tendency to give in too much." The therapists asked that these items be used in the session during the behavioral contracting.

The therapists introduced the concept of behavioral contracting by asking the group what they thought this term means. The discussion produced a working definition that included the following points:

1. One at a time, each family identifies problem areas that result from the demands of OC symptoms by considering the following questions: How does OCD impose on others? Do family members participate in rituals? Is criticism directed toward the patient by family? Do family members take over the patient's tasks and responsibilities? The problems are to be defined in very clear, specific behavioral terms.
2. The group leaders guide the family to focus on one problem area and define it (as in the example above).
3. Utilizing feedback from the group, family members explore behavioral response options and the possible consequences of each.
4. With principles of behavior therapy in mind, family members select the best response options.

5. The leaders facilitate a negotiation process between family members. This consists of direct dialogue of behavioral expectations among the family interspersed with group comments, suggestions, and feedback. At this point the family creates a contract that establishes the behavior therapy goal for the patient and the behavioral responses for family members.
6. The family, with the assistance of the group, assesses whether the solution is reasonable.
7. When possible, the family rehearses the behavioral contract during the treatment session.
8. The group evaluates the contract, adding suggestions based on observations of the family's ability to carry out the plan.
9. If necessary, the family negotiates any modifications in the planned contract before the next family takes its turn. All exposure homework is written on the homework sheets and contracts are to be recorded in the space provided.

Kim and Joe discussed the problems encountered over the weekend and how Kim would not touch the clothes that had been worn. She wanted Joe to do the laundry and throw out the makeup. The group encouraged Kim to touch the clothing and use the makeup. She balked—but then acknowledged that "it always works"; once she exposes herself, the discomfort decreases and her perspective improves.

With feedback from the group, Kim and Joe negotiated a behavioral contract stipulating that she was to use the makeup several times a day and touch the "contaminated" clothes to her "clean" clothes and then wear the touched garment. Kim agreed to this and to resisting reassurance-seeking from Joe. Also, she was to hold Lilly, or let Lilly touch the "contaminated" clothing. Joe raised the possibility that Kim would want to wash her hands, Lilly's toys, and anything else that came into contact with the "contaminants." Others in the group quickly responded that this would "defeat the purpose" and urged Kim to resist these compulsions. Anxious at the thought of this challenge, Kim said that she would try to complete the ERP, but what if she "slipped"? Another patient told Kim that she should expect to feel a strong urge to wash but should delay the compulsion and continue to touch contaminated objects. She reminded Kim of the alternatives of using positive self-help statements, thinking of others in the group, and distracting herself; in fact, she offered her phone number so that Kim could call her for encouragement rather than seek reassurance from Joe. The therapist reinforced these strategies and redirected the group back to the task of family contracting.

Thus far they had discussed Kim's exposure homework, but what exactly should Joe do to be supportive but not facilitate the OCD? Kim and Joe decided they would target reassurance-seeking, which had decreased but was still out of hand. The group discussed what was reasonable with regard to reassurance. One father asked, "But don't we all need reassurance?" One spouse responded that the kind of reassurance people with OCD ask for may seem reasonable at times but the repetitive questioning and urgency of the need for certainty are not "normal." Others agreed, and added that most times the questions do not have absolute answers and other times the patient already knows the answer. All families identified the process of giving reassurance as "futile," "exhausting," and "frustrating." Patients expressed feelings of shame about their behavior. One of the therapists led Kim and Joe through a detailed negotiation process to arrive at agreement on how Joe was expected to repond to Kim's requests for reassurance.

Kim "gave Joe permission" to label her questions as OCD and to remind her that she knows how he would answer the "OCD question." If she persisted, he was to suggest that she put the question on hold, even if it seemed urgent, and if it still bothered her they could talk about it later. If Kim continued to persist, Joe was to once more remind her this was a reassurance question; he knew what she was going through but it wouldn't help to talk about it. Kim agreed that at this point Joe would suggest that she do something else to distract herself because she always felt better over time. If this didn't work and the requests became very unreasonable, the couple agreed that Joe would leave the room— or house, if necessary—to remove himself from the situation. If Kim became very agitated, they agreed that Joe would answer her once and only once.

Other group members participated in the negotiation process to assist Kim and Joe in arriving at this behavioral contract, which seemed satisfying to the couple and feasible to the group. Other spouses coached Joe to be consistent and stick to the agreement. The therapist suggested to the families that it was often useful to remind the patient that they had made this agreement together and it was everyone's responsibility to carry it out. However, although the contracts are meant to provide guidelines for expectable behavior in any given situation, they should be amenable to renegotiation and modification as needed. All families left the session with a behavioral contract to practice and homework forms to record the progress. In a fashion similar to that of the preceding sessions, each patient committed to individual exposure homework, as well as the family contract. The therapists outlined the critical concepts in behavioral contracting:

1. Realistic expectations on the part of both patient and family are clearly defined.
2. The family learns how to be supportive in ways that are therapeutic to the patient.
3. The patient is given responsibility for therapy that enhances his or her sense of control, motivation, and confidence.
4. Limits of responsibility are clarified and family members are redirected to get involved in their own lives again.
5. A third party (or group) moderating the negotiations decreases emotional tension between family members, encourages objective feedback during the behavioral task negotiation, and teaches families how to engage in clear and direct communication.

Sessions 5–11

These sessions were devoted to in vivo and imaginal ERP, practice in family contracting, self-monitoring distress levels, and homework planning. Family responses to OCD were discussed in greater detail, and greater disclosure about symptoms emerged. Group interaction became highly personalized as families described the interpersonal conflict that interfered with their attempts to manage the OC symptoms. Each session began with the go-round of patients' and families' reporting on the previous week's exposure homework and compliance with the behavioral contract.

Families were supported by the therapists and group members in their efforts "to help." Many were unaware of how to negotiate a family approach with the patient's consent. One husband grasped the general concept of ERP, but tried a new response without discussing it with his wife. This backfired because the patient felt powerless and out of control. During these sessions, group members who complained about not having enough guidance or who tried to rush the group ahead to the contracting were often the ones who avoided committing themselves to a task. Such patients consumed group time. They were confronted about their behavior and given permission to pass or to work on an exposure challenge of their own without family involvement. Thus, the decision to change was placed on the patient. The group coached the family to accept that they could not make the patient participate in a treatment that the family chooses unless the family was ready to carry out the consequences. The exposure homework had to be the patient's choice. However, when a chosen task was not sufficiently challenging, the therapist used the group process to encourage a more meaningful one. Other patients and family members proved instrumental in helping an adolescent in the group to come to terms with accepting family limits as reasonable. The behavioral contract helped to limit parental responsibility for the carrying out of exposure homework, allowing the boy to engage in independent, responsible behavior.

In each of the sessions, the therapist asked which family wanted to initiate the contracting. This cross-family modeling appeared to be a therapeutic factor in MFBT. After hearing about the success Kim and Joe had with their contract, another woman with a 20-year OCD history decided to reduce unnecessary hand-washing when she entered the house or touched anything in the house she suspected of being "contaminated." She asked her husband to go about his business without accommodating her, and to avoid "hovering" around her. "Don't ask me how I do every day; I put enough pressure on myself. When you notice I've done well or that I've really tried, give me praise, a simple 'You're doing well. Keep it up.' " Her behavioral contracting helped her resume responsibility for her treatment and prevented a family struggle over control.

The question "How much should I push?" was a pervasive family concern. The therapists noted that using force or ultimatums in the midst of rituals would probably lead to more conflict, and possibly physical violence or destructive acts out of frustration and anger. Families were advised to encourage resistance and discourage avoidance as much as possible, but to recognize mounting tension, often manifested as an increase in OC symptoms, as a warning signal to "back off." No family in this group required crisis intervention and interruption of behavioral family contracting.

As each family in the group was guided through the behavioral contracting, they incorporated what they had observed from the families before. After participating in helping another couple resolve their conflict, an astute mother whose 18-year-old son had washing and checking rituals identified a conflict between her husband and herself that came out in the son: "It's not a matter of where Sam leaves his 'contaminated' towels. The problem of where to leave used towels in general is between my husband and me." This came out while the three negotiated the son's reducing the number of towels he used after showering and where the towels were to be placed. Apparently, the mother also objected to where the father put his used towels! This provided the family with an opportunity to separate out preexisting interpersonal issues, which are often magnified by the impact of the OC symptoms. In this case, the parents were asked to resolve their conflict about the towels before they could clearly communicate expectations to their son. Through this constant evaluation of the outcome of the behavioral con-

tract, families and patients became engaged in the processes of communication, problem-solving, and decision-making to learn more effective
behaviors to cope with the "demands" of OCD. Another biproduct of
behavioral contracting was the clarification of roles. Due to avoidance,
Kim had stopped doing the household tasks that had been hers before
she became symptomatic. To "help" Kim, Joe took over the tasks, but
this added to Kim's sense of herself as "inept." Through the behavioral
contracting and exposure, Kim slowly resumed her roles in the household.

   Throughout the later sessions, there was a growing emphasis on
independently initiating ERP challenges and behavioral contracting with
less therapist involvement. The therapists continually stressed the importance of self-instruction and patients' and families' ability to utilize
the techniques on their own. By session 11, the therapists ensured that
each family had reviewed their gains and the symptoms that needed
more intensive work. As in GBT, many patients expressed fear that they
would not be able to maintain their improvement once the group
ended. Again, the therapist, with feedback from other group members,
highlighted the symptomatic improvement and wealth of knowledge
and understanding gained through MFBT. Also, the therapist reminded
the group that one of the purposes of the monthly follow-up sessions
was to consolidate treatment gains. The therapists emphasized that if
patients anticipated stressors that might increase OCD symptoms (birth
of a baby, job change, etc.), troubleshooting and preventive planning
were needed.

Session 12

The last weekly session began with the go-round and practice of ERP
and family behavioral contracting. Throughout this session, families and
patients asked: "What will we do now?," "Does this group have to
end?," "Can't we extend it? We just got to know each other." The therapist addressed feelings of sadness and loss as part of ending the group.
Kim and Joe spoke about how much they would miss the encouragement and coaching from the group. Kim, like other patients, was well
aware of the importance of consistently practicing the strategies but
feared she would not continue to be so diligent without the accountability of the group. Joe responded that, with the behavioral contracting
and his better understanding, she didn't have to worry because he
wouldn't let her "get away with as much." Kim said that Joe used to try
to stop her by confronting her with statements like "that's irrational,"
which made her feel "pushed aside and small." Through MFBT, Joe had
learned to communicate understanding and to set limits at the same

time. Kim described a contract they made that, when they were in public and Kim got into an "OCD thing," Joe would gently squeeze her hand and wink at her as a signal that she was being unreasonable. This worked very well because no hostile, critical comments were made. Joe spoke for other family members in the group when he said that before MFBT "I thought I knew about OCD, but now I not only understand it intellectually, I understand it emotionally too."

SUMMARY

Clinical research has clearly demonstrated that behavioral treatment that offers a combination of exposure and response prevention is effective in reducing OC symptoms. Despite these promising findings, a large number of patients refuse or drop out of treatment, or remain symptomatic following treatment. In addition, the costs of providing individual behavioral treatment have spiraled upward. We have demonstrated the efficacy of two alternative, cost-effective forms of behavioral treatment that use a group modality. Group behavioral treatment (GBT) is for patients only. Multifamily behavioral treatment (MFBT) includes the patients' significant other(s). Both are 12-session groups held weekly, and include psychoeducation, exposure with modeling and response prevention, and homework assignments. Six monthly follow-up sessions are held after the active phase of behavioral treatment.

Based on our clinical impression and recent research findings, MFBT may offer hope for those not benefiting from standard individual treatment. Families of OCD patients are inevitably brought into rituals, and their responses are often countertherapeutic. MFBT incorporates the family into the behavioral treatment by teaching family members and patients to negotiate contracts with the goal of extracting others from the patient's compulsions in a supportive manner.

REFERENCES

1. American Psychiatric Association. Diagnostic and Statistical Manual of Mental Disorders. 4th ed. Washington, DC: American Psychiatric Association, 1994.
2. Yalom I. Theory and Practice of Group Psychotherapy. New York: Basic Books, 1975.
3. Budman S. Forms of Brief Therapy. New York: Guilford Press, 1981.
4. Hand I, Tichatzky M. Behavioral group therapy for obsessions and compulsions: first results of a pilot study. In: Sjoden PO, Bates D, Dockens WS, eds. Trends in Behavior Therapy. New York: Academic Press, 1979:269–297.

5. Epsie CA. The group treatment of obsessive-compulsive ritualizers: behavioral management of identified patterns of relapse. Behav Psychother 1986; 14:21–33.
6. Taylor CJ, Sholomskas DE. Group exposure and response prevention for OCD. Annual meeting of the Anxiety Disorders Association of America, Santa Monica, CA, March 1993.
7. Enright SJ. Group treatment for obsessive-compulsive disorder: an evaluation. Behav Psychother 1991; 19:183–192.
8. Krone KP, Himle JA, Nesse RM. A standardized behavioral group treatment program for obsessive-compulsive disorder: preliminary outcomes. Behav Res Ther 1991; 29:627–632.
9. Van Noppen B, Pato MT, Marsland R, Rasmussen S. A time-limited behavioral group for treatment of OCD. 1995. Submitted.
10. Van Noppen B, Steketee G, McCorkle BH, Pato M. Group and family behavioral treatment for obsessive compulsive disorder: a pilot study. 1996. Submitted.
11. Fals-Stewart W, Marks AP, Schafer J. A comparison of behavioral group therapy and individual behavior therapy in treating obsessive-compulsive disorder. J Nerv Ment Dis 1993; 181:189–193.
12. Calvocoressi L, Lewis B, Harris M, Trufan S, Goodman W, McDougle C, Price L. Family accommodation in obsessive-compulsive disorder. Am J Psychiatry 1995; 152:441–443.
13. Allsopp M, Verduyn C. Adolescents with obsessive compulsive disorder: a case note review of consecutive patients referred to a provincial regional adolescent psychiatry unit. J Adolesc 1990; 13:157–169.
14. Marks IM, Hodgson R, Rachman S. Treatment of chronic obsessive-compulsive neurosis with *in vivo* exposure, a 2 year follow-up and issues in treatment. Br J Psychiatry 1975; 127:349–364.
15. Black DW, Blum NS. Obsessive-compulsive disorder support groups: the Iowa model. Comp Psychiatry 1992; 33:65–71.
16. Cooper M. A group for families of obsessive-compulsive persons, Families in Society. J Contemp Human Serv, May 1993:301–307.
17. Tynes LL, Salins C, Skiba W, Winstead DK. A psychoeducational and support group for obsessive-compulsive disorder patients and their significant others. Comp Psychiatry 1992; 33:197–201.
18. Hafner RJ. Marital interaction in persisting obsessive-compulsive disorders. Aust NZ J Psychiatry 1982; 16:171–178.
19. Hafner R. Anxiety disorders and family therapy. Aust NZ J Fam Ther 1992; 13:99–104.
20. Cobb J, McDonald R, Marks IM, Stern R. Marital versus exposure therapy: psychological treatments of co-existing marital and phobic obsessive problems. Behav Analysis Mod 1980; 4:3–16.
21. Dalton P. Family treatment of an obsessive-compulsive child: a case report. Fam Process 1983; 22:99–108.
22. Hafner RJ, Gilchrist P, Bowling J, Kalucy R. The treatment of obsessional neurosis in a family setting. Aust NZ J Psychiatry 1981; 15:145–151.

23. Hoover C, Insel T. Families of origin in obsessive-compulsive disorder. J Nerv Ment Dis 1984; 172:207–215.
24. Emmelkamp PMG, de Haan E, Hoogduin CAL. Marital adjustment and obsessive-compulsive disorder. Br J Psychiatry 1990; 156:55–60.
25. Emmelkamp PMG, DeLange I. Spouse involvement in the treatment of obsessive-compulsive patients. Behav Res Ther 1983; 21:341–346.
26. Emmelkamp PMG, Kloek J, Blaauw E. Obsessive-compulsive disorders in principles and practice of relapse prevention. In: Wilson PH, ed. New York: Guilford Press, 1992:213–234.
27. Mehta M. A comparative study of family-based and patient-based behavioral management in obsessive-compulsive disorder. Br J Psychiatry 1990; 157:133–135.
28. Thornicroft G, Colson L, Marks I. An in-patient behavioural psychotherapy unit: description and audit. Br J Psychiatry 1991; 158:362–367.
29. Brown GW, Birley JLT, Wing JK. Influence of family life on the course of schizophrenic disorders: a replication. Br J Psychiatry 1972; 121:241–258.
30. Falloon IRH, Boyd J, McGill CW. Family Care of Schizophrenia. New York: Guilford Press, 1984.
31. Hooley JM, Orley J, Teasdale JD. Levels of expressed emotion and relapse in depressed patients. Br J Psychiatry 1986; 148:642–647.
32. Hibbs ED, Hamburger SD, Lenane M, Rapoport JL, Kruesi MJ, Keysor CS, Goldstein MJ. Determinants of expressed emotion in families of disturbed and normal children. J Child Psychol Psychiatry 1991; 32(5):757–770.
33. Leonard H, Swedo S, Lenane M, Rettew D, Rappoport J. A prospective follow-up study of 54 obsessive-compulsive children and adolescents. Arch Gen Psychiatry 1993; 50.
34. Steketee G. Social support and treatment outcomes of obsessive compulsive disorder at 9-month follow up. Behav Psychother 1993; 21:81–95.
35. Anderson C, Hogarty G, Reiss D. Family treatment of adult schizophrenic patients: a psychoeducational approach. Schiz Bull 1980; 6:490–505.
36. McFarlane WR, Lukens E, Link B, Dusay R, Deakins SA, Newmark M, Dunne EJ, Horen B, Toran J. Multiple-family groups and psychoeducation in the treatment of schizophrenia. Arch Gen Psychiatry 1995; 52:679–687.
37. Hogarty GE, Anderson CM, Reiss DJ, Kornblith SJ, Greenwald DP, Javna CS, Madonia MJ. Family psychoeducation, social skills training and maintenance chemotherapy in the aftercare treatment of schizophrenia. Arch Gen Psychiatry 1986; 43:633–642.
38. Falloon IRH, Liberman RP, Lillie IFJ, Vaugh ICE. Family therapy of schizophrenics coping with the high risk of relapse. Fam Process 1984; 20:211–221.
39. Steketee G, White K. When Once is Not Enough: help for obsessive compulsives. Oakland, CA: New Harbinger Publications, 1990.
40. Van Noppen B, Pato M, Rasmussen S. Learning to Live with OCD. 3rd ed. Milford, CT: OC Foundation, 1993.

41. Van Noppen B, Rasmussen S, Eisen J, McCartney L. A multi-family group approach as an adjunct to treatment of obsessive-compulsive disorder. In: Current Treatments of Obsessive Compulsive Disorder. Pato M, Zohar J, eds. Washington, DC: American Psychiatric Press, 1991:118.

14

Support Groups

A Valuable Ingredient in Recovery

James W. Broatch
Obsessive-Compulsive Foundation
Milford, Connecticut

> My worst moments have been when I felt totally alone with my problems, that no one could ever understand me, that I was a failure as a human being, that I was crazy (1).

INTRODUCTION

According to a 1992 Gallup survey, one American in three belongs to some kind of small support or self-help group (2). More people are involved in self-help groups than in any other form of therapy. As many as 500,000 mutual-help support groups are thought to exist in the United States (3). This chapter discusses the essential role that a self-help group (SHG) or professionally led or assisted support group plays in the treatment and recovery of individuals with obsessive-compulsive disorder (OCD). Various support group models are presented.*

The Obsessive-Compulsive Foundation is a worldwide organization dedicated to providing information and support to individuals with OCD and related spectrum disorders, their family members, and the mental health profession. To contact the OCF, write: Obsessive-Compulsive Foundation, P.O. Box 70, Milford, CT 06460-0070.

*Throughout this chapter, I use *self-help* and *mutual-help* interchangeably when referring to support groups headed by laypeople. Mutual-help is the preferred term because it im-

A common fear experienced by individuals with OCD is that if others discover their secret obsessions or observe their rituals, they will be labeled "crazy." They strive to conceal their disorder because OCD is still classified as a "mental illness." One SHG facilitator, concerned about declining attendance, surveyed group members who did not return to her group. She discovered that "a large number would attend a group if they could come as anonymous observers only" (4).

In a 1991 Gallup Poll commissioned by the Obsessive-Compulsive Foundation (OCF), individuals disclosed that the fear of others discovering their symptoms often prevented them from making friends (5). Researchers since as early as 1980 have reported that individuals with OCD experience greater problems in social impairment than schizophrenics, acute depressives, and alcoholics (6). The significance of these findings is that, while researchers increasingly cite strong social support as crucial to the maintenance of physical and mental health, individuals with OCD frequently have poor social support networks.*

OCD support groups can be a vehicle for decreasing the social isolation caused by this disorder. A support group often serves as the doorway to treatment and the starting point on the path to recovery. This door-opening function is very important because it is estimated that less than 20% of those with neurobiological disorders such as OCD are in treatment (8). Some individuals with OCD who are currently not in treatment may have previously been in ineffectual or inappropriate treatment prior to the development of the newer serotonin-reuptake inhibitor antidepressants (SRIs) and the widespread use of exposure and response prevention (ERP) to treat OCD (9). An OCD support group can inform these individuals about advances in treatment and help motivate them to take the risk to re-enter treatment.

Patricia Perkins-Doyle, a founder of the OCF and an experienced SHG facilitator, has written that "the support and encouragement of people who have successfully dealt with OCD is incredibly effective

---

plies that helping is a mutual process. Each person in a mutual-help group is both a helper and helpee. I also use *leader* and *facilitator* interchangeably. Facilitator is the preferred term because the group process of a mutual-help group is the catalyst for change. The success of the group is the shared responsibility of all group members.

*In a 10-year study, Dr. David Spiegel of Stanford University found that women with advanced breast cancer who attended a professionally led support group in addition to receiving treatment lived twice as long as women with breast cancer who did not attend a similar support group and only received medical treatment. Researchers studing other diseases have uncovered similar findings (7).

in getting sufferers through the rough spots in treatment" (9). Participation in an SHG can have immediate benefits for individuals with OCD and their family members and significant others. The OCD sufferer realizes that he or she is not alone, that others experience similar symptoms, and that there is now hope. Barbara Breuer, quoted in an interview in *The Women's Times*, described these benefits well: "When I feel myself starting to spiral, it's important to be able to reach out to somebody even just to say, 'I'm having a really bad day today. I hate this disease. I don't want to have it anymore' . . . and have someone respond, 'I understand, I don't blame you. I'm really sorry that you have it too and have to be going through this' " (10). Epidemiological studies consistently find that between 1% and 2% of the general public have OCD at any given time (8) yet some individuals with OCD have never met another person with the same disorder! In a support group, individuals can discover that what they thought were "unique" symptoms are also experienced by others. Group members have the opportunity to gauge their symptom severity in comparison to others. Some members make excellent progress while most members continue to struggle.

As mentioned above, most individuals with OCD strive to conceal it because OCD is still classified as a "mental illness." If members continue to attend the SHG, social isolation may begin to decrease. OCF SHG facilitators have observed that some individuals with OCD attended their group for at least 6 months prior to entering or re-entering treatment. Others, sadly, do not choose to begin treatment and leave the group.

Although there are a number of OCD support group models, a review of support group listings maintained by the OCF reveals that the most common OCD support group format available for individuals with OCD or their support people is the self-help or mutual help group (see the characteristics listed in Table 1). A consistent problem is that most of these groups stay in existence for no more than 2 years. Some groups limit attendance to individuals with OCD, and only occasionally conduct open meetings. The OCF is currently exploring funding options to conduct a certification workshop for OCD SHG leaders, with the objectives of establishing an OCD SHG in every state, reducing the failure rate of existing and new groups, and increasing the overall number of OCD SHGs by one-fourth. Participants in the certification workshop will "start, advise, and nuture three or more SHGs in their state or nearby" (11).

Table 1   Characteristics of a Mutual-Help Group

No fees are charged. Nominal donations may be requested to cover expenses.
Participation is voluntary.
It is a gathering of people who share common experiences, situations, or problems, and
   offer one another emotional and practical support based on the unique perspective
   available only to those who have shared these experiences.
Self-help groups are run by and for members.
Professionals may participate in the self-help process at the request and sanction of the
   group.

Source: *Adapted from A Self-Help Group Is . . . , Michigan Self-Help Clearinghouse Newsletter.*

EDUCATIONAL/SUPPORT SELF-HELP MODEL

The primary objective of an educational/support SHG model is to create a safe, supportive atmosphere in which members can: share feelings and common experiences, hear the latest information about treatment and recovery, provide mutual support and encouragement, socialize, and accomplish whatever other objectives the group members decide on. Since 1987, the OCF has sponsored an SHG based on the above model. Although mental health professionals sometimes observe or are guest speakers, the group facilitators conduct the meetings.

A typical group meeting may focus on a particular topic, agreed on in advance, such as perfectionism, the controlling aspects of the disorder, behavior therapy, taking risks, managing side effects of anti-OCD medications, and the role of family members in supporting recovery. The Richmond, Virginia, SHG meetings begin with the facilitator's announcing the group's ground rules: "Know what we share is confidential and that we have the right to remain anonymous; we listen, explore options, express feelings; we don't prescribe, diagnose, judge, or give advice; and we each share in the responsibility for making the group work. Having benefited from the help of others, we recognize the need to offer our help to others" (12).

Group members usually then begin the meeting by "checking in." This procedure gives everyone an opportunity to share something that has occurred or is occurring in his or her life related to OCD. "Check-in" time is monitored so that all members have an equal opportunity to participate, although no one is pressured to speak (13).

The atmosphere of some SHGs can become "contaminated" by individuals who focus only on the negative aspects of their past week or on their present circumstances. One veteran group facilitator counteracted this phenomenon by repeating the "check-in" and requiring members to share at least one positive event (T. Peters, personal communication). In successful groups, members learn that one's attitude is important—that constant whining and repetition of the refrain "why me?" and myopic focusing on the negatives do not help. Successful groups emphasize that the first step in recovery is the acceptance of OCD as a chronic, lifelong illness and that recovery is hard work, not accomplished simply by swallowing a pill. It is the patient's responsibility to work on his recovery; medication is a tool to facilitate the recovery work.

In some cases, a group's attitude toward treatment is flavored by the treatment history of its founder(s). If an SHG facilitator has been in behavior therapy, the group may adopt weekly behavior goals for its members. Group facilitators often engage in a delicate process—encouraging newcomers to share their feelings and histories while ensuring that the needs of other group members are met. One successful strategy used in Al-Anon groups is to schedule an introductory newcomer meeting prior to the regular meeting. There, newcomers can ask "old-timers" questions about OCD without monopolizing too much of the regular group's time.

The Obsessive-Compulsive Foundation periodically publishes *Check It Out*, a newsletter for OCD support group leaders. The newsletter's objectives are to link up group leaders to share their successful techniques and strategies to maintain a vibrant group; to disseminate the latest information about OCD's 3 Rs: research, resources, and recovery; to announce legislative alerts, upcoming seminars, and research studies; and to encourage group members to participate in fund-raising and awareness-generating events. Local SHG activities are highlighted to encourage other groups to participate. One SHG in Wilkes-Barre, Pennsylvania, raised funds for the OCF's award-winning video, "The Touching Tree," by redeeming soda cans. An Oregon SHG invited its local congressperson's health aide to attend a meeting, where the members voiced their concerns about "Medicare Part B not paying for the expensive medications we need and also about the time it has been taking to go through the process to receive disability" (14).

Recently, an Austin, Texas, SHG got very involved in asking over 200 mental health agencies, doctors' offices, counseling centers, supporters of public radio, and friends and relatives of individuals with OCD to ask the local Public Broadcasting Service station to broadcast the documentary "The Mind's Eye" (15). A goal of the OCF is to develop a "grass roots" SHG advocacy network that will respond quickly to both local and national issues. Self-help groups in California are advocating that the California state legislature pass a bill that will end discrimination by insurers in health care coverage against those with "mental and nervous disorders." Individuals with neurobiological disorders remain the last minority still in the closet.

In my conversations with SHG leaders, I have frequently learned that most of their members have not had adequate trials of behavior therapy. The members of one SHG, recognizing this discrepancy, purchased copies of Reid and Wilson's book *Stop Obsessing*, which outlines how to design and implement a self-help behavioral program. The OCF is planning to conduct 3-day behavior therapy institutes for clinicians in order to increase the availability of behavior therapists. Another option for SHG members is to pool their financial resources and contract with a local behavior therapist for group therapy sessions (16).

The OCF sometimes attempts to help start a family-members-only SHG, but most such groups are organized with the assistance of mental health professionals. In a 1994 OCF/Fordham University study of OCD family members, half the respondants said that support groups were needed. According to Dr. Marlene Cooper, author of the study, support groups "can help families manage difficult OC behaviors, express and handle their anger, grief, and sense of loss, and minimize the disruption that OCD causes to family life" (17). Family members learn that OCD is a neurobiological disorder, that it's nobody's fault, and that there are specific ways in which they can support their relative's recovery.

The OCF provides free to all its members the booklet *Learning to Live with OCD*, written especially for OCD family members (18). The booklet outlines 14 comprehensive and supportive guidelines. Dr. Gail Steketee of Boston University has found that "poor functioning within the family and unpleasant family interactions such as anger and criticism were associated with fewer gains in OCD symptom reduction 9 months after treatment" (19). Clearly, research is pointing to the importance of addressing family issues, and a professionally assisted family-member support group could be the venue.

THE OBSESSIVE-COMPULSIVE ANONYMOUS MODEL

Obsessive-Compulsive Anonymous (OCA) is another OCD SHG model. This program is an adaptation of the 12 steps originated by Alcoholics Anonymous in 1935 (see Table 2). OCA meetings usually begin with a formal opening statement defining the group and its goals: "An individual in recovery shares how it was before OCA and how he implements the OCA program for recovery. . . . other variations include step meetings (reading and discussion of one of the 12 steps) or meetings [on topics] such as resentment, control, perfectionism, willfulness, Higher

Table 2 The Twelve Traditions of Obsessive Compulsive Anonymous

1	Our common welfare should come first; personal recovery depends on OCA unity.
2	For our group purpose there is but one ultimate authority—a loving God as He may express Himself in our group conscience. Our leaders are but trusted servants; they do not govern.
3	The only requirement for OCA membership is a desire to recover from Obsessive Compulsive Disorder.
4	Each group should be autonomous except in matters affecting other groups or OCA as a whole.
5	Each group has but one primary purpose—to carry its message to those who still suffer from Obsessive Compulsive Disorder.
6	An OCA group ought never endorse, finance, or lend the OCA name to any related facility or outside enterprise, lest problems of money, property and prestige divert us from our primary purpose.
7	Every OCA group ought to be fully self-supporting, declining outside contributions.
8	Obsessive Compulsive Anonymous should remain forever nonprofessional, but our service centers may employ special workers.
9	OCA, as such, ought never be organized; but we may create service boards or committees directly responsible to those they serve.
10	Obsessive Compulsive Anonymous has no opinion on outside issues; hence the OCA name ought never be drawn into public controversy.
11	Our public relations policy is based on attraction rather than promotion; we need always maintain personal anonymity at the level of press, radio, and films.
12	Anonymity is the spiritual foundation of all our traditions, ever reminding us to place principles before personalities.

Source: Adapted from Alcoholics Anonymous World Services, Inc., and Obsessive Compulsive Anonymous.

Power, etc." (20). Meetings are usually held weekly. OCA group members do not spend time comparing symptoms or complaining about their OCD. OCA emphasizes the individuals's acceptance of his or her OCD, the use of the 12 steps as the ingredients for recovery, and the surrender to a Higher Power of the member's own choosing in order to change.

Roy C., one of the orginators of OCA, has written a companion volume to his OCA manual, *Obsessive Compulsive Disorder: A Survival Guide for Family Members and Friends*. The OCA SHGs are a fast-growing phenomonon. As of March 1995, 50 OCA SHGs had been started in the United States. OCA groups have greater longevity than the educational/support SHGs. OCA is a simple prototype that can be easily replicated anywhere. OCA facilitators are usually experienced, generally having been in other 12-step groups. The program is not dependent on one individual. Facilitators change. The OCA program is the constant.

LIMITATIONS OF EDUCATIONAL/SUPPORT SHGs

Too often, the development of an educational/support SHG is the work of one individual, who may never have participated in a mutual-support group. He or she becomes the leader. If group leadership is not encouraged, members will not assume a shared responsibility for the group's success. The members will look to the leader for the answers and become dependent. The leader may also serve as the phone contact, which can be a strong stressor. Research has shown that 60% of individuals referred to an SHG by professionals never attend a meeting, and dropout rates from 30% to over 50% are reported for those who do attend (21). Leaders may relapse, move, go back to work, or just "flame out," and then the group often dissolves.

Rotating the facilitation of the group among its members can reduce the stress on just one person and prevent a leader from becoming the "superstar" who is totally responsible for the success of the group. In a "true" mutual-help group, there are no distinctions between the helper and the helpee. Members, including facilitators, are equals (22).

The OCF provides to individuals interested in starting an SHG how-to materials that stress the importance of forming a core group of others also interested in starting a new group prior to "going public." We also suggest that potential SHG facilitators 1) contact a regional self-help group clearinghouse to determine whether a group facilitation workshop will be offered in the near future, 2) locate a mental health professional who will serve as treatment consultant, and 3) join the OCF.

We also include in our introductory materials a letter written by a veteran SHG facilitator, Wally Green, to people interested in starting an OCD SHG. His message is blunt: "Are you starting an SHG to relieve your own feelings of isolation? . . . it's not for the super-sensitive . . . often OCD sufferers attend once and you never see them again. That hurts." His ending, though, says it all: "A self-help group has a definite chemistry to it. It is, somehow, more than the sum of its members. When it really starts cooking, such a group is quite wonderful. It is definitely worth doing if you think you are up for it" (23). Addicted physicians participating in a 1990 Impaired Physicians Program rated the peer-led, self-help group component (Alcoholics Anonymous) as more important to their recovery than professional treatment (24).

ON-LINE SUPPORT GROUPS

A recent phenomenon has been the appearance of cyberspace SHGs, in which members connect through their computer modems. Individuals with OCD and related disorders "meet" on specialized medical bulletin boards. The OCF has been active on Prodigy (a national commercial computer information network) via a medical bulletin board (Depression'Anx/OCD) since 1994. The Prodigy group has about 50 active members nationwide, but many other people "lurk" and monitor postings. There are many advantages to on-line SHGs not available to "live" SHGs. For example, on-line support groups have no set meeting times; members can "meet" around the clock. Meetings aren't canceled in inclement weather. Individuals with severe OCD, imprisoned by their contamination fears or unable to drive out of fear of becoming a "car killer," can log on and receive support and encouragement without leaving their house. As in a "live" group, members are not obligated to participate, but an on-line member may be more likely to share in this relatively anonymous forum.

Another distinct advantage over "live" groups is that information can be communicated instantaneously by e-mail, which is usually offered by the Internet service provider at no extra charge. For example, the OCF immediately communicated the FDA's recent approval of fluvoxamine (Luvox) on Prodigy, and individuals who had been in fluvoxamine research protocols logged on and shared their experiences, both good and bad. Newly diagnosed individuals receive accurate, "free" information about resources and treatment. Individuals who have successfully embraced behavior therapy serve as role models and cheerleaders for those hesitant about entering behavior therapy, fearful of taking the risk. Individuals can even receive referrals to "live" groups in their area. There are also OCD sites on the World Wide Web.

A major impediment to participation, of course, is cost: you must have a computer system with a modem and subscribe to a commercial on-line service or have access to the Internet. An article in the *Wall Street Journal* highlighted the risk that consumers will receive erroneous information. The article traced the spectacular increase in the use of an epilepsy medication, Neurontin, to treat amyotrophic lateral sclerosis (ALS) after its curative benefits had been touted by ALS patients on Prodigy. ALS sufferers participating in other medication research trials demanded to be put on the commercially available Neurontin. A double-blind, placebo-controlled trial of the drug is now being designed to test its effectiveness in treating ALS, although researchers are concerned that participants will break their promise not to discuss their drug reac-

tions with other trial participants and post their progress on Prodigy
(25).

ROLE OF MENTAL HEALTH PROFESSIONALS AND SHGs

Although SHG research is very limited, a consistent finding is that when
professionals are involved in SHGs, there is an increase in "professionally toned helping activities and a decrease in the supportive atmosphere
characteristic of SGHs" (21). Mental health professionals can help SHGs
without compromising their integrity by linking up individuals interested in starting a SHG; writing a "Dear Colleague" letter introducing
the SHG to fellow professionals; donating in-kind services such as meeting space, an answering machine, access to copying facilities, and coffee;
serving as the group's treatment consultant and troubleshooter or as a
guest presenter; assisting in fund-raising and advocacy; and assuming
any other roles negotiated with the SHG.

Professional involvement with an SHG is a two-way relationship.
Although some "psychiatrist-bashing" does occur, SHGs can be an important source of referrals for mental health professionals. Research has
shown that participation in an SHG increases the utilization of professional services by its members (26). Members of SHGs can also exert
political clout. OCF SHG facilitators and group members have testified
twice before the Connecticut state legislature to protest threatened cuts
to the research and services budget of the Connecticut Mental Health
Center. The National Alliance of the Mentally Ill (NAMI) is an excellent
example of a national self-help organization that has forged alliances
with mental health professionals and their professional associations and
state and national politicians to ensure that individuals with severe and
chronic neurobiological disorders receive the comprehensive wrapa-
around services they desperately need.

THE PROFESSIONALLY ASSISTED SUPPORT GROUP

Almost half of all the OCD support groups listed by the OCF involve a
mental health professional as either facilitator or cofacilitator with a patient or family member. Some professionals start a support group with
the hope that a group member will eventually emerge and assume facilitation of the group. Group formats vary; some are based on the
educational/support model (similar to the previously discussed SHG
format).

An immediate advantage to involving a professional facilitator is
that he or she can screen potential group members for their appropriate-

ness for the group. A common problem faced by all OCD SHGs is that many individuals misinterpret a compulsive or impulsive problem as obsessive-compulsive disorder. Dr. Claghorn, a professional consultant to the OCF's Texas affiliate, has likened an open SHG meeting to a "lamp in the woods." Unwelcome guests may appear, monopolizing sessions and offending genuine OCDers (27). An initial interview with a mental-health professional can filter out inappropiate self-referrals.

Dr. Marlene Cooper, the author of the OCF/Fordham University Family Member Study, has led an OCD family-member support group for a number of years. A key finding of her study was that support groups can "help families manage difficult OC behaviors, express and handle their anger, grief, and sense of loss, and minimize the disruption that OCD causes to family life" (17). However, families seeking support discover that OCD family support groups are very rare. OCF staff often refer families seeking support to Al-Anon groups. Most professionally led OCD support groups, such as Dr. Cooper's group, have a didactic or therapeutic orientation. Another key difference between an SHG and a professionally led support group is that a fee for membership is usually charged in the latter, although sometimes the fee is reimbursed by insurance companies.

Since 1981, Dr. Jon Grayson, a founding member of the Philadelphia OCF affiliate, has co-led the affiliate's GOAL group (Giving Obsessive-Compulsives Another Lifestyle). A GOAL group meeting is divided into three parts. The first is a general discussion of an OCD-related topic selected prior to the meeting. Lay facilitators keep the group focused on the agreed-upon topic. Approximately an hour and a half later, the members divide into smaller groups. The objective of these five- to nine-member groups is for each person to devise a behavioral goal that will be accomplished before the next meeting. The goal usually has an exposure or response prevention focus. Group members report back at the next meeting. If an individual has not succeeded, the small group will help redesign the goal so that it can be accomplished. Failure is not recognized. Sometimes group members will offer to support a member who is difficulty between meetings (28).

Dr. Grayson, his colleagues at Rosemont Counseling Associates, and Gayle Frankel, President of the OCF—Philadelphia, presented the GOAL model at the OCF's 1995 membership meeting. After a brief introduction of the model, individuals with OCD broke up into small groups and, with the help of a GOAL facilitator, selected a behavioral goal to accomplish during the remaining day and a half of the conference. Each individual was given the opportunity to write his or her goal on a large posterboard, which was displayed throughout the conference.

Members were encouraged to check off their goal when it was accomplished. One remarked to me, "This has been the first time I've experienced success in resisting my compulsions." The OCF is exploring funding options to develop a GOAL manual and videotape to distribute to its support group network and affiliates.

Kenneth Kobak, a Research Scientist at the Dean Foundation in Madison, Wisconsin, also discovered that "setting goals in a group appears to be an important motivational factor, as clients are aware that they will share with other group members their progress at the next session" (26). The final part of the GOAL meeting is set aside for socialization, which builds the group's cohesiveness.

Professionally assisted OCD support groups are often started by institutions or practitioners specializing in treating anxiety disorders, and membership may be restricted to individuals currently in treatment at that institution or with that therapist.

SUMMARY

SHGs or professionally facilitated support groups are valuable resources for individuals with OCD and their support people struggling with this chronic, relapsing illness. A support group can be a crucible for metamorphosis. A recent member of the OCF succinctly captured this magic by writing, "The conference in Boston this past weekend was one of the greatest times in my life because this was the first time I've met another OCD 'sufferer' with similar obsessions and compulsions. This reinforces the fact that support groups play a significant role in recovery. Unfortunately, it took me 51 years to know this."

REFERENCES

1. Foster CH. Funny, You Don't Look Crazy. Ellsworth, ME: Dilligaf Publishing, 1993.
2. Rupprecht R. George Gallup, Jr., Princeton pollster. New Jersey Monthly, January 1992:32.
3. Leerhsen C. Unite and conquer. Newsweek, February 5, 1990.
4. Lohmann S. A response to letters. Check It Out 1993; 4:1.
5. A Gallup Study of Obsessive Compulsive Disorder Sufferers. Princeton, NJ: The Gallup Organization, December 1993.
6. Khanna S, et al. Social adjustment in obsessive-compulsive disorder. Int J Soc Psych 1988; 34(2):118–122.
7. Can Your Mind Heal Your Body? Consumer Reports, February 1993.
8. Rasmussen S, Eisen J. The Epidemiology and Clinical Features of Obsessive Compulsive Disorder. Psychiatr Clin North Am 1992; 14(4):743–758.

9. Perkins P. Foundations of an OCD Self-Help Group. Check It Out 1990; 1:1.
10. Black M. Being well. The Women's Times Jan/Feb 1995.
11. Broatch J. A proposal to conduct a certification workshop for obsessive-compulsive disorder support group leaders. December 1993. Unpublished.
12. Cribbs L. Groundrules for OCD Support Group of Richmond. Unpublished.
13. Lees A. Leadership is key to self-help groups. National Mental Health Consumers' Self-Help Clearinghouse. Fall–winter 1993–1994.
14. Moffett B, Salman V. Letter to the editor. Check It Out 1995; 5:1.
15. Weldon Y. Letter to the editor. Check It Out 1995; 5:2.
16. Pollard CA. Proposal for a Behavior Therapy Institute. December 1994. Unpublished.
17. Cooper M. Report on the findings of study of OCD family members. OCD Newsletter 1994; 8:4.
18. Van Noppen B, et al. Learning to Live with OCD. 3rd ed. Milford, CT: Obsessive-Compulsive Foundation, 1993.
19. Steketee G. Family Treatment for OCD? OCD Newsletter 1995; 9:3.
20. R. C. Obsessive Compulsive Anonymous. New York: Alden Graphics, 1990.
21. Wollert R. The role of self-help groups in the delivery of mental health services. Self-Help Mental Health Services Workshop, Washington, DC, March 1990.
22. Young T. Clearinghouse advisor: foundations of a self-help group. Helping Ourselves 1991.
23. Green W. To people thinking of starting a self-help group for OCD. Personal correspondence, 1989.
24. Galanter. Addicted MDs rate self-help groups most helpful. Intern Med News 1990; 23:7.
25. Bulkeley W. Untested treatments, cures find stronghold on on-line services. Wall Street Journal, March 6, 1995.
26. Kobak K, et al. Group behavior therapy for obsessive-compulsive disorder. Unpublished.
27. Claghorn J. Questions & answers. Check It Out 1990; 1:1.
28. Grayson J. Making goals. OCD Newsletter 1994; 8:2.

Index

About the Editors

Eric Hollander is a Professor of Psychiatry; the Director of Clinical Psychopharmacology as well as of the Anxiety, Compulsive, Impulsive Disorders Program; and the Clinical Director of the Seaver Autism Research Center at The Mount Sinai School of Medicine, New York, New York. The editor or coeditor of six books and the author or coauthor of over 250 journal publications and book chapters, he is a member of the American Psychiatric Association, the American Medical Association, and the American Psychopathological Association, among others. Dr. Hollander received the B.A. degree (1978) from Brandeis University, Waltham, Massachusetts, and the M.D. degree (1982) from the State University of New York Downstate Medical College, Brooklyn.

Dan J. Stein is the Director of Research, Department of Psychiatry, University of Stellenbosch, Tygerberg, South Africa. The editor or coeditor of five books and the author or coauthor of over 150 journal publications and book chapters, he is a member of the American Psychiatric Association, the society of Biological Psychiatry, and the Society of Psychiatrists of South Africa, among others. Dr. Stein received the B.Sc. degree (1983) in biochemistry and psychology, and the M.B., Ch.B. degree (1986) from the University of Cape Town, Rondebosch, South Africa.